Update of Gynecologic Oncology

Guest Editor

CAROLYN Y. MULLER, MD

OBSTETRICS AND GYNECOLOGY CLINICS OF NORTH AMERICA

www.obgyn.theclinics.com

Consulting Editor
WILLIAM F. RAYBURN, MD, MBA

June 2012 • Volume 39 • Number 2

SAUNDERS an imprint of ELSEVIER, Inc.

W.B. SAUNDERS COMPANY
A Division of Elsevier Inc.

Elsevier, Inc. • 1600 John F. Kennedy Blvd. • Suite 1800 • Philadelphia, PA 19103-2899

http://www.theclinics.com

OBSTETRICS AND GYNECOLOGY CLINICS OF NORTH AMERICA Volume 39, Number 2
June 2012 ISSN 0889-8545, ISBN-13: 978-1-4557-3901-1

Editor: Stephanie Donley

Obstetrics and Gynecology Clinics (ISSN 0889-8545) is published quarterly by Elsevier Inc., 360 Park Avenue South, New York, NY 10010-1710. Months of issue are March, June, September, and December. Periodicals postage paid at New York, NY, and additional mailing offices. Subscription price per year is $293.00 (US individuals), $498.00 (US institutions), $146.00 (US students), $353.00 (Canadian individuals), $628.00 (Canadian institutions), $214.00 (Canadian students), $428.00 (foreign individuals), $628.00 (foreign institutions), and $214.00 (foreign students). To receive student/ resident rate, orders must be accompanied by name of affiliated institution, date of term, and the signature of program/ residency coordinator on institution letterhead. Orders will be billed at individual rate until proof of status is received. Foreign air speed delivery is included in all *Clinics* subscription prices. All prices are subject to change without notice. POSTMASTER: Send address changes to *Obstetrics and Gynecology Clinics*, Elsevier Health Sciences Division, Subscription Customer Service, 3251 Riverport Lane, Maryland Heights, MO 63043. **Customer Service: Telephone: 1-800-654-2452 (U.S. and Canada); 314-447-8871 (outside U.S. and Canada). Fax: 314-447-8029. E-mail: journalscustomerservice-usa@elsevier.com (for print support); journalsonlinesupport-usa@elsevier.com (for online support).**

Reprints. For copies of 100 or more of articles in this publication, please contact the Commercial Reprints Department, Elsevier Inc., 360 Park Avenue South, New York, New York 10010-1710. Tel.: 212-633-3818; Fax: 212-462-1935; E-mail: reprints@elsevier.com.

Obstetrics and Gynecology Clinics of North America is also published in Spanish by McGraw-Hill Interamericana Editores S.A., P.O. Box 5-237, 06500, Mexico; in Portuguese by Reichmann and Affonso Editores, Rio de Janeiro, Brazil; and in Greek by Paschalidis Medical Publications, Athens, Greece.

Obstetrics and Gynecology Clinics of North America is covered in *MEDLINE/PubMed (Index Medicus)*, *Excerpta Medica*, *Current Concepts/Clinical Medicine*, *Science Citation Index*, *BIOSIS*, *CINAHL*, and *ISI/BIOMED*.

Printed and bound by CPI Group (UK) Ltd, Croydon, CR0 4YY
Transferred to Digital Print 2012

GOAL STATEMENT

The goal of *Obstetrics and Gynecology Clinics of North America* is to keep practicing physicians up to date with current clinical practice in OB/GYN by providing timely articles reviewing the state of the art in patient care.

ACCREDITATION

The *Obstetrics and Gynecology Clinics of North America* is planned and implemented in accordance with the Essential Areas and Policies of the Accreditation Council for Continuing Medical Education (ACCME) through the joint sponsorship of the University of Virginia School of Medicine and Elsevier. The University of Virginia School of Medicine is accredited by the ACCME to provide continuing medical education for physicians.

The University of Virginia School of Medicine designates this enduring material activity for a maximum of 15 *AMA PRA Category 1 Credit*(s)™ for each issue, 60 credits per year. Physicians should only claim credit commensurate with the extent of their participation in the activity.

The American Medical Association has determined that physicians not licensed in the US who participate in this CME enduring material activity are eligible for a maximum of 15 *AMA PRA Category 1 Credit*(s)™ for each issue, 60 credits per year.

Credit can be earned by reading the text material, taking the CME examination online at http://www.theclinics.com/home/cme, and completing the evaluation. After taking the test, you will be required to review any and all incorrect answers. Following completion of the test and evaluation, your credit will be awarded and you may print your certificate.

FACULTY DISCLOSURE/CONFLICT OF INTEREST

The University of Virginia School of Medicine, as an ACCME accredited provider, endorses and strives to comply with the Accreditation Council for Continuing Medical Education (ACCME) Standards of Commercial Support, Commonwealth of Virginia statutes, University of Virginia policies and procedures, and associated federal and private regulations and guidelines on the need for disclosure and monitoring of proprietary and financial interests that may affect the scientific integrity and balance of content delivered in continuing medical education activities under our auspices.

The University of Virginia School of Medicine requires that all CME activities accredited through this institution be developed independently and be scientifically rigorous, balanced and objective in the presentation/discussion of its content, theories and practices.

All authors/editors participating in an accredited CME activity are expected to disclose to the readers relevant financial relationships with commercial entities occurring within the past 12 months (such as grants or research support, employee, consultant, stock holder, member of speakers bureau, etc.). The University of Virginia School of Medicine will employ appropriate mechanisms to resolve potential conflicts of interest to maintain the standards of fair and balanced education to the reader. Questions about specific strategies can be directed to the Office of Continuing Medical Education, University of Virginia School of Medicine, Charlottesville, Virginia.

The faculty and staff of the University of Virginia Office of Continuing Medical Education have no financial affiliations to disclose.

The authors/editors listed below have identified no professional or financial affiliations for themselves or their spouse/partner:

Mostafa Ahmed, BS; Ahmed N AL-Niaimi, MD; Lori L. Ballinger, MS; Shazia Bashir, MD; Jori S. Carter, MD; Koen De Geest, MD; J. Dodge, MD, FRCSC, MEd; Stephanie Donley, (Acquisitions Editor); Levi S. Downs, Jr., MD, MS; Laurie Elit, MD, MSc, FRCS(C); Michael J. Goodheart, MD; William Irvin, MD (Test Author); Mario Javier Pineda, MD; Yichen Jia; Jayanthi S. Lea, MD; Kimberly K. Leslie, MD; Ken Y. Lin, MD, PhD; Carolyn Y. Muller, MD (Guest Editor); Chase B. Petersen, MD; William F. Rayburn, MD, MBA (Consulting Editor); Clare Reade, MD, FRCS(C); Teresa Rutledge, MD; Maria B. Schiavone, MD; Diljeet K. Singh, MD, DrPH; Kristina W. Thiel, PhD; and Shujie Yang, PhD.

The authors/editors listed below identified the following professional or financial affiliations for themselves or their spouse/partner:

Barbara A. Goff, MD is a consultant for Fujirebio, and is on the Speakers' Bureau for Qiagen.

Thomas J. Herzog, MD is a consultant for Morphotek, Roche, and J&J.

R. Osborne, MD, FRCSC, MBA owns stock in Pfizer, Inc. and Abbott Laboratories.

Disclosure of Discussion of non-FDA approved uses for pharmaceutical products and/or medical devices:

The University of Virginia School of Medicine, as an ACCME provider, requires that all faculty presenters identify and disclose any off-label uses for pharmaceutical and medical device products. The University of Virginia School of Medicine recommends that each physician fully review all the available data on new products or procedures prior to clinical use.

TO ENROLL

To enroll in the Obstetrics and Gynecology Clinics of North America Continuing Medical Education program, call customer service at 1-800-654-2452 or visit us online at www.theclinics.com/home/cme. The CME program is available to subscribers for an additional fee of $180.00

Contributors

CONSULTING EDITOR

WILLIAM F. RAYBURN, MD, MBA
Randolph Seligman Professor and Chair, Department of Obstetrics and Gynecology;
Chief of Staff, University Hospital, University of New Mexico Health Science Center,
Albuquerque, New Mexico

GUEST EDITOR

CAROLYN Y. MULLER, MD
Professor of Obstetrics and Gynecology, Director, Gynecologic Oncology, Department
of Obstetrics and Gynecology, University of New Mexico Cancer Center, Albuquerque,
New Mexico

AUTHORS

MOSTAFA AHMED, BS
University of Wisconsin School of Medicine and Public Health, Madison, Wisconsin

AHMED N. AL-NIAIMI, MD
Assistant Professor, Division of Gynecologic Oncology, Department of Obstetrics and
Gynecology, University of Wisconsin School of Medicine and Public Health, Madison,
Wisconsin

LORI L. BALLINGER, MS
Senior Genetic Counselor, Hereditary Cancer Assessment Program, University of New
Mexico Cancer Research and Treatment Center, Albuquerque, New Mexico

SHAZIA BASHIR, MD
Department of Gynecologic Oncology, Columbia University College of Physicians and
Surgeons, New York Presbyterian Hospital, New York, New York

JORI S. CARTER, MD
Division of Gynecologic Oncology, Department of Obstetrics, Gynecology, and
Women's Health, University of Minnesota, Minneapolis, Minnesota

KOEN DE GEEST, MD
Professor, Division of Gynecologic Oncology; Department of Obstetrics and
Gynecology, University of Iowa, Iowa City, Iowa

J. DODGE, MD, FRCSC, MEd
Division of Gynecologic Oncology, Princess Margaret Hospital, Toronto, Ontario,
Canada

LEVI S. DOWNS JR, MD, MS
Division of Gynecologic Oncology, Department of Obstetrics, Gynecology, and
Women's Health, University of Minnesota, Minneapolis, Minnesota

LAURIE ELIT, MD, MSc, FRCS(C)
Department of Clinical Epidemiology and Biostatistics, Health Research Methodology
Program; Department of Obstetrics and Gynecology, Division of Gynecologic Oncology;
Department of Oncology, McMaster University, Hamilton, Ontario, Canada

BARBARA A. GOFF, MD
Director, Gynecologic Oncology, Department of Obstetrics and Gynecology, University of Washington School of Medicine, Seattle, Washington

MICHAEL J. GOODHEART, MD
Assistant Professor, Division of Gynecologic Oncology; Department of Obstetrics and Gynecology, University of Iowa, Iowa City, Iowa

THOMAS J. HERZOG, MD
Department of Gynecologic Oncology, Columbia University College of Physicians and Surgeons, New York Presbyterian Hospital, New York, New York

MARIO JAVIER PINEDA, MD, PhD
Division of Gynecologic Oncology, Northwestern University Feinberg School of Medicine, Chicago, Illinois

YICHEN JIA
Undergraduate Research Assistant, Department of Obstetrics and Gynecology, University of Iowa, Iowa City, Iowa

JAYANTHI S. LEA, MD
University of Texas Southwestern School of Medicine, Dallas, Texas

KIMBERLY K. LESLIE, MD
Professor and Chair, Department of Obstetrics and Gynecology, University of Iowa, Iowa City, Iowa

KEN Y. LIN, MD, PhD
University of Texas Southwestern School of Medicine, Dallas, Texas

R. OSBORNE, MD, FRCSC
Division of Gynecologic Oncology, Odette Cancer Centre, Toronto, Ontario, Canada

CHASE B. PETERSEN, MD
Department of Obstetrics and Gynecology, University of Wisconsin School of Medicine and Public Health, Madison, Wisconsin

CLARE READE, MD, FRCS(C)
Division of Gynecologic Oncology, University of Toronto, Toronto; Department of Clinical Epidemiology and Biostatistics, Health Research Methodology Program, McMaster University, Hamilton, Ontario, Canada

TERESA L. RUTLEDGE, MD
Assistant Professor, Department of Obstetrics and Gynecology, Division of Gynecologic Oncology, 1 University of New Mexico Albuquerque, New Mexico

MARIA B. SCHIAVONE, MD
Department of Obstetrics and Gynecology, Columbia University College of Physicians and Surgeons, New York Presbyterian Hospital, New York, New York

DILJEET K. SINGH, MD, DrPH
Division of Gynecologic Oncology, Northwestern University Feinberg School of Medicine, Chicago, Illinois

KRISTINA W. THIEL, PhD
Assistant Research Scientist, Department of Obstetrics and Gynecology, University of Iowa, Iowa City, Iowa

SHUJIE YANG, PhD
Postdoctoral Scholar, Department of Obstetrics and Gynecology, University of Iowa, Iowa City, Iowa

Contents

> This article reviews population-based studies addressing structures and processes influencing outcomes in women with ovarian, uterine, cervical, or vulvar cancer. Treatment of ovarian cancer in specialized high-volume centers improved outcomes. Structural and process variables did not significantly impact outcome for uterine cancer. Cervical cancer studies showed no significant association between structural variables and outcomes. Vulvar cancer studies suggested that high-volume surgeons were more likely to achieve adequate negative margins. Population-based data confirm the importance of centralized care for ovarian cancer, but currently do not support recommendations for or against centralizing care for women with uterine, cervical, and vulvar cancer.

> Personalized medicine in tumor treatment identifies and targets a specific protein or pathway. Treatment of gynecologic tumors has relied on surgical cytoreduction and cytotoxic chemotherapy; however, relapse and survival rates have improved only modestly. Research has focused on molecular-based oncologic transformation and cell growth. Treatment possibilities have encompassed stromal, vasculature, and cell signaling targets. Antiangiogenic agents have had success, and other agents are being investigated. Results have been mixed, yet great promise remains. This article focuses on the main categories of molecular targeting for ovarian, uterine, and cervical cancers and highlights recently completed and current clinical trials.

> The surgical management of gynecologic malignancy is the cornerstone of the subspecialty. As technology advances, surgical care is changing rapidly. New devices, surgical instruments, and understandings of the

disease process have all improved the surgical management of gynecologic malignancies. This article summarizes some of the recent advances
in the surgical management of gynecologic malignancies.

Gynecologists and gynecologic oncologists have a major role in identifying patients at increased risk of inherited cancer syndromes. Awareness of the biological and familial risk factors can assist in navigating
follow-up. Large consortia are invaluable resources with massive
datasets requiring herculean analyses that will continue to rapidly
advance our present knowledge and management of women with
hereditary cancer syndromes.

Currently, ovarian cancer screening is not recommended for woman at
average risk. Studies evaluating screening in high-risk women have
been disappointing. Therefore, risk-reducing surgery is recommended
for women with genetic mutations when childbearing is complete. The
best way to detect ovarian cancer is for both the patient and the
clinician to have a high index of suspicion when the patient is symptomatic. There have been numerous studies showing that ovarian
cancer patients often have symptoms 3 to 6 months before diagnosis.
It is important for practitioners to be aware of these symptoms to avoid
potentially harmful delays in diagnosis.

Trophoblastic neoplasms are a set of diseases that arise from a failed
gestation. A molar pregnancy is an allograft of fetal tissue typically
containing only paternal chromosomes that may invade the maternal
tissues. Most molar pregnacies spontaneously resolve but a subset of
patients will develop trophoblastic neoplasia and will require treatment.
Patients with low risk disease are usually cured with single agent
chemotherapy but a small number of patients develop high risk disease
and require combination chemotherapy. This article reviews the current
diagnosis and management of gestational trophoblastic neoplasms.

Vulvar cancer is becoming more common as the population ages and
is primarily a disease of the elderly. Most vulvar cancers are diagnosed

at a localized stage and can be cured with surgery and adjuvant radiotherapy. The most important prognostic factor for survival is the assessment of metastatic disease within the groin lymph nodes. Vaginal cancer is a rare cancer that also affects elderly women. Prognosis is poor; however, adequate treatment can be delivered with a combination of external beam radiotherapy and brachytherapy, and with surgical resection for a select group of patients.

oncology to improve both the quality and quantity of our patients' lives. Whereas substantial work remains in clarifying the ultimate value of many integrative techniques, clear evidence for their benefit can be found in the arena of symptom management. Quality of life has become increasingly important both as an outcome itself and as it contributes to survival. Integrative approaches have been used to improve quality of life and can be incorporated into the routine approach of the gynecologic oncologist.

OBSTETRICS AND GYNECOLOGY

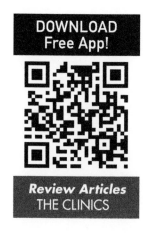

Foreword

Gynecologic Oncology

This issue, guest edited by Carolyn Muller, MD, provides a comprehensive update of gynecologic oncology clinics. Remaining current can be challenging, and gynecologic oncology is no exception. As Dr Muller mentions in her preface, the field of gynecologic oncology has undergone remarkable evolution since our last issue pertaining to this subject—five years ago.

This issue provided readers with data-driven, up-to-date information about the nonsurgical and surgical management of women with trophoblastic disease and cancers of the vulva, vagina, cervix, uterus, and ovary. By way of example, terms or expressions not mentioned in the prior issue now include the following: genome sequencing, personalized targeted therapeutics, germline genetic risk, robotic surgical technology, complementary therapies, and quality-of-life analysis.

The issue begins with a description of trends in cancer care and appropriately ends with a perspective on quality of life for affected persons. The roles of cancer genetics and hereditary risk are brought to the reader's attention in an understandable manner. Certain guidelines have changed about early detection and screening of gynecologic malignancies and are updated here. Along with a description of advances in surgical care, certain articles deal with biological therapies and complementary medicine.

It is my desire that this issue activates attention to subjects of cutting-edge interest in gynecologic oncology. On behalf of Dr Muller and her excellent group of knowledgeable contributors, I hope that the practical information provided herein will aid in the implementation of evidence-based and well-planned approaches to evaluating and recommending treatment of our patients with these maladies.

William F. Rayburn, MD, MBA
Department of Obstetrics and Gynecology
University of New Mexico School of Medicine
MSC10 5580; 1 University of New Mexico
Albuquerque, NM 87131-0001, USA

E-mail address:
wrayburn@salud.unm.edu

Obstet Gynecol Clin N Am 39 (2012) xiii–xiii
http://dx.doi.org/10.1016/j.ogc.2012.04.004
0889-8545/12/$ – see front matter © 2012 Elsevier Inc. All rights reserved.

obgyn.theclinics.com

Preface

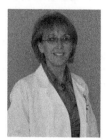

Carolyn Y. Muller, MD
Guest Editor

I grew up watching the original Star Trek, amazed at the level of medical technology utilized in many episodes. Captain Kirk and Mr Spock loaded samples into a complex machine able to sequence the DNA of their alien enemies. I also watched the Jetsons, intrigued at the futuristic "phone calls", communication that was visual on a portable screen and their robot Rosie that took care of the kids, cleaned the house and served as the family caretaker. Never in my youthful imagination did I think I would live and work in a world with such technology. DNA sequencing is commonplace, now automated and a core facility at every major cancer center and medical research industry. Affordable whole genome sequencing is here, providing the ability to truly personalize medicine. New fields in bioinformatics have emerged in order to handle the insurmountable data derived from these technologies. And "robots" now do our surgery.

This edition of the *Obstetrics and Gynecology Clinics of North America* will indeed focus on the advances in gynecologic oncology that have emerged within the last decade. With increasing technology comes increasing cost and Dr Elit has provided an outstanding comprehensive chapter on the challenges, disparities and delivery of gynecologic cancer care throughout North America with the impact on patient outcomes. This chapter addresses differences in gynecologic oncology care between our own health systems and our Canadian and Mexican neighbors. A chapter by Dr Herzog is dedicated to the advances in personalized treatment of gynecologic cancer with a glimpse of present day and future targeted therapeutics for our disease states. The impact of whole genome sequencing of tumors will radically change how we choose treatment strategies in the next few decades. The field of cancer genetics is reviewed by Ms Ballinger, as this field moves quickly involving germline genetic risk, testing and prevention strategies for women at high risk for developing gynecologic cancers. Dr Rutledge addresses surgical advances in our field, providing evidence-based data on minimally invasive surgery including the rapid utilization of robotic surgical technology, allowing us to perform extremely complex surgery in less fit surgical candidates with better outcome measures.

This edition of the *Obstetrics and Gynecology Clinics of North America* will update the reader on further advances across the tumor sites that make up our field of

Obstet Gynecol Clin N Am 39 (2012) xv–xvi
http://dx.doi.org/10.1016/j.ogc.2012.04.003

obgyn.theclinics.com

gynecologic oncology. Experts in ovarian, endometrial, cervical. vulvovaginal cancers and gestational trophoblastic disease will concisely review the key components of the disease site and concentrate on pivotal clinical trials that have changed the practice of gynecologic cancer care in the 21st century. Lastly, Dr Singh has provided a comprehensive chapter on complimentary therapies that are being utilized at a significant rate by women affected by gynecologic cancers. She debunks the mystery of complimentary medicinals, provides an outstanding review on risk and drug interaction of the commonly used agents and reviews the data on quality of life analyses linked to many complimentary and alternative therapy trials.

Science moves fast, perhaps now at "warp speed". Keeping current is challenging for all of us in gynecologic oncology and health care in general. But these are exciting times, with paradigms being challenged due to the "information revolution". It will not take a decade before this update in gynecologic oncology will need to be written again. I challenge the reader to review the data of the present and think about the challenges of the future for our field. New strategies in clinical trials are paramount for rapid drug and technology development that will improve gynecologic cancer cure and better the lives of our patients in a fiscally responsible way. As a "mid-century" provider, I see this as the greatest challenge for our young innovative generation of physicians and scientists. I want to thank this vast group of expert authors for providing exceptional chapters that highlight these issues, Dr Rayburn for the opportunity to put together this collection of articles and lastly Ms Stephanie Donley at Elsevier who worked tirelessly to publish this work for your enjoyment.

Carolyn Y. Muller, MD
Department of Obstetrics and Gynecology,
University of New Mexico Cancer Center,
1201 Camino De Salud
MSC 07 4025,
Albuquerque, NM 87131, USA

E-mail address:
cmuller@salud.unm.edu

Trends in Gynecologic Cancer Care in North America

Clare Reade, MD, FRCS(C)[a,b], Laurie Elit, MD, MSc, FRCS(C)[b,c,d],*

KEYWORDS

- Structures • Processes • Quality of care • Outcomes

KEY POINTS

- Quality of care in medicine is described by how structures and processes impact on outcome(s).
- In ovarian cancer, treatment at specialized high volume centers has been shown to improve outcomes.
- In vulvar cancer, treatment by high volume surgeons has been shown to improve the disease margin on the operative specimen.
- Population based studies in cervical and endometrial cancer have currently not shown a significant association between structures and outcomes.

In 2011, the United Nations World Health Organization (WHO) put forward a six-point agenda within which it operates to meet the increasingly complex landscape of public health. Within its mandate of promoting health development, WHO stresses the ethical principle of equity. It recommends that access to life-saving or health-promoting interventions should not be denied for unfair reasons, including those with economic or social roots.[1] Globally, an individual's access to health care varies based on the system available in the jurisdiction where he or she lives.

NORTH AMERICAN HEALTH CARE SYSTEMS: CONTEXTUALIZING CANCER CARE

Health care systems vary across the three jurisdictions that comprise North America: Canada, the United States, and Mexico. Because cancer care is provided within a health care system, it is important to understand the context of this care.

The authors have nothing to disclose.
[a] Division of Gynecologic Oncology, University of Toronto, Toronto, Ontario, Canada M5S 2S2;
[b] Department of Clinical Epidemiology and Biostatistics, Health Research Methodology Program, McMaster University, Hamilton, Ontario, Canada L8V 5C2; [c] Department of Obstetrics and Gynecology, Division of Gynecologic Oncology, McMaster University, Hamilton, Ontario, Canada L8V 5C2; [d] Department of Oncology, McMaster University, Hamilton, Ontario, Canada L8V 5C2
* Juravinski Cancer Centre, 699 Concession Street, Hamilton, Ontario, Canada, L8V 5C2.
E-mail address: Laurie.elit@jcc.hhsc.ca

Obstet Gynecol Clin N Am 39 (2012) 107–129
doi:10.1016/j.ogc.2012.02.003
0889-8545/12/$ – see front matter © 2012 Elsevier Inc. All rights reserved.

Health care in Mexico is a combination of private health care, which is generally paid for out-of-pocket by individuals, and a complex system of government-funded programs. One third of hospital beds are privately operated, and physicians often work in both the public and private sectors. Public programs serve different parts of the population and are not interconnected. Approximately half of the Mexican population (those who are employed in salaried positions) are covered by Social Security Institute programs. For Mexicans who are unemployed or uninsured, the Ministry of Health and State Health Service provide public health care, although this varies in availability and quality depending on region.[2] Significant inequalities exist in the Mexican system in terms of access to medical care; however, recent reforms aim to improve equity and quality.[3]

In Mexico in 2009, the most recent year for which Organisation for Economic Cooperation and Development (OECD) data are available, the proportion of total health expenditure that was publicly funded was 48.3%. Public per-capita health care expenditure was US$443 and total per-capita expenditure was US$918. Mexico spent 6.4% of its Gross Domestic Product (GDP) on health care in 2009, the lowest of the three North American countries.[4]

In Canada, health care is provincially administered and financed, with regulatory oversight by the federal government through the Canada Health Act.[5] All Canadian citizens have comprehensive health coverage provided for medically necessary hospital and physician services. Individuals are able to purchase private insurance funding to cover outpatient medication costs, private rooms in the hospital, and allied health services. The main "access" issue affecting Canadians is lengthy wait times for services. Several provinces now have strategies to reduce wait times for targeted procedures; however, wait times remain one of the largest concerns about the Canadian health care system.[6]

In the Canadian publicly funded health system in 2009, 70.6% of all health care spending was financed by the government. The public per-capita spending on health care in Canada in 2009 was US$3081 and total per-capita health care spending was US$4363. As a percentage of Canada's GDP, health care consumed 11.4% of all resources in 2009.[4]

In the United States, health care is provided by many separate legal entities. Health care facilities are largely owned and operated by the private sector. Health insurance is provided by private insurance often tied to employment or by the government in the public sector through programs such as Medicare, Medicaid, and the Veterans Health Administration. The proportion of Americans with private health insurance has been decreasing steadily since 2001. In 2010, 16.3% of the U.S. population, or 49.9 million people, were uninsured, and must pay out-of-pocket for health services.[7] Consequently, in 2010 more than one in six Americans delayed or did not receive the medical care they needed in.[8]

In the United States in 2009, 47.7% of all health care spending was financed by the government. In that year, public per-capita expenditure on health care was US$3795 and total per-capita spending was US$7960. This accounts for 17.4% of U.S. GDP in 2009.[4] Of the three North American countries, the United States spends the most on health care, both on a per-capita basis and as a percentage of GDP.

Although studies vary in their conclusions about health outcomes across jurisdictions, the 2000 WHO rating of "overall health service performance" ranked Mexico as 61st, Canada as 30th, and the United States as 37th among 191 member nations.[9] The 2007 life expectancy at birth figures for the female population in the three countries were 77.4 years, 83 years, and 80.4 years, respectively. As health care spending continues to increase in each country, there is concern regarding whether the dollars spent are procuring the desired results.

QUALITY OF CARE

The concept of quality of care was originally described by Donabedian.[10,11] This model describes how structures and processes impact on outcomes. **Structure** involves those variables that reflect the setting in which care is delivered (ie, measures that relate to staff expertise, coordination, and organization). The most commonly cited variables describing structure are hospital or physician case volumes.[12] **Process** variables describe the care journey that patients actually experience (ie, diagnostic tests, procedures, adjuvant therapies). **Outcome** refers to the endpoint of interest such as overall survival or 30-day mortality. Surrogate outcomes could be progression-free survival or overall survival.

To understand trends in gynecologic cancer care in North America, we have chosen to look at population-based studies. This allows us to look at outcomes for the whole population in a region and avoid the biases inherent with single institution studies (ie, related to socioeconomic status, race, or comorbidities). As well, population-based studies allow us the opportunity to identify where variations in care may lead to superior outcomes for the population, and so provide insight as to how to improve care.

This article discusses the epidemiologic trends of gynecologic cancers in North America. It also reviews the outcomes research completed in various global jurisdictions over the last decade. Within this objective, where the literature allows, the article discusses the sociodemographic variations identified within different population-based health care delivery contexts. It also discusses the process and structural factors that influence health care delivery.

METHODS

A systematic search of the published English-language literature from January 1, 2000 to July 26, 2011 was undertaken to present an unbiased view of the current population-based literature in the field of quality of health care. Several key articles were identified,[13–16] and Medical Subject Heading terms within these references were used to create a search strategy for PubMed MEDLINE (**Fig. 1**).

The search yielded 980 articles, of which 159 were identified as potentially relevant by article title. Inclusion and exclusion criteria (**Table 1**) were then applied to the abstracts of the 159 publications, and 42 abstracts met the criteria. In addition, 11 articles were identified by searching the reference lists of included articles, and 1 article was identified using the PubMed related articles feature. This produced a total of 54 articles for full-text review, of which 12 were excluded at the full-text stage. This left a total of 42 published articles, reporting on 40 unique studies meeting the inclusion and exclusion criteria. Two gynecologists reviewed the manuscripts.

> http://www.ncbi.nlm.nih.gov/entrez/query.fcgi?CMD=search&term=(genital neoplasms, female[mh]+AND+(th[sh]+OR+su[sh]+OR+rt[sh]+OR+dt[sh]+OR+surgery[tiab]+OR+surgical *[tiab]))+AND+(health planning[mh]+OR+"health care quality, access, and evaluation"[mh]+OR+"outcome and process assessment (health care)"[mh])+AND+(outcome*[ti]+OR+population*[ti]+OR+treatment outcome[majr])+AND+2000:2011[dp]+AND+english[la]&db=PubMed

Fig. 1. Search strategy.

Table 1
Inclusion and exclusion criteria

Inclusion Criteria	Exclusion Criteria
Population-based data collection	Not population-based data
Reporting structure or process in relation to outcomes of care	Studies on screening, precancerous or benign conditions
	Studies focusing solely on quality of life, biologic therapies, biomarkers, and personalized medicine, which are addressed in subsequent articles
	Studies not reporting clinical outcomes and practice patterns (process or structure)
	Studies focusing on cancer survivors or palliative care
	Studies focusing on breast or nongynecologic cancers

RESULTS
Ovarian Cancer

Epidemiologic trends

Globocan is a database of cancer incidence and mortality produced by the International Agency for Research on Cancer (IARC).[17] Incidence and mortality rates are presented as crude numbers for each country as well as age-standardized rates, which can be used for comparisons between countries. The incidence and mortality rates for ovarian cancer in 2008 (the most recent year for which data are available) are presented in **Table 2**.

Ovarian cancer occurs at a median age of 63 years, and the lifetime risk for women born today is 1.4%, or 1 in 72. The incidence of ovarian cancer has remained relatively stable with slight decreases over the last 20 years.[19] Despite advances in the treatment of ovarian cancer, overall mortality rates have not improved.[20] This may be due, in part, to the fact most patients are diagnosed with advanced disease, and there are no effective screening tests currently available to detect early ovarian cancer.[21]

In the United States, there are racial disparities in 5-year relative survival (a measurement of the survival of cancer patients compared to survival in the general population). The Surveillance Epidemiology and End Results (SEER) data report white women with ovarian cancer have a 5-year relative survival of 43.7% compared to 34.9% for African American women.[19] This may be due to different tumor biology, access to care and consequent differences in stage at presentation, and differential

Table 2
Ovarian cancer incidence and mortality rates

Country	Incidence		Mortality	
	Number of Cases in 2008	Age-Standardized Rate (per 100,000)	Number of Deaths in 2008	Age-Standardized Rate (per 100,000)
Canada	2235	7.9	1672	5.1
United States	21,652	8.8	15,519	5.4
Mexico	2910	5.6	1851	3.6

The standard population used for the age-standardized rate is the World Standard Population.[18]

Table 3 Type of structural variables reported		
Structural Variable	Number of Studies Demonstrating an Improvement in Survival	Number of Studies Demonstrating an Improvement in Surrogate Outcomes
Physician volume	2	6
Hospital volume	6	9
Physician type	5	12
Hospital type	4	9

treatment.[22–26] A single-institution study from the University of Chicago showed that African American women who had equal access to care and were treated by gynecologic oncologists according to current recommendations had the same survival as white women treated at the same institution. Their conclusion, "equal care yields equal outcomes," points to differential access and treatment as the major contributor to the difference in outcomes seen at the population level.[25] Thus, regional outcomes vary considerably, so significant improvements in survival could be possible by concentrating efforts to improve the quality of care provided to patients with ovarian cancer. This section focuses on epithelial ovarian cancer, which is the most common and deadly form of the disease.

Quality of care population-based literature: ovarian cancer

The vast majority of studies identified by our search reported on ovarian cancer. This is likely because treatment of this disease requires specialized surgical skills and knowledge of the disease process. The surgical procedures required to manage this disease include general gynecologic operations, pelvic and para-aortic lymphade-nectomy as part of staging for early stage disease, debulking of advanced disease, as well as bowel resections and upper abdominal procedures as appropriate. The medical knowledge of the disease process required for the treatment of ovarian cancer includes a familiarity with the natural history of the disease and experience with the use of chemotherapy. The clinical outcomes reported in these articles are measures of survival (overall survival, disease-free survival, 30-day postoperative mortality). Structural variables are also reported in association with important surrogate outcomes such as adequate surgery, appropriate chemotherapy, and need for reoperation. These same markers of appropriate care are reported as process variables in other studies.

Structural variables that influence health care outcomes

Twenty-three unique studies reported structural variables in relation to clinical outcomes for ovarian cancer (**Table 3**). This represents population-based data on 45,130 patients, with a spectrum of stages of ovarian cancer. Out of the 18 studies reporting survival as an outcome, 14 (78%) demonstrated an improvement in survival related to structural outcomes. Physician volume, hospital volume, physician type (ie, specialization), and hospital type (ie, teaching, community) were the structural variables reported in these studies.

Invariably, studies demonstrating an association between physician volume and outcomes showed physicians with higher volumes had improved outcomes. This relationship was seen in studies investigating surgeon volume; for the single study evaluating oncologist volume of chemotherapy given, no such relationship was demonstrated.[27] This reinforces the findings of a large study showing improved outcomes in many types of cancers from centralization of specialized care for complex and rarely performed operations, but not from those that are more common or less complex.[28]

Hospitals treating a high volume of patients with ovarian cancer and teaching hospitals or academic centers had improved patient survival and other clinical outcomes in several studies (**Table 4**). Studies reporting on physician type generally found patients treated by gynecologic oncologists had the best outcomes, followed by those treated by gynecologists, and then lastly by general surgeons. Some of the difference in survival and outcomes in patients of general surgeons are likely related to the fact that general surgeons are more likely to perform emergency surgeries; however, the difference in outcomes persisted after adjusting for prognostic factors. A detailed knowledge of the disease process is an important factor in providing optimal care, in addition to surgical skill.

These results demonstrate improved patient outcomes when care is provided by specialized high-volume physicians at specialized high-volume centers. No study demonstrated improved outcomes for patients treated by low-volume or less specialized care providers. Centralization of care for ovarian cancer patients therefore seems to be a sensible objective to improve patient outcomes at a population level.

There are important limitations in these data. Not all studies were able to obtain individual data to allow adjustment for every important confounding variable that impacts survival or other outcomes. Also, because the majority of these studies were retrospective or dependent on accurate data entry into databases, it is possible some of the advantages seen for type or volume of provider may in fact be due to more diligent data entry and recording of patient demographics, stage, and treatment received. For example, teaching hospitals may have more accurate and detailed documentation of the surgical procedures provided to patients, which may lead to an assumption they provided more complete surgical care when in fact the differences were in documentation only. Also, the use of reoperation as a surrogate outcome is questionable when discussing physician type because more specialized physicians are typically the ones making the decision to perform a second operation, and this decision may be more likely if the primary surgery was performed by a less specialized surgeon.

Process variables that influence health care outcomes: ovarian cancer

The concept of process of care is the provision of procedures and therapy known to improve outcomes. This can be thought of as providing the best quality care as per evidence-based guidelines. There are a number of reasons patients may not receive treatment known to be beneficial: (1) the patient may decline, fearing side effects or financial repercussions; (2) the physician may not offer care because of patient comorbidities and performance status, age, or ability to pay; or (3) the physician may not be aware of or believe in the evidence for the most effective treatment strategies.

There is evidence that older patients and nonwhite patients may receive effective treatment less often,[23,25,26,51,52,56–58] and have decreased survival as a result.[59] The "mix" of reasons for differential treatment is unclear and likely includes a combination of the three aforementioned reasons. What is known, however, is that chemotherapy or surgery should not be withheld simply because of a patient's chronologic age, as older patients can tolerate chemotherapy for ovarian cancer with rates of complications

Table 4
Structural variables in relation to outcomes for ovarian cancer

Study	Country	Data Source	Number of Patients	Did Structure Impact Survival?	Did Structure Impact Surrogate Outcomes?	Which Surrogate Outcomes Were Used?
Stockton & Davies[29]	United Kingdom	Retrospective database	989	Yes	n/a	n/a
Olaitan et al[30]	United Kingdom	Prospective cohort	595	n/a	Yes	Adequate surgery
Carney et al[31]	United States	Retrospective database	734	Yes	n/a	n/a
Elit et al[32]	Canada	Retrospective database	3815	Yes	Yes	Reoperation rates
Grossi et al[33]	Australia	Retrospective database + chart review	434	No	Yes	Adequate surgery
Kumpulainen et al[34]	Finland	Retrospective database	3851	Yes	Yes	Appropriate chemotherapy
Cress et al[35]	United States	Retrospective database	1088	n/a	Yes	Appropriate chemotherapy
Harlan et al[23]	United States	Retrospective database	1167	n/a	Yes	Adequate surgery, appropriate chemotherapy
Ioka et al[36]	Japan	Retrospective database	2450	Yes	Yes	Adequate surgery
Diaz-Montes et al[37]	United States	Retrospective database	2417	n/a	No	30-day post-operative mortality
Bailey et al[38]	United Kingdom	Prospective cohort	361	No[a]	Yes	Adequate surgery
Earle et al[39]	United States	Retrospective database	3067	Yes	Yes	Adequate surgery, reoperation rates, appropriate chemotherapy
Elit et al[27]	Canada	Retrospective database	2502	No	n/a	n/a
Engelen et al[40]	Netherlands	Retrospective database + chart review	632	Yes	Yes	Adequate surgery, appropriate chemotherapy

Study	Country	Data Source	Number of Patients	Did Structure Impact Survival?	Did Structure Impact Surrogate Outcomes?	Which Surrogate Outcomes Were Used?
Goff et al[41,42]	United States	Retrospective database	10,432	n/a	Yes	Adequate surgery
Kumpulainen et al[43,44]	Finland	Prospective cohort	275	Yes	Yes	Adequate surgery, appropriate chemotherapy
Oberaigner & Stuhlinger[45]	Austria	Retrospective database	911	Yes	n/a	n/a
Paulsen et al[46]	Norway	Prospective registry	198	Yes	Yes	Adequate surgery, appropriate chemotherapy
Schrag et al[47]	United States	Retrospective database	2952	Yes	Yes	Appropriate chemotherapy
Elit et al[48]	Canada	Retrospective database	1341	No	Yes	Reoperation rates
Bristow et al[49]	United States	Retrospective database	1894	Yes	Yes	Adequate surgery
Marth et al[28]	Austria	Prospective cohort	1948	Yes	No	Adequate surgery
Vernooij et al[50]	Netherlands	Retrospective cohort	1077	Yes	Yes	Adequate surgery

[a] The authors report this study was underpowered for this outcome. The definition of adequate surgery varies by study, but generally includes hysterectomy, bilateral salpingo-oophorectomy, plus staging for early stage disease or an attempt at debulking for advanced disease. Similarly, the definition of appropriate chemotherapy varies by study, but generally includes at least six cycles of a combination of platinum and taxane for patients deemed to have an accepted indication for chemotherapy.

Abbreviation: n/a, not evaluated in the study.

similar to those of younger patients.[55,60] This is of critical importance for improving outcomes in ovarian cancer because almost 50% of patients are diagnosed at or after 65 years of age.[61]

The mainstays of treatment for ovarian cancer include comprehensive surgical staging for disease apparently confined to the ovaries, aggressive cytoreductive (debulking) surgery for advanced disease to leave as little residual tumor as possible,[62] and at least six cycles of combination chemotherapy[63] with platinum and a taxane for patients with at least stage 2 disease. It does not appear to matter whether primary debulking or interval debulking surgery is performed; debulking to microscopic disease is an important prognostic factor regardless of which treatment strategy is used.[64]

Not surprisingly, these factors were the processes found to improve survival at a population level. Twelve population-based studies were identified, linking processes of care to improved survival (**Table 5**). These reports include 21,779 patients across three continents. Improving adherence to evidence-based processes that improve survival is a key component of improving the quality of care for ovarian cancer.

Uterine Cancer

Epidemiologic trends
Globocan incidence and mortality rates[17] are presented as crude numbers for each country as well as age-standardized rates, which can be used for comparisons between countries. The incidence and mortality rates for uterine cancer in 2008 (the most recent year for which data are available) are presented in **Table 6**.

Endometrial cancer is the most common gynecologic malignancy, and occurs at a median age of 61 years. Women born today will have a 2.5%, or 1 in 39, chance of developing uterine cancer in their lifetimes.[19] Although the age-adjusted incidence of uterine cancer in the United States had increased from 1988 to 1997, this was followed by a slight decrease from 1997 to 2006 and a period of relative stability from 2006 to 2008. The mortality rates for uterine cancer in the United States had been decreasing from 1975 to 1997, but have now been increasing significantly since 1997.[65]

In the United States, there remains a significant difference in survival by race, with the 5-year relative survival (a measurement of the survival of cancer patients compared to survival in the general population) at 83.7% for white women and 60.2% for African American women.[18] This may be due to differing rates of aggressive histologies, differing access to care resulting in delays in diagnosis and more advanced stage at diagnosis, and differential treatment.[66,67]

Quality of care population-based literature for uterine cancer
Table 7 outlines the population-based studies identified for uterine cancer. They represent a spectrum of stages. These women all underwent surgery as the initial part of their care; however, surgery that included removal of the uterus may or may not have involved pelvic or para-aortic node dissection.

Structural variables that influence health care outcomes: uterine cancer
Structural variables were reported in only four studies on uterine cancer from 2000 to 2011. Of these, only one found an association between a structural factor and survival, and one found an association between a structural variable and a surrogate outcome. Diaz-Montes and colleagues[71] reported a significant reduction in 30-day postoperative mortality in women older than 80 years of age with treatment in a high-volume hospital. Improved short-term survival in this case likely reflects

Table 5
Process variables in relation to outcomes for ovarian cancer

Study	Country	Data Source	Number of Patients	Did Process Impact Survival?	Which Process Variables Affected survival?
Grossi et al[33]	Australia	Retrospective database + chart review	434	Yes	Adequate surgery
Hershman et al[51]	United States	Retrospective database	236	Yes	Appropriate chemotherapy
Maas et al[52]	Netherlands	Retrospective database	1116	Yes	Multimodality therapy (surgery + chemotherapy)
Bailey et al[38]	United Kingdom	Prospective cohort	361	Yes	Adequate surgery
Elit et al[27]	Canada	Retrospective database	2502	Yes	1. Multimodality therapy (surgery + chemotherapy), 2. Multiagent chemotherapy
Engelen et al[40]	Netherlands	Retrospective database + chart review	632	Yes	Adequate surgery
Paulsen et al[46]	Norway	Prospective registry	198	Yes	1. Adequate surgery, 2. Appropriate chemotherapy
Petignat et al[53]	Switzerland	Retrospective database	50	Yes	Adequate surgery
Chan et al[54]	United States	Retrospective database	8372	Yes	Adequate surgery
Elit et al[48]	Canada	Retrospective database	1341	Yes	1. Adequate surgery, 2. Appropriate chemotherapy
Marth et al[28]	Austria	Prospective cohort	1948	Yes	Adequate surgery
Fairfield et al[55]	United States	Retrospective database	4589	Yes	Adequate surgery

The definition of adequate surgery varies by study, but generally includes hysterectomy, bilateral salpingo-oophorectomy, plus staging for early stage disease or an attempt at debulking for advanced disease. Similarly, the definition of appropriate chemotherapy varies by study, but generally includes at least six cycles of a combination of platinum and taxane for those patients deemed to have an accepted indication for chemotherapy.

Abbreviation: n/a, not evaluated in the study.

Table 6 Uterine cancer incidence and mortality rates	Incidence		Mortality	
Country	Number of Cases in 2008	Age-Standardized Rate (per 100,000)	Number of deaths in 2008	Age-Standardized Rate (per 100,000)
Canada	4535	16.3	606	1.7
United States	40,102	16.5	7469	2.5
Mexico	2606	5.4	1142	2.3

The standard population used for the age-standardized rate is the World Standard Population.[18]

improvements in overall perioperative care provided, rather than simply surgical factors. Crawford and colleagues,[68] Oberaigner and Stuhlinger,[45] and Kwon and colleagues[73] did not find any difference in survival related to physician or hospital type or volume (see **Table 7**). Crawford and colleagues reported patients operated by gynecologic oncologists were more likely to receive surgical staging. They view this as a surrogate outcome reflecting quality of care; however, the value of lymphadenectomy in uterine cancer is a topic of considerable controversy.[74–76] Overall, structural factors do not seem to have much impact on clinical outcomes for uterine cancer. This is likely due to the fact that uterine cancer is often found in early stages and is highly curable with surgery alone, and hysterectomy is a relatively common and uncomplicated procedure. It stands to reason, therefore, that centralization of surgical care for uterine cancer would not necessarily improve outcomes.

Process variables that influence health care outcomes: uterine cancer
A total of five articles reported process variables in relation to survival in patients with uterine cancer. Four of these found process variables had an impact on survival. Crawford and coworkers[68] reported surgical staging and postoperative radiotherapy were associated with improved survival. Truong and colleagues[69] reported treatment with both surgery and radiotherapy improved survival. Similarly, Chan and coworkers[70] found patients receiving hysterectomy had improved survival. They also found that lymphadenectomy improved survival for patients with stage 1 grade 3 disease, as well as more advanced stages. Kwon and colleagues[73] in 2008 found surgical staging improved 5-year overall survival in a population-based cohort of all patients with uterine cancer. However, in 2007, Kwon and colleagues[72] did not find any survival advantage for surgical staging or postoperative radiotherapy in women with intermediate risk and high risk stage 1 and stage 2 disease.

These findings are difficult to interpret in the context of the ASTEC (A Study in the Treatment of Endometrial Cancer) randomized controlled trials (RCTs), which have demonstrated no survival benefit for lymphadenectomy[74] and postoperative radiotherapy[77] in early stage uterine cancer. In addition, one other RCT has been published in patients with clinical stage 1 endometrial cancer evaluating the benefit of lymphadenectomy. Five hundred and fourteen patients were randomized to either systematic pelvic lymphadenectomy or no systematic lymphadenectomy. All patients received the standard treatment of total abdominal hysterectomy and bilateral salpingoophorectomy, and removal of clinically enlarged nodes. There were no differences in 5-year disease-free or overall survival, and patients in the lymphadenectomy arm had increased rates of postoperative complications.[78] There is also a

Table 7
Structure and process variables in relation to outcomes in uterine cancer

Study	Country	Data Source	Number of Patients	Did Structure Variables Impact Survival?	Did Structure Variables Impact Surrogate Outcomes?	Did Process Variables Impact Survival?
Crawford et al[68]	Scotland	Retrospective database	703	No	Yes	Yes
Truong et al[69]	Canada	Retrospective database	401	n/a	n/a	Yes
Oberaigner & Stuhlinger[45]	Austria	Retrospective database	907	No	n/a	n/a
Chan et al[70]	United States	Retrospective database	39,396	n/a	n/a	Yes
Diaz-Montes et al[71]	United States	Retrospective database	6181	Yes	n/a	n/a
Kwon et al[72]	Canada	Retrospective database	995	n/a	n/a	No
Kwon et al[73]	Canada	Retrospective database	3875	No	n/a	Yes

Abbreviation: n/a, not evaluated in the study.

Table 8
Cervical cancer incidence and mortality rates

Country	Incidence		Mortality	
	Number of Cases in 2008	Age-Standardized Rate (per 100,000)	Number of Deaths in 2008	Age-Standardized Rate (per 100,000)
Canada	1419	6.6	544	1.9
United States	11,069	5.7	3869	1.7
Mexico	10,186	19.2	5061	9.7

The standard population used for the age-standardized rate is the World Standard Population.[17]

systematic review and meta-analysis of four RCTs reporting no survival benefit from radiotherapy.[79] Despite the availability of high-quality evidence, whether lymphadenectomy or radiotherapy improves survival in early stage uterine cancer remains highly controversial.[75] Unfortunately, population-based data may not contain adequate information on demographics or other confounding variables, which may impact survival. Also, surgical staging or radiotherapy may simply reflect other differences in the care provided (not accounted for in administrative databases), which could be driving the results. The population-based literature will not resolve the debate over management of uterine cancer. More research is needed to determine if various subpopulations of patients with uterine cancer may have a survival benefit from radiotherapy or lymphadenectomy.

Cervical Cancer

Epidemiologic trends

Worldwide, cancer of the uterine cervix is the third most common cancer in women; however, more than 85% of these cancers occur in developing countries.[17] Virtually all cervical cancer is a result of human papillomavirus (HPV) infection.

Globocan incidence and mortality rates[17] are presented as crude numbers for each country as well as age-standardized rates, which can be used for comparisons between countries. The incidence and mortality rates for cervical cancer in 2008 (the most recent year for which data are available) are presented in **Table 8**.

Cervical cancer occurs at a median age of 48 years, and the lifetime risk of cervical cancer for women born in the United States today is 0.7%, or 1 in 147. The incidence of cervical cancer has been decreasing since 1990, and the mortality rate in the United States has followed a similar trend.[19] As HPV vaccination programs become established, there is the potential for further decreases in incidence in North America.[80] Organized, population-based screening programs also have the potential to reduce the incidence of cervical cancer further.[81,82]

As with ovarian and uterine cancers, the SEER database shows significant racial disparities in survival exist for cervical cancer. White women have a 5-year relative survival of 70% compared to 58.4% in African American women.[19] Again, this may be due to genetics, tumor biology, stage at presentation, access to care, and differing treatment.[83–86] A single-institution study from the University of Pennsylvania found African American women were more likely to be diagnosed with cervical cancer than white women, and that they were diagnosed at a more advanced stage. The authors suggested access to screening and preventative health services may have accounted for the differences.[87] Special attention should be paid to promoting screening and

HPV vaccination in high-risk and minority groups to decrease the burden of cervical cancer in North America.[88]

Quality of care population-based literature for cervical cancer

Table 9 shows the population-based studies of women diagnosed with cervical cancer. These women represent a spectrum of stages; some were treated initially with surgery[89] while others were treated only with radiation[90] depending on the inclusion criteria for the study.

Structural variables that influence health care outcomes: cervical cancer

Only three studies reported structural variables in relation to survival or clinical surrogate endpoints. Downing and coworkers[91] did not find an association between surgeon volume or radiation oncologist volume and survival after multivariate analysis was used to adjust for differences in patient demographics and disease stage. Denton and coworkers[90] did not find an association between hospital volume and either survival or late severe radiation complications in a population-based cohort of cervical cancer patients who had primary radiotherapy. Oberaigner and Stuhlinger[45] reported that patients treated in low-volume hospitals actually had improved survival compared to those treated in high-volume centers, even after controlling for age, stage, and histology. This finding is unexpected, and is contrary to findings of improved outcomes in larger centers in many other disease sites that require complex surgery.[28] The authors state that more cases in the small centers were of unknown stage, and therefore the effect of stage may not have been fully adjusted for in the multivariate analysis. This unexpected finding deserves further study in other population-based cohorts. Overall, however, there does not appear to be a significant association between structural variables and outcomes in cervical cancer based on the current population-based literature.

Process variables that influence health care outcomes: cervical cancer

The process variables addressed by the four studies from **Table 9** are varied, and depend on the nature of the population under study. Denton and coworkers[90] did not find any association between the type of surgery performed or the type of radiation therapy provided (external beam vs brachytherapy vs combination treatment) and late severe radiation complications. They suggested their sample size may have been too small to find these differences, given the rarity of these late severe complications (6.1% in the entire cohort). They did not report information on survival.

Webb and colleagues[89] evaluated a population of patients with stage 1A1 or 1A2 adenocarcinoma of the cervix, and found the type of hysterectomy performed (radical vs. simple hysterectomy) did not affect survival. They also state they believe the study was underpowered to find such a difference, and therefore more study is required.

Downing and colleagues[91] found improved survival in patients who were treated surgically, rather than with radiotherapy or multimodality treatment, but this effect was no longer significant after adjusting for patient age and stage, and likely simply reflects the fact that patients undergoing surgical management have earlier stage disease.

Pearcey and colleagues[92] found that the use of chemoradiation improved survival of cervical cancer patients compared to radiotherapy alone. They did not find any evidence of increasing toxicity from the use of chemotherapy as judged by hospital admissions.

Because the publications on cervical cancer examine a wide range of populations and outcomes, it is impossible to draw broad conclusions. More study is needed to

Table 9
Structure and process variables in relation to outcomes in cervical cancer

Study	Country	Data Source	Number of Patients	Did Structure Variables Impact Survival?	Did Structure Variables Impact Surrogate Outcomes?	Did Process Variables Impact Survival?
Denton et al[90]	United Kingdom	Retrospective chart review	1993	No	No	No
Webb et al[89]	United States	Retrospective database	301	n/a	n/a	No
Oberaigner & Stuhlinger[44]	Austria	Retrospective database	804	Yes	n/a	n/a
Downing et al[91]	United Kingdom	Retrospective database	1500	No	n/a	No
Pearcey et al[92]	Canada	Retrospective database	4069	n/a	n/a	Yes

Abbreviation: n/a, not evaluated in the study.

identify processes that improve outcomes at a population level and patterns of care in cervical cancer.

Vulvar Cancer

Epidemiologic trends

Vulvar cancer is a rare disease, representing only 3% to 5% of gynecologic malignancies. Because of its rarity, vulvar cancer epidemiology is not reported by the International Agency for Research on Cancer (IARC) or the World Health Organization (WHO) mortality database. The incidence and mortality data reported here are from the National Cancer Institute's SEER Cancer Statistics Review.[19]

The median age of patients diagnosed with vulvar cancer is 68 years, and the lifetime risk for women born today in the United States is 0.3%, or 1 in 387. In the United States, approximately 3900 women are diagnosed with vulvar cancer annually, and 920 will die of this disease. The age-adjusted incidence is 2.3 per 100,000 women per year and the age-adjusted mortality rate is 0.5 per 100,000 women per year based on the 2000 U.S. standard population. The incidence of vulvar cancer has been increasing steadily since 1975.[19] Most of the increase in incidence has been attributed to HPV infection,[93] and HPV-related cases are thought to occur more often in younger women.[94,95]

Similar to other gynecologic cancers, there are racial disparities in relative survival. White women with vulvar cancer have a relative 5-year survival of 72.8% compared to 66.7% for African American women.[19] Again, this may be due to different tumor biology, access to care, and differential treatment.[96]

Quality of care population-based literature for vulvar cancer

Table 10 outlines the two population-based vulvar cancer studies identified from the literature.

Structural variables that influence health outcomes: vulvar cancer

Of the gynecologic cancer disease sites, the fewest population-based publications on quality of care focused on vulvar cancer, with only two articles identified.[96,97] Neither article reported on patient survival in terms of structural variables, although one article[97] reported that high-volume surgeons were more likely to achieve adequate negative margins (a surrogate endpoint). Margins less than 8 mm after formalin fixation are associated with an increased risk of recurrence.[98] Neither study evaluated the impact of surgeon specialization or hospital type or volume.

Process variables that influence health care outcomes: vulvar cancer

The small number of studies makes a full evaluation of processes of care impossible at a population level. Although the study by Falconer and coworkers[97] did outline practice patterns in relation to clinical practice guidelines, the processes of care were not compared to clinical outcomes. The study by Rad and Ogunyemi[96] reported surgical management of vulvar cancer improved survival, but did not specify if this was in comparison to radiation therapy or no therapy, and did not adjust for important covariates.

SUMMARY

Overall, there has been tremendous movement over the last decade toward centralization of cancer care into specialized centers. This comes from the recognition that multidisciplinary care, including access to opinions from gynecologic, medical, and radiation oncologists, can improve patient outcomes. In addition to this input, it is

Table 10
Structure and process variables in relation to outcomes for vulvar cancer

Study	Country	Data Source	Number of Patients	Did Structure Variables Impact Survival?	Did Structure Variables Impact Surrogate Outcomes?	Did Process Variables Impact Survival?
Falconer et al[97]	United Kingdom	Prospective collection	436	n/a	Yes	n/a
Rad & Ogunyemi[96]	United States	Retrospective administrative database	1566	n/a	n/a	Yes

Abbreviation: n/a, not evaluated in the study.

important to have access to subspecialty pathology, diagnostic radiology, oncology nursing, and other disciplines as necessary.[99] The population-based literature on quality of care in gynecologic cancers reflects this movement, with many articles evaluating outcomes in terms of structural variables. However, the continued presence of regional and sociodemographic variation in outcomes suggests it is still possible to achieve significant improvements in survival by concentrating efforts to improve the quality of care provided to gynecologic cancer patients. Improved outcomes for patients with ovarian cancer can be achieved by continued centralization of gynecologic cancer care and provision of care by gynecologic oncologists in high-volume centers. Further study is needed to determine if cervical cancer and vulvar cancer outcomes can be improved with centralization. For uterine cancer, at this time there do not appear to be significant improvements in outcomes related to centralization.

For all gynecologic cancers, more attention should be paid to the processes of care and their impact on patient outcomes. An appropriate goal for all health care systems is to ensure all women have access to evidence-based care. This is particularly important for high-risk women, older women, and minority women, who suffer a disproportionate amount of the gynecologic cancer–related mortality and often do not receive evidence-based care.[35,87] Clinical practice guidelines exist to provide guidance to clinicians as to what constitutes evidence-based care and to make recommendations concerning current best practices. Adherence to guidelines can help to reduce variations in care due to sociodemographic factors.[22] As the provision of cancer care becomes more and more centralized, outcomes at the population level will be improved only by focusing on the processes of care.

A look at the three North American health care systems shows there are issues with women having access to high-quality, timely care. This fundamental problem must be addressed to systematically improve health at the population level. Governments should strive toward the WHO goal of promoting health development in their populations by reducing inequalities in the access to health care and health promotion activities.

ACKNOWLEDGMENTS

The authors thank Michelle Marcotte for her contribution to this chapter.

REFERENCES

1. WHO. The WHO agenda. Available at: http://www.who.int/about/agenda/en.index.html. Accessed August 5, 2011.
2. OECD. OECD reviews of health systems: Mexico. Paris: OECD Publishing; 2005. Available at: http://www.oecdbookshop.org/oecd/display.asp?langEN&sf1identifiers&st1812005081e1. Accessed October 11, 2011.
3. Ruelas E. Health care quality improvement in Mexico: challenges, opportunities, and progress. Proc Bayl Univ Med Cent 2002;15(3):319–22.
4. OECD Health Data 2011. Frequently requested data. Available at: www.oecd.org/health/healthdata. Accessed August 10, 2011.
5. Public Information. Available at: http://www.health.gov.on.ca/en/ministry/. Accessed August 5, 2011.
6. Glynn PA. Timely and appropriate access to healthcare. The way forward—the roles of the players. Healthc Q 2006;9(4):30–6, 32.
7. DeNavas C, Proctor B, Smith J. Income, poverty, and health insurance coverage in the United States. In: Current population reports. Washington, DC: United States Census Bureau. 2010. Available at: http://www.census.gov/prod/2011pubs/p60-239.pdf. Accessed October 11, 2011.

8. Boukus ER, Cunningham PJ. Mixed signals: trends in Americans' access to medical care, 2007–2010. Track Rep 2011(25):1–6.

9. Ajay Tandon, Murray CJ, Lauer JA, et al. Measuring overall health system performance for 191 countries. GPE Discussion Paper Series No. 30. 2000. Available at: http://www.who.int/healthinfo/paper30.pdf. Accessed October 11, 2011.

10. Donabedian A. Evaluating the quality of medical care. Milbank Mem Fund Q 1966; 44(3 Suppl):166–206.

11. Birkmeyer JD, Dimick JB, Birkmeyer NJ. Measuring the quality of surgical care: structure, process, or outcomes? J Am Coll Surg 2004;198(4):626–32.

12. Hillner BE, Smith TJ, Desch CE. Hospital and physician volume or specialization and outcomes in cancer treatment: importance in quality of cancer care. J Clin Oncol 2000;18(11):2327–40.

13. Elit L, Schultz S, Prysbysz R, et al. Patterns of care in the initial management of women with vulvar cancers in Ontario. Eur J Gynaecol Oncol 2009;30(5):503–5.

14. Elit L, Schultz S, Prysbysz R, et al. Patterns of care for the initial management of cervical cancer in Ontario. Eur J Gynaecol Oncol 2009;30(5):493–6.

15. Elit L, Schultz S, Prysbysz R, et al. Patterns of surgical care for uterine cancers in Ontario. Eur J Gynaecol Oncol 2009;30(3):255–8.

16. Elit L, Schultz S, Prysbysz R, et al. Patterns of care in the initial management of women with ovarian cancer in Ontario. Eur J Gynaecol Oncol 2009;30(4):361–4.

17. Ferlay J, Shin H, Bray F, et al. GLOBOCAN 2008 v1.2, Cancer incidence and Mortality Worldwide: IARC CancerBase No. 10. Available at: http://globocan.iarc.fr. Accessed August 17, 2011.

18. Doll R, Payne P, Waterhouse JAH, eds. Cancer incidence in five continents. Geneva: Union Internationale Contre le Cancer; 1966; No. I.

19. Howlader N, Noone A, Krapcho M, et al. SEER Cancer statistics review, 1975–2008. Bethesda, MD: National Cancer Institute. Available at: http://seer.cancer.gov/csr/1975_2008/index.html. Accessed September 30, 2011.

20. Engel J, Eckel R, Schubert-Fritschle G, et al. Moderate progress for ovarian cancer in the last 20 years: prolongation of survival, but no improvement in the cure rate. Eur J Cancer 2002;38(18):2435–45.

21. Buys SS, Partridge E, Black A, et al. Effect of screening on ovarian cancer mortality: the Prostate, Lung, Colorectal and Ovarian (PLCO) Cancer Screening Randomized Controlled Trial. JAMA 2011;305(22):2295–303.

22. Brewster WR. The complexity of race in the disparate outcome and treatment of minority patients. Gynecol Oncol 2008;111(2):161–2.

23. Harlan LC, Clegg LX, Trimble EL. Trends in surgery and chemotherapy for women diagnosed with ovarian cancer in the United States. J Clin Oncol 2003;21(18): 3488–94.

24. Farley JH, Tian C, Rose GS, et al. Race does not impact outcome for advanced ovarian cancer patients treated with cisplatin/paclitaxel: an analysis of Gynecologic Oncology Group trials. Cancer 2009;115(18):4210–7.

25. Terplan M, Temkin S, Tergas A, et al. Does equal treatment yield equal outcomes? The impact of race on survival in epithelial ovarian cancer. Gynecol Oncol 2008; 111(2):173–8.

26. Bristow RE, Zahurak ML, Ibeanu OA. Racial disparities in ovarian cancer surgical care: a population-based analysis. Gynecol Oncol 2011;121(2):364–8.

27. Elit L, Chartier C, Oza A, et al. Outcomes for systemic therapy in women with ovarian cancer. Gynecol Oncol 2006;103(2):554–8.

28. Marth C, Hiebl S, Oberaigner W, et al. Influence of department volume on survival for ovarian cancer: results from a prospective quality assurance program of the Austrian Association for Gynecologic Oncology. Int J Gynecol Cancer 2009;19(1):94–102.

29. Stockton D, Davies T. Multiple cancer site comparison of adjusted survival by hospital of treatment: an East Anglian study. Br J Cancer 2000;82(1):208–12.

30. Olaitan A, Weeks J, Mocroft A, et al. The surgical management of women with ovarian cancer in the south west of England. Br J Cancer 2001;85(12):1824–30.

31. Carney ME, Lancaster JM, Ford C, et al. A population-based study of patterns of care for ovarian cancer: who is seen by a gynecologic oncologist and who is not? Gynecol Oncol 2002;84(1):36–42.

32. Elit L, Bondy SJ, Paszat L, et al. Outcomes in surgery for ovarian cancer. Gynecol Oncol 2002;87(3):260–7.

33. Grossi M, Quinn MA, Thursfield VJ, et al. Ovarian cancer: patterns of care in Victoria during 1993–1995. Med J Aust 2002;177(1):11–6.

34. Kumpulainen S, Grenman S, Kyyronen P, et al. Evidence of benefit from centralised treatment of ovarian cancer: a nationwide population-based survival analysis in Finland. Int J Cancer 2002;102(5):541–4.

35. Cress RD, O'Malley CD, Leiserowitz GS, et al. Patterns of chemotherapy use for women with ovarian cancer: a population-based study. J Clin Oncol 2003;21(8): 1530–5.

36. Ioka A, Tsukuma H, Ajiki W, et al. Influence of hospital procedure volume on ovarian cancer survival in Japan, a country with low incidence of ovarian cancer. Cancer Sci 2004;95(3):233–7.

37. Diaz-Montes TP, Zahurak ML, Giuntoli RL 2nd, et al. Surgical care of elderly women with ovarian cancer: a population-based perspective. Gynecol Oncol 2005;99(2): 352–7.

38. Bailey J, Murdoch J, Anderson R, et al. Stage III and IV ovarian cancer in the South West of England: five-year outcome analysis for cases treated in 1998. Int J Gynecol Cancer 2006;16(Suppl 1):25–9.

39. Earle CC, Schrag D, Neville BA, et al. Effect of surgeon specialty on processes of care and outcomes for ovarian cancer patients. J Natl Cancer Inst 2006;98(3):172–80.

40. Engelen MJ, Kos HE, Willemse PH, et al. Surgery by consultant gynecologic oncologists improves survival in patients with ovarian carcinoma. Cancer 2006; 106(3):589–98.

41. Goff BA, Matthews BJ, Wynn M, et al. Ovarian cancer: patterns of surgical care across the United States. Gynecol Oncol 2006;103(2):383–90.

42. Goff BA, Matthews BJ, Larson EH, et al. Predictors of comprehensive surgical treatment in patients with ovarian cancer. Cancer 2007;109(10):2031–42.

43. Kumpulainen S, Kuoppala T, Leminen A, et al. Surgical treatment of ovarian cancer in different hospital categories—a prospective nation-wide study in Finland. Eur J Cancer 2006;42(3):388–95.

44. Kumpulainen S, Sankila R, Leminen A, et al. The effect of hospital operative volume, residual tumor and first-line chemotherapy on survival of ovarian cancer—a prospective nation-wide study in Finland. Gynecol Oncol 2009;115(2):199–203.

45. Oberaigner W, Stuhlinger W. Influence of department volume on cancer survival for gynaecological cancers—a population-based study in Tyrol, Austria. Gynecol Oncol 2006;103(2):527–34.

46. Paulsen T, Kjaerheim K, Kaern J, et al. Improved short-term survival for advanced ovarian, tubal, and peritoneal cancer patients operated at teaching hospitals. Int J Gynecol Cancer 2006;16(Suppl 1):11–7.

47. Schrag D, Earle C, Xu F, et al. Associations between hospital and surgeon procedure volumes and patient outcomes after ovarian cancer resection. J Natl Cancer Inst 2006;98(3):163–71.
48. Elit LM, Bondy SJ, Paszat LP, et al. Surgical outcomes in women with ovarian cancer. Can J Surg 2008;51(5):346–54.
49. Bristow RE, Zahurak ML, Diaz-Montes TP, et al. Impact of surgeon and hospital ovarian cancer surgical case volume on in-hospital mortality and related short-term outcomes. Gynecol Oncol 2009;115(3):334–8.
50. Vernooij F, Heintz AP, Coebergh JW, et al. Specialized and high-volume care leads to better outcomes of ovarian cancer treatment in the Netherlands. Gynecol Oncol 2009;112(3):455–61.
51. Hershman D, Fleischauer AT, Jacobson JS, et al. Patterns and outcomes of chemotherapy for elderly patients with stage II ovarian cancer: a population-based study. Gynecol Oncol 2004;92(1):293–9.
52. Maas HA, Kruitwagen RF, Lemmens VE, et al. The influence of age and co-morbidity on treatment and prognosis of ovarian cancer: a population-based study. Gynecol Oncol 2005;97(1):104–9.
53. Petignat P, de Weck D, Goffin F, et al. Long-term survival of patients with apparent early-stage (FIGO I-II) epithelial ovarian cancer: a population-based study. Gynecol Obstet Invest 2007;63(3):132–6.
54. Chan J, Fuh K, Shin J, et al. The treatment and outcomes of early-stage epithelial ovarian cancer: have we made any progress? Br J Cancer 2008;98(7):1191–6.
55. Fairfield KM, Lucas FL, Earle CC, et al. Regional variation in cancer-directed surgery and mortality among women with epithelial ovarian cancer in the Medicare population. Cancer 2010;116(20):4840–8.
56. Sundararajan V, Hershman D, Grann VR, et al. Variations in the use of chemotherapy for elderly patients with advanced ovarian cancer: a population-based study. J Clin Oncol 2002;20(1):173–8.
57. Petignat P, Fioretta G, Verkooijen HM, et al. Poorer survival of elderly patients with ovarian cancer: a population-based study. Surg Oncol 2004;13(4):181–6.
58. Thrall MM, Gray HJ, Symons RG, et al. Trends in treatment of advanced epithelial ovarian cancer in the Medicare population. Gynecol Oncol 2011;122(1):100–6.
59. Vercelli M, Capocaccia R, Quaglia A, et al. Relative survival in elderly European cancer patients: evidence for health care inequalities. The EUROCARE Working Group. Crit Rev Oncol Hematol 2000;35(3):161–79.
60. Gronlund B, Hogdall C, Hansen HH, et al. Performance status rather than age is the key prognostic factor in second-line treatment of elderly patients with epithelial ovarian carcinoma. Cancer 2002;94(7):1961–7.
61. Yancik R. Cancer burden in the aged: an epidemiologic and demographic overview. Cancer 1997;80(7):1273–83.
62. Bristow RE, Tomacruz RS, Armstrong DK, et al. Survival effect of maximal cytoreductive surgery for advanced ovarian carcinoma during the platinum era: a meta-analysis. J Clin Oncol 2002;20(5):1248–59.
63. Advanced Ovarian Cancer Trialists Group. Chemotherapy for advanced ovarian cancer. Cochrane Database Syst Rev 2000;2:CD001418.
64. Vergote I, Trope CG, Amant F, et al. Neoadjuvant chemotherapy or primary surgery in stage IIIC or IV ovarian cancer. N Engl J Med 2010;363(10):943–53.
65. Surveillance Research Program. Fast Stats: An interactive tool for access to SEER cancer statistics. National Cancer Institute; 2011. Available at: http://seer.cancer.gov/faststats. Accessed October 11, 2011.

66. Randall TC, Armstrong K. Differences in treatment and outcome between African-American and white women with endometrial cancer. J Clin Oncol 2003;21(22): 4200–6.
67. Tammemagi CM. Racial/ethnic disparities in breast and gynecologic cancer treatment and outcomes. Curr Opin Obstet Gynecol 2007;19(1):31–6.
68. Crawford SC, De Caestecker L, Gillis CR, et al. Staging quality is related to the survival of women with endometrial cancer: a Scottish population based study. Deficient surgical staging and omission of adjuvant radiotherapy is associated with poorer survival of women diagnosed with endometrial cancer in Scotland during 1996 and 1997. Br J Cancer 2002;86(12):1837–42.
69. Truong PT, Kader HA, Lacy B, et al. The effects of age and comorbidity on treatment and outcomes in women with endometrial cancer. Am J Clin Oncol 2005;28(2):157–64.
70. Chan JK, Wu H, Cheung MK, et al. The outcomes of 27,063 women with unstaged endometrioid uterine cancer. Gynecol Oncol 2007;106(2):282–8.
71. Diaz-Montes TP, Zahurak ML, Giuntoli RL 2nd, et al. Concentration of uterine cancer surgical care among the elderly: a population-based perspective. Gynecol Oncol 2007;107(3):436–40.
72. Kwon JS, Carey MS, Cook EF, et al. Patterns of practice and outcomes in intermediate- and high-risk stage I and II endometrial cancer: a population-based study. Int J Gynecol Cancer 2007;17(2):433–40.
73. Kwon JS, Carey MS, Cook EF, et al. Are there regional differences in gynecologic cancer outcomes in the context of a single-payer, publicly-funded health care system? A population-based study. Can J Public Health 2008;99(3):221–6.
74. Kitchener H, Swart AM, Qian Q, et al. Efficacy of systematic pelvic lymphadenectomy in endometrial cancer (MRC ASTEC trial): a randomised study. Lancet 2009; 373(9658):125–36.
75. Creasman WT, Mutch DE, Herzog TJ. ASTEC lymphadenectomy and radiation therapy studies: are conclusions valid? Gynecol Oncol 2010;116(3):293–4.
76. Lee TS, Kim JW, Seong SJ, et al. Benefit of lymphadenectomy in endometrial cancer: can the truth be obtained by randomized controlled trial after ASTEC? Int J Gynecol Cancer 2009;19(8):1467.
77. Blake P, Swart AM, Orton J, et al. Adjuvant external beam radiotherapy in the treatment of endometrial cancer (MRC ASTEC and NCIC CTG EN.5 randomised trials): pooled trial results, systematic review, and meta-analysis. Lancet 2009; 373(9658):137–46.
78. Benedetti Panici P, Basile S, Maneschi F, et al. Systematic pelvic lymphadenectomy vs. no lymphadenectomy in early-stage endometrial carcinoma: randomized clinical trial. J Natl Cancer Inst 2008;100(23):1707–16.
79. Kong A, Simera I, Collingwood M, et al. Adjuvant radiotherapy for stage I endometrial cancer: systematic review and meta-analysis. Ann Oncol 2007;18(10):1595–604.
80. Finn OJ, Edwards RP. Human papillomavirus vaccine for cancer prevention. N Engl J Med 2009;361(19):1899–901.
81. Nieminen P, Kallio M, Anttila A, et al. Organised vs. spontaneous Pap-smear screening for cervical cancer: a case-control study. Int J Cancer 1999;83(1):55–8.
82. HPV Consensus Guidelines Committee. Canadian consensus guidelines on human papillomavirus. J Obstet Gynaecol Can 2007;28(8 Suppl 3):S5–S6.
83. Brooks SE, Chen TT, Ghosh A, et al. Cervical cancer outcomes analysis: impact of age, race, and comorbid illness on hospitalizations for invasive carcinoma of the cervix. Gynecol Oncol 2000;79(1):107–15.

84. Downs LS, Smith JS, Scarinci I, et al. The disparity of cervical cancer in diverse populations. Gynecol Oncol 2008;109(2 Suppl):S22–30.
85. Leath CA 3rd, Straughn JM Jr, Kirby TO, et al. Predictors of outcomes for women with cervical carcinoma. Gynecol Oncol 2005;99(2):432–6.
86. Patel DA, Barnholtz-Sloan JS, Patel MK, et al. A population-based study of racial and ethnic differences in survival among women with invasive cervical cancer: analysis of Surveillance, Epidemiology, and End Results data. Gynecol Oncol 2005;97(2):550–8.
87. Morgan MA, Behbakht K, Benjamin I, et al. Racial differences in survival from gynecologic cancer. Obstet Gynecol 1996;88(6):914–8.
88. Downs LS Jr, Scarinci I, Einstein MH, et al. Overcoming the barriers to HPV vaccination in high-risk populations in the US. Gynecol Oncol 2010;117(3):486–90.
89. Webb JC, Key CR, Qualls CR, et al. Population-based study of microinvasive adenocarcinoma of the uterine cervix. Obstet Gynecol 2001;97(5 Pt 1):701–6.
90. Denton AS, Bond SJ, Matthews S, et al. National audit of the management and outcome of carcinoma of the cervix treated with radiotherapy in 1993. Clin Oncol (R Coll Radiol) 2000;12(6):347–53.
91. Downing A, Mikeljevic JS, Haward B, et al. Variation in the treatment of cervical cancer patients and the effect of consultant workload on survival: a population-based study. Eur J Cancer 2007;43(2):363–70.
92. Pearcey R, Miao Q, Kong W, et al. Impact of adoption of chemoradiotherapy on the outcome of cervical cancer in Ontario: results of a population-based cohort study. J Clin Oncol 2007;25(17):2383–8.
93. Judson PL HE, Baxter NN, Durham SB, et al. Trends in the incidence of invasive and in situ vulvar carcinoma. Obstet Gynecol 2006;107(5):1018–22.
94. Al-Ghamdi A, Freedman D, Miller D, et al. Vulvar squamous cell carcinoma in young women: a clinicopathologic study of 21 Cases. Gynecol Oncol 2002;84(1):94–101.
95. Hampl M, Deckers-Figiel S, Hampl JA, et al. New aspects of vulvar cancer: changes in localization and age of onset. Gynecol Oncol 2008;109(3):340–5.
96. Rad S, Ogunyemi D. An analysis of the demographics and outcome of vulvar cancer in California. Gynecol Oncol 2007;105(3):828–9.
97. Falconer AD, Hirschowitz L, Weeks J, et al. The impact of improving outcomes guidance on surgical management of vulval squamous cell cancer in southwest England (1997–2002). BJOG 2007;114(4):391–7.
98. Heaps JM, Fu YS, Montz FJ, et al. Surgical-pathologic variables predictive of local recurrence in squamous cell carcinoma of the vulva. Gynecol Oncol 1990;38(3):309–14.
99. Multidisciplinary Cancer Conferences. Available at: https://www.cancercare.on.ca/cms/one.aspx?portalId=1377&pageId=8256. Accessed October 26, 2011.

Biologic Therapies and Personalized Medicine in Gynecologic Malignancies

Maria B. Schiavone, MD[a],*, Shazia Bashir, MD[b],
Thomas J. Herzog, MD[b]

KEYWORDS

- Biologic therapies • Personalized medicine • Malignancies • Gynecology

KEY POINTS

- Personalized medicine has been championed as the next frontier in solid tumor treatment development.
- Through advances in human genomic sequencing, multiple cellular and molecular pathways have been identified to potentially serve as targets for drug development for gynecologic malignancies on an individualized basis.
- Currently, treatment studies have focused on stromal, vascular and cell signaling targets.
- Although results to date for biologic therapies have been mixed, great promise remains.

The concept of personalized medicine has been championed as the next frontier in solid tumor treatment development. The goal is to identify and then target a specific protein or pathway that is upregulated or overexpressed in tumors. Traditionally, treatment of gynecologic tumors has relied on the combination of surgical cytoreduction and cytotoxic chemotherapy to improve outcomes for patients with pelvic malignancies. Unlike many other oncologic subspecialties, however, rates of relapse and overall survival (OS) have improved only modestly over the past couple of decades despite the continued pursuit for novel chemotherapeutic regimens. As such, research in the field of female cancers has more recently focused on the highly

[a] Department of Obstetrics and Gynecology, Columbia University College of Physicians and Surgeons, New York Presbyterian Hospital, 622 West 168th Street, PH16-29, New York, NY 10032, USA; [b] Department of Gynecologic Oncology, Columbia University College of Physicians and Surgeons, New York Presbyterian Hospital, 161 Fort Washington Avenue, New York, NY 10032, USA
* Corresponding author.
E-mail address: ms4013@columbia.edu

Obstet Gynecol Clin N Am 39 (2012) 131–144
doi:10.1016/j.ogc.2012.02.004
0889-8545/12/$ – see front matter © 2012 Elsevier Inc. All rights reserved.

obgyn.theclinics.com

variable molecular-based causes of oncologic transformation and cell growth. Through advances in human genomic sequencing, multiple cellular and molecular pathways have been identified to potentially serve as targets for drug development on an individualized basis. A better understanding of the biology of gynecologic malignancies has also led to a greater appreciation of the interconnectedness of the numerous cell signaling pathways that work together to produce states of heath and disease.

Not surprisingly, myriad treatment possibilities have encompassed stromal, vasculature, and cell signaling targets. Early success with antiangiogenic agents has become well-known in the field of ovarian cancer, but many other lesser known agents are being investigated in preclinical and early phase trials for not only ovarian but also cervical and uterine cancers. Results to date for biologic therapy development have been mixed, yet great promise remains. In this review the authors focus on the main categories of molecular targeting for ovarian, uterine, and cervical cancers and highlight key recently completed and current clinical trials.

CELL SIGNALING PATHWAYS

One of the most exciting new areas of research and drug development is in the area of cell signaling pathways. Although it is well-known that the initial insult of many malignancies results from numerous genetic and epigenetic circumstances, it is the maintenance of such neoplastic conditions that has prompted researchers to focus on the numerous cell signaling pathways that exist to maintain and perpetuate the survival of a malignant phenotype.[1] One such pathway that has been targeted as an important player in numerous solid organ malignancies is that of the phosphatidylinositide 3-kinase (PI3K)/AKT/mammalian target of rapamycin (mTOR) cell signaling pathway.[2-6] This pathway has been noted in recent years to be a key regulator of cell cycle initiation and survival, as well as protein synthesis and glucose metabolism.[1]

AKT is often seen as the central agent in the pathway, with multiple downstream pathways and feedback loops that make it an integral part of normal cell growth and proliferation.[2-6] Upstream from the AKT complex lies P13K, an active kinase that is encoded by PIK3CA that in turn activates AKT in the signaling cascade, thereby mediating survival signals that protect cells from apoptosis. Not surprisingly, many studies have demonstrated high rates of AKT hyperactivation in various cancers including ovarian malignancies. Yuan and colleagues[4] demonstrated AKT activation in 36% of ovarian cancer specimens assessed for AKT and PI3K activity. The majority of these cancers were histologically high grade and late stage tumors. In nearly half of these cases, high levels of PI3K were also noted, with the majority also exhibiting AKT amplification. Similarly, other amplifications and mutations have been observed in PIK3CA, with rates as high as 15% in various cancers.[1] Various aberrations have been found in uterine, cervical, and ovarian cancers, with particular overrepresentation in endometrioid and clear cell histologies.[7]

Another key player in the PI3K/AKT/mTOR pathway is PTEN that serves to inhibit PI3K signaling through dephosphorylation of the second messenger PIP3.[3,5,6] Inhibition of PI3K thus results in a breakdown of the normal apoptotic mechanisms necessary for preventing neoplastic proliferation. The second most commonly mutated tumor suppressor gene after p53, PTEN is often inactivated through various mechanisms in a number of malignancies including endometrial cancers.[2] More specifically, inactivation of P13K signaling through either PIK3CA or PTEN mutations is seen in approximately 40% of endometrial cancers in comparison with less than 5% of ovarian malignancies.[8]

A number of drugs targeting the PI3K/AKT/mTOR pathway have begun to emerge. Inhibitors of P13K are now ongoing in early clinical development, whereas AKT and mTOR inhibiting agents such as KRX-0401 and everolimus have reported phase II studies.[9] Although the majority of trials involve the inhibitors as single-agent treatments, a few have been paired with standard chemotherapeutic regimens to assess the potential synergistic effects of such combinations given the hypothesized interplay between the PI3K/AKT/mTOR pathway and chemoresistance in cancer cells.[10] Earlier studies have established that pretreatment of hyperactive AKT mutated neoplasms with a P13K inhibitor could augment cell death from cisplatin.[11] Similar results have been noted with inhibition of the PI3K/AKT pathway and improvement in docetaxel-induced apoptosis in ovarian cancer cells.[12]

As such, proponents of molecular-targeted treatment modalities have also exploited recent advances in florescent in situ hybridization, both genomic-wide and specific mutation sequencing, and immunohistochemistry to better classify malignant subtypes.[2] However, despite the hope of improved side effect profiles of biologic agents, unique side effects have been observed including hyperglycemia and glucose intolerance such as with PI3K/AKT pathway inhibition.[1]

Another cell signaling pathway whose overexpression has been noted in gynecologic malignancies is that of the Ras/Raf/MEK/ERK pathway. Similar to the PI3K/AKT/mTOR pathway, multiple studies have clearly demonstrated the presence of activated Ras/Raf/MEK/ERK in ovarian cancers.[2,8,9,13] Various molecular components of this chain work through successive phosphorylation and subsequent activation of each downstream target which ultimately activate ERK1 and ERK2, otherwise known as mitogen-activated protein kinase (MAPK).[8] MAPK in turn produces multiple cytosolic and nuclear substrates through mRNA transcription and translation, which ultimately serve as the backbone for cell growth and proliferation.[13] As such, hyperactivation of this pathway has been shown to be associated with specific mutations in BRAF and KRAS proteins.[8] Not surprisingly, some of the most frequent genetic abnormalities in ovarian cancers are mutations in these proteins. In one study, a total of 12 of 58 ovarian malignancies (21%) demonstrated BRAF/KRAS mutation.[8] Interestingly, in this Japanese cohort, these mutations were more often found in low-grade serous and nonserous histologies. Of the 31 tumors with KRAS/BRAF mutation, approximately 32% were of nonserous histology. Similarly, these mutations positively correlated with early stage tumors (8/9 tumors stage I/II). Such data have supported the important concept that different histologic types of ovarian cancer represent discrete entities with distinct genetic abnormalities that should guide treatment.[14]

Various agents have been assessed that target KRAS/BRAF mutations. In the same study by Nakayama and colleagues,[8] an MEK-specific inhibitor, CI-1040, was used to theoretically block the activation of MAPK in patients with known KRAS and BRAF mutations.[8] Significant growth inhibition and apoptosis were noted after MAPK inhibition in cells with KRAS and BRAF mutations versus wild-type sequences. MAPK pathway suppression with an exogenous inhibiting agent illustrates a potential individualized treatment strategy for patients with BRAF/KRAS mutations. Currently, a number of phase II trials are ongoing with c-raf and MEK/MAPK inhibitors (ie, ISIS 5132, selumetinib); however, results have been mixed with some showing no real clinical results.[9] Others have investigated the efficacy of synergistic inhibiting agents, including a 2007 study that examined combination P13K and MEK inhibition for ovarian cancer.[15] Enhanced paclitaxel sensitivity and prolonged survival were noted using mouse models.

Another significant cell signaling pathway that has generated clinical interest in the past decade is that of the epidermal growth factor receptor inhibitors. These proto-oncogenes consist of four transmembrane receptors: EGFR, ErbB2, ErbB3, and ErbB4 that play important physiologic roles in regulating cell growth and survival as well as invasion and angiogenesis. The frequency of mutations in these genes in solid tumors including gynecologic malignancies positions this pathway as a particularly relevant target for molecularly based treatments.[2] Similar to the mTOR and MAPK pathways, cell signaling cascades that are initiated through the EGFR family are also prone to amplification and mutation on the molecular level. In a study of 97 patients with ovarian tumors, 70% of those found to be malignant overexpressed EGF receptor mRNA versus 33% of those with benign masses.[16] Furthermore, Lafky and colleagues[17] demonstrated that EGFR overexpression was an independent poor prognostic factor rather than any singular mutation in this group of receptor kinases.

A combination of monoclonal antibodies (cetuximab, matuzumab) and small molecule inhibitors (gefitinib, erlotinib) are currently in single-agent phase II trials for targeting against epidermal growth factor receptors.[9] A National Institutes of Health study of gefitinib in 24 women with relapsed ovarian cancer showed that despite causing decreased total and phosphorylated EGF receptor expression, no significant clinical response was observed.[18] More favorable results were observed with erlotinib, and it is currently being studied in a phase III European Organization for Research and Treatment of Cancer trial.[9,19] Single-agent cetuximab also has shown poor results, with objective response rates of approximately 4% in women with relapsed ovarian cancer.[20] Similarly, unremarkable results in front-line therapy were seen when combining cetuximab with carboplatin and paclitaxel, because progression-free survival (PFS) was not improved.[21]

Of the remaining EGFR family receptors, HER2 (ErbB2) has been of particular interest given its relevance in the management of breast and lung cancers.[9] Similar to EGFR/HER1, ovarian malignancies have been seen to overexpress HER2, and its presence has been seen as an independent poor prognostic factor.[16,22] The Gynecologic Oncology Group (GOG) evaluated trastuzumab, a monoclonal antibody inhibitor of HER2 commonly used in breast cancer, in women with relapsed ovarian and primary peritoneal malignancies.[23] Of the 837 patients screened for HER2 expression, 11% demonstrated 2/3+ overexpression, and only 7% of those patients who overexpressed receptor had an objective response. A randomized phase II trial evaluated pertuzumab, another monoclonal antibody with activity against HER2, in combination with gemcitabine in patients with platinum-resistant ovarian, fallopian tube, and primary peritoneal cancer (PPC), and whereas a trend toward improved PFS was demonstrated, it was not statistically significant (hazard ratio [HR] = .67 [95% confidence interval (CI) .43–1.02], $P = 0.06$).[24] Overall, however, the use of targeted treatments for EGFR abnormalities has demonstrated minimal activity in gynecologic malignancies. The hope is that activating mutations may be identified in the future that will identify candidates for EGFR axis treatment.

HOMOLOGOUS RECOMBINATION PATHWAYS

From its discovery in 1990, the BRCA gene, and later its mutation, have elicited a tremendous amount of interest and subsequent research regarding their role in neoplastic transformation as well as their potential utility in individually targeted therapies. Traditionally, the BRCA1 and 2 genes have been associated with regulatory mechanisms of cell proliferation and DNA repair through the process of homologous recombination.[25] Cells with either mutations or deficiencies in either of these tumor suppressor genes lose their ability to repair double-stranded DNA breaks by homologous recombination, and instead are relegated to using less robust mechanisms of repair including nonhomologous end joining and single strand annealing.[26] It is thus through the accumulation of errors that malignant transformation occurs, often resulting in breast and/or ovarian cancers. To date, many studies have sought to illustrate the myriad of characteristics that are associated with BRCA mutations. Clinically, patients with hereditary BRCA mutations have been noted to be younger at time of initial diagnosis, more often with a concurrent malignancy and with a strong family history of breast and/or ovarian cancer.[25] Pathologically, ovarian cancers with BRCA mutations present more often at advanced stages with high grade serous histologies.[27]

Initial observations of ovarian cancer patients with germ-line BRCA1 or 2 mutations versus clinically matched controls demonstrated statistically significant superior rates of both overall (95.5% vs 59.1%) and complete (81.8% vs 43.2%) response rates with front-line platinum-based therapy, as well as higher response rates to second- and third-line platinum-based therapies.[25] This result has led to the belief that BRCA-positive tumors are particularly platinum-sensitive. Multiple studies have demonstrated cells with BRCA mutations have an inability to repair the DNA damage caused by platinum-based agents.[27] Contrarily, ovarian cancers that demonstrate BRCA mutations have been associated with resistance to taxane-based chemotherapy. This observation is likely secondary to the role that BRCA is believed to play in cellular checkpoints, including its activation of the mitotic spindle.[27] As a result, BRCA positivity has begun to be viewed by many as a new biomarker in guiding chemotherapy selection and predicting treatment response.

Most recently, the loss of homologous repair mechanisms has also proved to be an opportunistic target for molecular-based treatment. Poly (ADP-ribose)-polymerase, or PARP, inhibitors have emerged as a potent new therapy for patients with existing BRCA mutations.[28] On the cellular level, PARP is a nuclear enzyme that functions in base excision repair.[25] It binds to sites of DNA damage and promotes repair through modification of key proteins. Inhibitors of the PARP enzyme compromises cellular repair mechanisms. As such, a deficiency in homologous recombination, as seen in BRCA mutations, serves to further sensitize the cell to the functions of PARP inhibitors, thereby causing enhanced cytotoxicity.[29,30,31] Current clinical trials have placed risk reduction with PARP inhibitors at approximately 33% to 41% in patients with the BRCA mutation.[32] Clearly, although efficacious as single agents, combination therapy has been shown to have synergistic effects. Thus, similar to its role in evaluating standard chemotherapeutic options, the use of the BRCA mutation status as a biomarker may better individualize treatment options.

Given the favorable results from PARP inhibitors seen in hereditary and somatic BRCA-mutated tumors, many researchers have begun to isolate other possible candidates for their use. Specifically, patients who demonstrate a "BRCAness" phenotype, namely those who seem to have similar appearance and response to individuals with known mutations despite testing negative themselves.[25,33] Similarly, recognition of BRCA-deficient states in sporadic tumors has been described that results in similar response profiles to platinum-based chemotherapy.[34] Given the prevalence of patients with some element of BRCA positivity or manifesting synthetic lethality, PARP inhibition seems to be a promising targeted strategy.

OTHER MOLECULAR TARGETS OF INTEREST

Although the previously mentioned cellular pathways and stromal agents are currently among the most promising in targeted biologic therapies, many other preclinical and early phase developmental programs feature a myriad of promising agents and potential biomarkers. Src inhibitors have been used to block kinases that mediate signaling between multiple growth factor receptors and their targets.[2] Two of the agents are currently in phase II trials.[35] Other small molecules and receptor targets such as lysophosphatidic acid, endothelin, nuclear factor-ĸB, and NOTCH-3 are also under study.

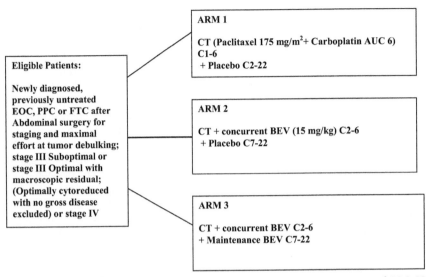

Fig. 1. GOG 218 was a phase III trial of bevacizumab in the primary treatment of EOC, PPC, and FTC. This placebo-controlled trial consisted of three arms combining standard front-line chemotherapy with placebo versus bevacizumab either with or following chemotherapy. BEV, bevacizumab; CT, chemotherapy.

ANTIANGIOGENESIS AGENTS

One of the key players in the progression of cancer is angiogenesis, which is the formation of new blood vessels.[36] Neovascularization is necessary in order for a tumor growth to exceed 2 mm^3.[37] Thus, therapies that target angiogenesis and inhibit the formation of new blood vessels will limit tumor growth. The process of angiogenesis involves a complex interaction of endothelial precursor cells, metalloproteins, and proangiogenic factors.

The most potent and well-characterized promoting molecule is vascular endothelial growth factor (VEGF).[38] Many tumors have an overexpression of VEGF, such as ovarian tumors. There is a poor prognosis associated with ovarian tumors with high levels of VEGF. These malignancies have carcinomatosis, more advanced stage, decreased survival, and distant metastases.[39] The first antiangiogenesis agent to be evaluated in epithelial ovarian cancer (EOC) has been bevacizumab, a recombinant humanized monoclonal antibody directed against VEGF-A.[36]

There have been many trials evaluating the therapeutic value of bevacizumab. The first significant trial that highlighted the clinical potential of this compound was GOG 170-D, which consisted of 62 eligible patients with recurrent or persistent ovarian cancer, or PPC. Thirteen patients demonstrated a clinical response, a 21% objective response rate. Twenty-five patients (40.3%) had a PFS rate observed at 6 months in a mixed population of platinum-sensitive and resistant recurrent ovarian cancer patients.[40] The median PFS was 4.7 months and the OS was 17 months. Another phase II trial was performed on single-agent bevacizumab in 44 patients with recurrent ovarian cancer patients who had predominately platinum-resistant disease.[41] The median PFS was 4.4 months and median survival at the termination of the study was 10.7 months. The most common side effect in these two studies was grade 3 to 4 hypertension (9.1%–9.4%); however, it was well-controlled with antihypertensives.[40,41] Other major complications included proteinuria

Table 1
Ovarian cancer: GOG 170 series—Recurrent ovarian cancer in mixed platinum-sensitive and platinum-resistant population

Protocol	PI	Agent	N	RR (%)	PFS at 6 Mo (%)
170-B	Hurteau	IL-12	26	4	Not reported
170-C	Schilder	Iressa	27	4	15
170-D	Burger	Bevacizumab	62	21	40
170-E	Schilder	Gleevac	26	2	40
170-F	Matei	Bay 43-9006 (raf kinase-I)	68	3	24
170-G	Garcia	Lapatinib	28	15	8
170-H	Modesitt	Vorinostat	27	4	7
170-I	Behbakht	Temsirolimus	44	9	24
170-J	Usha, L	Enzastaurin	27	7	11
170-L	Schilder	AMG-706	34	5	Too toxic
170-M	Schilder	Dasatinib (Sprycel)	34	0	21
170-N	Gold, M	Urokinase-derived peptide	31	0	7
170-P	Martin	AMG-102	31- closed		
170-Q	Alvarez	EGEN-001 IL-12 plasmid IP	Pending		

Abbreviation: IL, interleukin; PI, principal investigator; RR, relative risk.

(1.6%–15.9%) and thromboembolic disease (3%–7%). The Cannistra study was closed early because of the high rate of gastrointestinal perforation (11.4%). A third phase II trial was conducted with bevacizumab and metronomic (frequent administration of low doses) oral cyclophosphamide in 70 patients with recurrent ovarian cancer.[42] The PFS at 6 months was 56%. A partial response was recorded in 17 patients (24%). The median time to progression was 7.2 months and median survival was 16.9 months. The most common toxicities related to bevacizumab were hypertension (39%) and proteinuria (44%).

The significant activity seen in the recurrent setting generated enthusiasm for studying bevacizumab in the front-line setting. GOG 218 was a phase III trial of bevacizumab in the primary treatment of EOC, PPC, and fallopian tube cancer (FTC).

Table 2
Endometrial cancer: GOG 229 series—biologics in endometrial cancer

Protocol	PI	Agent	N	RR (%)	PFS at 6 Mo (%)
229-B	McMeekin	Thalidomide	25	12	8
229-C	Leslie, K	Gefitinib	26	3.8	15
229-D	Leslie, K	Lapatinib	30	3.3	10
229-E	Arghaianian	Bevacizumab	53	13.5	40
229-F	Coleman	VEGF-TRAP	44	7	41
229-G	Alvarez	Bevacizumab + temsirolimus	48 - closed		
229-H	Coleman	AZD6244 (MEK)	25 - closed		
229-I	Powell	Brivanib	45 - closed		
229-J	Bender, D	Cedarinib	31		
229-L	Moore, K	AMG-386	Open 6/11		

Table 3
Cervical Cancer: GOG 227 series—biologics in cervical cancer

Protocol	PI	Agent	N	RR (%)	PFS at 6 Mo (%)
227-C	Monk, B	Bevacizumab	46	11	24
227-D	Schilder	OSI-774	25	0	4
227-E	Santin, A	Cetuximab	33	0	14
227-G	Chan, J	Brivanib	Pending		

This placebo-controlled trial consisted of three arms combining standard front-line chemotherapy with placebo versus bevacizumab either with or following chemotherapy (**Fig. 1**). Patients in arm three treated with standard chemotherapy plus maintenance bevacizumab demonstrated a benefit in the hazard of first progression or death, .717 (95% CI: .625–.824, $P<.0001$) relative to arm 1, which was standard chemotherapy plus placebo.[43] The investigators reported complications of grade 3 or greater hypertension, gastrointestinal perforation, hemorrhage, or fistula.

A second phase III trial, ICON7, evaluated bevacizumab in addition to standard chemotherapy with carboplatin and paclitaxel, followed by maintenance bevacizumab. ICON7 also showed that bevacizumab improved PFS by 28%, from 18 to 23 months, in patients with EOC, PPC, and FTC and reported similar adverse effects.[44] A subset analysis from ICON7 also demonstrated an OS advantage for patients with advanced staged disease.

A third phase III trial, the OCEANS trial, evaluated bevacizumab in the recurrent disease setting in combination with chemotherapy. Patients were randomized to

Table 4
Active non-GOG trials featuring biologics

Cancer	PI	Phase	Agent	N	Completion Date
Ovarian					
	Poole, C	II	AZD0530	211	5/2012
	Konecny, G	II	AMG 479	61	8/2012
	Boehringer	II	BI 6727	110	9/2012
	Weil, S	III	MORAb-003 (farletuzumab)	1080	9/2012
	Kaye, S	II	AZD2281	97	12/2012
	Boehringer	III	BIBF 1120 (nintedanib)	1300	7/2016
Endometrial					
	Myers, A	II	MK2206	90	7/2012
	Sanofi-Aventis	II	XL147 (SAR245408)	88	3/2013
	Pfizer	II	PF-04691502, PF-05212384	252	9/2013
	Novartis	II	BEZ235	140	10/2013
	Novartis	II	TKI258	80	9/2014
Cervical					
	Zeimet, A	II	Panitumumab	50	3/2013
	Novartis	I	RAD001 (everolimus)	9	5/2013

Table 5
Ovarian cancer: completed phase II non-GOG trials

PI	Agent	N	RR (%)	PFS at 6 Mo (%)
Cannistra	Bevacizumab (Bev)	44	15.9	27.8
Garcia	Bev + cyclophosphamide	70	24	56

receive bevacizumab versus placebo until disease progression along with carboplatin and gemcitabine. OCEANS showed a significantly significant improvement in PFS when bevacizumab is used concurrently with carboplatin and gemcitabine followed by bevacizumab alone until progression compared with carboplatin and gemcitabine alone (HR = .484, $P<.0001$) in recurrent EOC, PPC, and FTC.[45] The objective response increased by 21%. Toxicities were similar to previous bevacizumab trials.

There are also several ongoing or recently completed trials that evaluate the therapeutic effect of bevacizumab in EOC, PPC, and FTC. GOG 213 is a phase III trial, in patients with recurrent EOC, PPC, and FTC who were first randomized to secondary cytoreduction or no surgery.[46] These platinum-sensitive patients were then randomized to receive carboplatin and paclitaxel with or without bevacizumab. The primary outcome measure is OS, and the secondary outcome measures are PFS and adverse events. GOG 252 is another phase III trial evaluating bevacizumab and intravenous chemotherapy compared with bevacizumab and intraperitoneal chemotherapy in patients with stage II, stage III, or stage IV EOB, PPC, and FTC.[47] The primary outcome is PFS, and the secondary outcomes are OS, adverse effects, and quality of life. GOG 262 is also a phase III ongoing trial studying two dose schedules of paclitaxel in combination with carboplatin with or without bevacizumab in stage III or stage IV EOC, PPC, and FTC.[48] The primary outcome is PFS, and the secondary outcomes are OS, response rate, toxicity, translational research, and quality of life.

A new antiangiogenesis agent called AMG 386 is currently being studied in two phase III trials. AMG 386 works on the angiopoietin axis by inhibiting the interaction between angiopoietin-1, angiopoietin-2, and their receptor Tie2. The first study is TRINOVA-1, which is comparing weekly paclitaxel plus AMG 386 to weekly paclitaxel and placebo in patients with recurrent partially platinum-sensitive or resistant EOC, PPC, and FTC.[49] The primary objective is PFS, and secondary objectives are OS, response rate, safety, pharmacokinetics, toxicities, and quality of life. The second phase III trial is TRINOVA-2, which is comparing pegylated liposomal doxorubicin

Table 6
Ovarian cancer: completed phase III trials

Protocol	PI	Agent	N	PFS HR	PFS P-Value
GOG 218	Burger	Paclitaxel + carboplatin +/− concurrent Bev +/− Maintenance Bev	1873	Relative to R1: R2 = 0.908 R3 = 0.717	R2 = 0.16 R3 = <.001
ICON 7	Perren	Paclitaxel + carboplatin +/− Bev	1528	+ Bev = 0.81	0.0041
OCEANS	Aghajanian	Carboplatin + gemcitabine +/− Bev	484	+ Bev = 0.484	<.0001

(PLD) plus AMG 386 to PLD plus placebo.[50] The primary objective is PFS, and the secondary objective is OS.

Three newer antiangiogenesis agents have been recently studied in phase II trials. Cediranib maleate is a selective inhibitor of the VEGF receptor tyrosine kinase. GOG 229-J studied the efficacy and side effects of cediranib maleate in patients with persistent or recurrent endometrial cancer.[51] The primary objective was PFS for at least 6 months, objective tumor response rate, and adverse effects. The secondary objectives were PFS and OS, and response. Another inhibitor of VEGF receptors is sorafenib, which also targets RAF kinases. A phase II trial was completed comparing sorafenib with placebo as maintenance therapy for patients with advanced ovarian cancer or PPC in complete remission after surgery and one regimen of chemotherapy.[52] The primary objective was PFS. The secondary objectives were time to first pathologic CA125 levels, OS, ovarian cancer symptom response rate, and general health status. The third inhibitor of VEGF receptor, pazopanib, also targets platelet-derived growth factor and c-Kit. A phase II trial has been completed and published evaluating pazopanib in patients with recurrent ovarian cancer.[53] The investigators found a 31% CA125 response rate, 29 days median time to response, and 113 days median response duration. In patients with initial measurable disease, the overall response rate was 18%. The most common toxicity was grade 3 elevations of ALT (8%) and AST (8%).

Antiangeogenesis agents are a very promising treatment strategy for ovarian, primary peritoneal, and fallopian tube cancers. Agents such as bevacizumab have been shown to be effective in first-line treatment and in recurrent disease. Nonetheless, the proper dose, cost effectiveness, length of treatment, and molecular profile of responders require further clarification. Other agents that exploit alternative targets in the angiogenic pathway are also promising. Trials are currently ongoing to determine how antiangiogenics are most favorably combined with chemotherapy and other novel biologics. Additionally, other means of inhibiting angiogenesis will continue to evolve. Agents such as Notch inhibitors and vascular disrupting agents will play increasingly prominent roles. Blocking alternative redundant pathways may be necessary to realize the full potential of antiangiogenic strategies.

SUMMARY

Through advances in human genomic sequencing, the unique molecular biology that predisposes certain individuals to either health or disease has now been illuminated. Although many malignancies behave similarly on a phenotypic level, biologically there exist multiple layers of interconnected molecular and cellular pathways that may make each patient's disease significantly more unique than previously appreciated. In gynecologic oncology, the most progress in developing targeted biologics has been in the treatment of ovarian cancers. Future investigations will see further development in endometrial and cervical cancers. Technology such as whole genome sequencing can theoretically identify the individual tumor's genetic profile; however, identifying the priority pathways for therapeutic interventions and subsequent complex interactions remains a significant challenge. New therapeutic technologies such as siRNA and immune modulators will also play a promising role in the movement toward individualized therapies. It is hoped that the identification and use of targeted agents will lead to individualized care that in turn will lead to significantly improved outcomes manifested by more cures and better quality of life through amelioration of toxicities (**Tables 1–6**).

REFERENCES

1. Yap TA, Garrett MD, Walton MI, et al. Targeting the PI3K-AKT-mTOR pathway: progress, pitfalls, and promises. Curr Opin Pharmacol 2008;8:393–412.

2. Blagden S, Gabra H. Promising molecular targets in ovarian cancer. Curr Opin Oncol 2009;21(5):412–9.
3. Nakayama K, Nakayama N, Kurman RJ, et al. Sequence mutations and amplification of PIK3CA and AKT2 genes in purified ovarian serous neoplasms. Cancer Biol Ther 2006;5:779–85.
4. Yuan ZQ, Sun M, Feldman RI, et al. Frequent activation of AKT2 and induction of apoptosis by inhibition of phosphoinositide-3-OH kinase/Akt pathway in human ovarian cancer. Oncogene 2000;19:2324–30.
5. Carpten JD, Faber AL, Horn C, et al. A transforming mutation in the pleckstrin homology domain of AKT1 in cancer. Nature 2007;448:439–44.
6. Trinh XB, Tjalma WA, Vermeulen PB, et al. The VEGF pathway and the AKT/mTOR/p70S6K1 signalling pathway in human epithelial ovarian cancer. Br J Cancer 2009; 100:971–8.
7. Levine DA, Bogomolniy F, Yee CJ, et al. Frequent mutation of the PIK3CA gene in ovarian and breast cancers. Clin Cancer Res 2005;11(8):2875–8.
8. Nakayama N, Nakayama K, Yeasmin S, et al. KRAS or BRAF mutation status is a useful predictor of sensitivity to MEK inhibition in ovarian cancer. Br J Cancer 2008;99:2020–8.
9. Kalachand R, Hennessy BT, Markman M. Molecular targeted therapy in ovarian cancer: what is on the horizon? Drugs. 2011;71(8):947–67.
10. Fraser M, Bai T, Tsang BK. Akt promotes cisplatin resistance in human ovarian cancer cells through inhibition of p53 phosphorylation and nuclear function. Int J Cancer 2008;122(3):534–46.
11. Altomare DA, Wang HQ, Skele KL, et al. AKT and mTOR phosphorylation is frequently detected in ovarian cancer and can be targeted to disrupt ovarian tumor cell growth. Oncogene 2004;23:5853–7.
12. Xing H, Weng D, Chen G, et al. Activation of fibronectin/PI-3K/Akt2 leads to chemore-sistance to docetaxel by regulating survivin protein expression in ovarian and breast cancer cells. Cancer Lett 2008;261:108–19.
13. Estep AL, Palmer C, McCormick F, et al. Mutation analysis of BRAF, MEK1 and MEK2 in 15 ovarian cancer cell lines: implications for therapy. PLoS ONE 2007;2:e1279.
14. Marquez RT, Baggerly KA, Patterson AP, et al. Patterns of gene expression in different histotypes of epithelial ovarian cancer correlate with those in normal fallopian tube, endometrium, and colon. Clin Cancer Res. 2005;11(17):6116–26.
15. Kigawa J, Kawaguchi W, Itamochi H, et al. Effect of simultaneous inhibition of MEK and PI3K/Akt pathways on paclitaxel sensitivity in ovarian cancer [abstract #16046]. J Clin Oncol 2007;25 (18S).
16. Bartlett JM, Langdon SP, Simpson BJ, et al. The prognostic value of epidermal growth factor receptor mRNA expression in primary ovarian cancer. Br J Cancer 1996;73:301–6.
17. Lafky JM, Wilken JA, Baron AT, et al. Clinical implications of the ErbB/epidermal growth factor (EGF) receptor family and its ligands in ovarian cancer. Biochim Biophys Acta 2008;1785:232–65.
18. Posadas EM, Liel MS, Kwitkowski V, et al. A phase II and pharmacodynamic study of gefitinib in patients with refractory or recurrent epithelial ovarian cancer. Cancer 2007;109:1323–30.
19. Gordon AN, Finkler N, Edwards RP, et al. Efficacy and safety of erlotinib HCl, an epidermal growth factor receptor (HER1/EGFR) tyrosine kinase inhibitor, in patients with advanced ovarian carcinoma: results from a phase II multicenter study. Int J Gynecol Cancer 2005;15:785–92.

20. Schilder RJ, Pathak HB, Lokshin AE, et al. Phase II trial of single agent cetuximab in patients with persistent or recurrent epithelial ovarian or primary peritoneal carcinoma with the potential for dose escalation to rash. Gynecol Oncol 2009;113:21–7.

21. Konner J, Schilder RJ, DeRosa FA, et al. A phase II study of cetuximab/paclitaxel/carboplatin for the initial treatment of advanced-stage ovarian, primary peritoneal, or fallopian tube cancer. Gynecol Oncol 2008;110:140–5.

22. Bast RC Jr, Pusztai L, Kerns BJ, et al. Coexpression of the HER-2 gene product, p185HER-2, and epidermal growth factor receptor, p170EGF-R, on epithelial ovarian cancers and normal tissues. Hybridoma 1998;17:313–21.

23. Bookman MA, Darcy KM, Clarke-Pearson D, et al. Evaluation of monoclonal human-ized anti-HER2 antibody, trastuzumab, in patients with recurrent or refractory ovarian or primary peritoneal carcinoma with overexpression of HER2: a phase II trial of the Gynecologic Oncology Group. J Clin Oncol 2003;21:283–90.

24. Makhija S, Glenn D, Ueland F, et al. Results from a phase II randomized, placebo-controlled, double-blind trial suggest improved PFS with the addition of pertuzumab to gemcitabine in patients with platinum-resistant ovarian, fallopian tube, or primary peritoneal cancer [abstract #5507]. J Clin Oncol 2007;25(18S).

25. Tan DS, Rothermundt C, Thomas K, et al. 'BRCAness' syndrome in ovarian cancer: a case-control study describing the clinical features and outcome of patients with epithelial ovarian cancer associated with BRCA1 and BRCA2 mutations. J Clin Oncol 2008;26:5530–6.

26. Sowter HM, Ashworth A. BRCA1 and BRCA2 as ovarian cancer susceptibility genes. Carcinogenesis 2005;26:1651–6.

27. Quinn JE, Carser JE, James CR, et al. BRCA1 and implications for response to chemotherapy in ovarian cancer. Gynecol Oncol 2009;113:134–42.

28. Chalmers AJ. The potential role and application of PARP inhibitors in cancer treat-ment. Br Med Bull 2009;89:23–40.

29. Yap TA, Boss DS, Fong PC, et al. First in human phase I pharmacokinetic (PK) and pharmacodynamic (PD) study of KU-0059436 (Ku), a small molecule inhibitor of poly ADP-ribose polymerase (PARP) in cancer patients (p), including BRCA1/2 mutation carriers [abstract #3529]. J Clin Oncol 2007;25(18S).

30. Fong PC, Boss DS, Carden CP, et al. AZD2281 (KU-0059436), a PARP (poly ADP-ribose polymerase) inhibitor with single agent anticancer activity in patients with BRCA deficient ovarian cancer: results from a phase I study [abstract #5510]. J Clin Oncol 2008;26(15S).

31. Farmer H, McCabe N, Lord CJ, et al. Targeting the DNA repair defect in BRCA mutant cells as a therapeutic strategy. Nature 2005;434(7035):917–21.

32. Audeh MW, Penson RT, Friedlander M. Phase II trial of the oral PARP inhibitor olaparib (AZD2281) in BRCA deficient advanced ovarian cancer [meeting abstract]. J Clin Oncol 2009;27(15S):5500.

33. Konstantinopoulos PA, Spentzos D, Karlan BY, et al. Gene expression profile of BRCAness that correlates with responsiveness to chemotherapy and with outcome in patients with epithelial ovarian cancer. J Clin Oncol 2010;28:3555–61.

34. Hennessy BT, Timms KM, Carey MS, et al. Somatic mutations in BRCA1 and BRCA2 could expand the number of patients that benefit from poly (ADP ribose) polymerase inhibitors in ovarian cancer. J Clin Oncol 2010;28:3570–6

35. Poole C, Lisyanskaya A, Rodenhuis S, et al. A randomized phase II clinical trial of the SRC inhibitor saracatinib (AZD0530) and carboplatin/paclitaxel (C+P) versus C+P in patients with advanced platinum sensitive epithelial ovarian cancer [meeting abstract]. Ann Oncol 2010;21(Suppl. 8):972O.

36. Barrena Medel, NI, Wright JD, Herzog TJ, et al. Targeted therapies in epithelial ovarian cancer. J Oncol 2010;2010:314326.

37. Folkman J. Tumor angiogenesis: therapeutic implications. N Engl J Med 1971; 285(21):1182–6.

38. Ma WW, Adjei AA. Novel agents on the horizon for cancer therapy. CA Cancer J Clin. 2009;59(2):111–37.

39. Burger RA. Experience with bevacizumab in the management of epithelial ovarian cancer. J Clin Oncol 2007;25(20):2902–8.

40. Burger RA, Sill MW, Monk BJ, et al. Phase II trial of bevacizumab in persistent or recurrent epithelial ovarian cancer or primary peritoneal cancer: a Gynecologic Oncology Group study. J Clin Oncol. 2007;25(33):5165–71.

41. Cannistra SA, Matulonis UA, Penson RT, et al. Phase II study of bevacizumab in patients with platinum-resistant ovarian cancer or peritoneal serous cancer. J Clin Oncol. 2007;25(33):5180–6.

42. Garcia AA, Hirte H, Fleming G, et al. Phase II clinical trial of bevacizumab and low-dose metronomic oral cyclophosphamide in recurrent ovarian cancer: a trial of the California, Chicago, and Princess Margaret Hospital phase II consortia. J Clin Oncol 2008;26(1):76–82.

43. Burger RA, Brady MF, Bookman MA, et al. Incorporation of bevacizumab in the primary treatment of ovarian cancer. N Engl J Med 2011;365(26):2473–83.

44. Perren TJ, Swart AM, Pfisterer J, et al. ICON7: a phase 3 trial of bevacizumab in ovarian cancer. N Engl J Med 2011;365(26):2484–96.

45. Aghajanian C, Finkler NJ, Rutherford T, et al. OCEANS: a randomized double-blinded, placebo-controlled phase III trial of chemotherapy with or without bevacizumab in patients with platinum-sensitive recurrent epithelial ovarian (EOC), primary peritoneal (PPC) or fallopian tube cancer (FTC) [abstract LBA 5007, 2011 ASCO annual meeting, oral abstract session]. J Clin Oncol 2011;(Suppl).

46. A phase III randomized controlled clinical trial of carboplatin and paclitaxel alone or in combination with bevacizumab (NSC #704865, IND #7921) followed by bevacizumab and secondary cytoreduction surgery in platinum-sensitive, recurrent ovarian, peritoneal primary and fallopian tube cancer [NLM identifier: NCT00565851]. ClinicalTrials.gov. Available at: http://www.clinicaltrials.gov/ct2/show/NCT00565851?term= Carboplatin+and+paclitaxel+with+or+without+bevacizumab&rank=5. Accessed December 1, 2011.

47. A phase III clinical trial of bevacizumab with IV versus IP chemotherapy in ovarian, fallopian tube, and primary peritoneal carcinoma NCI-supplied agent(s): bevacizumab (NSC #704865, IND #7921) [NLM identifier: NCT00951496]. ClinicalTrials.gov. Available at: http://www.clinicaltrials.gov/ct2/show/NCT00951496?term=nct0095 1496&rank=1. Accessed December 1, 2011.

48. A randomized phase III trial of every-3-weeks paclitaxel versus dose dense weekly paclitaxel in combination with carboplatin with or without concurrent and consolidation bevacizumab (NSC #704865, IND #7921) in the treatment of primary stage II, III or IV epithelial ovarian, peritoneal or fallopian tube cancer [NLM identifier: NCT01167712]. ClinicalTrials.gov. Available at: http://www.clinicaltrials.gov/ct2/ show/NCT01167712?term=nct01167712&rank=1. Accessed December 1, 2011.

49. A phase III, randomized, double-blind trial of weekly paclitaxel plus AMG 386 or placebo in women with recurrent partially platinum sensitive or resistant epithelial ovarian, primary peritoneal or fallopian tube cancers [NLM identifier: NCT01204749]. ClinicalTrials.gov. Available at: http://www.clinicaltrials.gov/ct2/show/NCT012047 49?term=NCT01204749&rank=1. Accessed December 1, 2011.

50. A phase III, randomized, double-blind trial of pegylated liposomal doxorubicin (PLD) plus AMG 386 or placebo in women with recurrent partially platinum sensitive or resistant epithelial ovarian, primary peritoneal, or fallopian tube cancer [NLM Identifier: NCT01281254]. ClinicalTrials.gov. Available at: http://www.clinicaltrials.gov/ct2/show/NCT01281254?term=trinova-2&rank=1. Accessed December 1, 2011.

51. A phase II Evaluation of cediranib (Recentin; AZD2171, IND# 72740, NSC# 732208) in the treatment of recurrent or persistent endometrial carcinoma [NLM identifier: NCT01132820]. ClinicalTrials.gov. Available at: http://www.clinicaltrials.gov/ct2/show/NCT01132820?term=NCT01132820&rank=1. Accessed December 1, 2011.

52. A double-blind, randomized phase II study evaluating the efficacy and safety of sorafenib compared to placebo in ovarian epithelial cancer or primary peritoneal cancer patients who have achieved a complete clinical response after standard platinum/taxane containing chemotherapy [NLM identifier: NCT00791778]. ClinicalTrials.gov. Available at: http://www.clinicaltrials.gov/ct2/show/NCT00791778?term=NCT00791778&rank=1. Accessed December 1, 2011.

53. A phase III study to evaluate the efficacy and safety of pazopanib monotherapy versus placebo in women who have not progressed after first line chemotherapy for epithelial ovarian, fallopian tube, or primary peritoneal cancer [identifier: ACTRN12609000591257]. WHO International Clinical Trials. Available at: http://apps.who.int/trialsearch/trial.aspx?trialid=ACTRN12609000591257. Accessed December 1, 2011.

Advances in Surgical Care

Teresa L. Rutledge, MD

KEYWORDS

- Gynecology • Gynecologic oncology • Malignancy • Surgical management

The surgical management of gynecologic malignancy is the cornerstone of the subspecialty. As technology advances, surgical care is changing rapidly. New devices, surgical instruments, and understandings of the disease process have all improved the surgical management of gynecologic malignancies. This article summarizes some of the recent advances in the surgical management of gynecologic malignancies.

HISTORICAL PERSPECTIVE

Although minimally invasive techniques are now commonplace for most surgical specialties, gynecologists actually pioneered the laparoscopic approach in the 1960s. Gynecologists began using laparoscopy primarily as a diagnostic tool that allowed direct visualization of the pelvic organs. As the technology and equipment improved, gynecologists led the field by first performing laparoscopic tubal ligations and then expanding the minimally invasive approach to include other pelvic surgeries. In 1988, the American gynecologist Harry Reich performed the first complete laparoscopic hysterectomy, removing the uterus through a colpotomy. which was performed and closed laparoscopically.[1]

With advances in laparoscopic techniques, it was a natural extension to use the laparoscopic technique in cancer surgery. Querleu and co-workers[2] were the first to report experience with laparoscopic transperitoneal lymphadenectomy as a staging procedure for patients with cervical cancer. The data on the first 39 operations were published in 1991.[2] After this early report, a number of surgeons began to apply minimally invasive techniques to the operative treatment of gynecologic malignancies, most commonly endometrial cancer. Childers and colleagues[3] and Spirtos and associates[4] both demonstrated the adequacy and safety of applying laparoscopic technique to endometrial cancer surgery in single-institution studies. These surgeons reported on the feasibility of the technique, but the field of gynecologic oncology adopted minimally invasive surgical techniques with caution. The safety, cost-effectiveness, and cancer survival outcomes were commonly cited areas of concern.

Department of Obstetrics and Gynecology, Division of Gynecologic Oncology, 1 University of New Mexico, MSC 07 4025, Albuquerque, NM 87131, USA
E-mail address: trutledge@salud.unm.edu

Obstet Gynecol Clin N Am 39 (2012) 145–163
doi:10.1016/j.ogc.2012.02.005
0889-8545/12/$ – see front matter © 2012 Elsevier Inc. All rights reserved.

With publication of research evaluating oncologic outcomes and improvements in equipment during the 2000s, minimally invasive approaches for the treatment of gynecologic malignancies have become more commonplace. The technology has infiltrated almost all aspects of surgical management for gynecologic malignancies with seemingly endless reports on minimally invasive outcomes. The introduction of robotic-assisted laparoscopic surgery has allowed even more applications to emerge and more surgeons to adopt the technology. Most recently, the field of minimally invasive surgical technique has seen further innovation with reports of single-port laparoscopic surgery. As the technology continues to advance, we can only expect continued evolution in our ability to perform surgery in a way that maximizes both oncologic outcome and quality of life.

UTERINE CANCER
Role of Minimally Invasive Surgery

Uterine cancer is common and requires comprehensive surgical staging, which historically has been performed via open laparotomy. Uterine cancer was a natural fit for the application of a minimally invasive technique. First, the majority of women with endometrial cancer have disease confined to the uterus; therefore, operative treatment usually involves hysterectomy, bilateral salpingo-oophorectomy, and pelvic/para-aortic lymphadenectomy. Second, the patient population who usually suffers from endometrial cancer includes high-risk surgical candidates, because obesity is so prevalent. Efforts to reduce operative morbidity in this patient population are needed. Childers and associates[4] were among the first to report on the use of laparoscopically assisted surgical staging for endometrial cancer in 1993. Their studies demonstrated the feasibility of the laparoscopic approach with a 93% success rate, acceptable blood loss at 200 mL and an average hospital stay of 2.9 days. Since this report, much research has been done to investigate the adequacy of minimally invasive staging, cost of the procedure, and effect on overall survival and recurrence rates.[5]

Laparoscopy Versus Laparotomy for Surgical Staging

Widespread adoption of laparoscopy for uterine cancer treatment did not gain acceptance until publication of studies establishing the safety of the procedure from a cancer treatment perspective. In this section, key studies comparing laparoscopy with the traditional open technique are reviewed.

Given the interest in a laparoscopic approach for the treatment of early stage endometrial cancer, randomized controlled trials were first reported in 2005 comparing the 2 surgical techniques. Tozzi and co-workers[6] were the first to report survival outcomes from a randomized, clinical trial of laparoscopic compared with open approaches in the management of endometrial cancer. With a median follow-up of 44 months, patients with stage I endometrial cancer had disease-free survival rates of 91% in the laparoscopic group and 94%, in the laparotomy group. The overall survival rates were 86% and 90%, respectively.[6] Malzoni and associates[7] randomized 159 patients with clinical stage I endometrial cancer to treatment with total laparoscopic hysterectomy versus abdominal hysterectomy with lymphadenectomy. After a 3-year follow-up period, the survival analysis showed no significant difference in overall and disease-free survival after laparoscopy or laparotomy.[7] Because the incidence of recurrence and death from clinical stage I uterine cancer is exceedingly rare, the true oncologic outcome equivalency was still questioned given the small numbers of patients enrolled in these first studies. Therefore more patients in a larger study were required to address the question of equivalency for the 2 techniques. In 1996, the Gynecologic Oncology Group opened

LAP2, a prospective, multi-institutional, randomized trial to assess whether laparoscopy could be considered noninferior to open laparotomy with regard to recurrence-free survival. Secondary endpoints were perioperative adverse events, conversion to laparotomy, length of hospital stay after surgery, operative time, quality of life, sites of recurrence, and survival.[8]

LAP2 evaluated 2516 patients with 1696 assigned to the laparoscopy group and 920 patients assigned to the laparotomy group. Laparoscopy was initiated in 1682 patients and completed in 1248 patients (74%). Conversion to laparotomy was advised when incomplete staging results would yield inadequate information for treatment planning. Factors associated with conversion were increasing body mass index (BMI), metastatic disease, and advancing patient age. As expected, the operative times were longer for the laparoscopy group (median, 204 vs 130 min). Despite longer operative times, laparoscopy had fewer moderate to severe postoperative adverse events than laparotomy (14% vs 21%, respectively; $P<.0001$). The length of hospital stay was shorter with laparoscopy; only 52% of patients who underwent laparoscopy stayed more than 2 days, compared with 94% of those who underwent laparotomy. No difference in positive cytology, node positivity rate, number of nodes removed, or detection of advanced stage could be attributed to the laparoscopic approach. The authors concluded that laparoscopic surgical staging for uterine cancer is feasible and safe in terms of short-term outcomes and results in fewer complications and shorter hospital stays.[8]

Multiple prospective and retrospective studies have shown laparoscopic surgery is equivalent to open surgery in terms of adequacy of surgical resection and lymph node counts with decreased risks of intraoperative and postoperative complications. **Table 1** summarizes the studies comparing robotic versus open versus laparoscopic approaches for uterine cancer surgical staging procedures.[9] Survival data from the LAP2 trial is anticipated in 2012, which are needed to validate the equivalency of the procedures from an oncologic outcome standpoint. Based on the available data, gynecologic oncologists should consider a minimally invasive surgical approach for the treatment of endometrial cancer when feasible.

Quality-of-Life Analysis

The laparoscopic approach has many potential benefits compared with laparotomy but, until recently, there was little information regarding improvement in patient quality-of-life outcomes. Two large prospective trials have now reported extensive quality-of-life analysis, which favors a minimally invasive approach. The first is the previously mentioned LAP2 trial, where 802 patients participated in the quality-of-life study. Patients in the laparoscopy group had better short-term quality-of-life outcomes compared with the laparotomy group up to 6 weeks after surgery. There was no difference at the 6-month assessment except for a better body image score in laparoscopy patients.[10] The LACE randomized trial compared total laparoscopic hysterectomy with abdominal hysterectomy for stage I endometrial cancer evaluated 332 patients in the quality-of-life substudy. Similar to the LAP2 trial, this prospective multi-institutional trial was conducted in Australia, New Zealand and Hong Kong. The investigators report quality-of-life improvements during early (up to 4 weeks) and late (up to 6 months) phases of recovery for total laparoscopic hysterectomy compared with abdominal hysterectomy for treatment of stage I endometrial cancer. The persistent improvement at 6 months in the LACE trial does differ from other studies. The authors attribute this longer lasting effect on quality-of-life measures to a very low conversion rate.[11]

Table 1
Comparative observational studies evaluating the da vinci robotic system (DRS) versus open surgery (OS) or laparoscopy (LSC) to perform uterine cancer staging procedures.

Surgery	N	DRS vs OS	DRS vs LSC	Control	Surgeon	OR Time (min)	EBL (mL)	Hospital Stay (days)	Lymph Node Count	Conversions	Bld Tx	Intraoperative Complications	Postoperative Complications
Uterine cancer staging													
Veljovich et al 2006–2007 Swedish Medical Center Seattle, WA	25 vs 131 / 25 vs 4	✓	✓	HC + CC Prospective HC + CC	DS	283 vs 139 / 283 vs 255	67 vs 198 / 67 vs 75	1.7 vs 5.3 / 1.7 vs 1.2	18 vs 13 / 18 vs 20	DRS: 1	NR	NR	DRS: Major: 8% Infection (1), cuff dehiscence (1) Minor: 12% OS: Major 21% Cardiac (5), pulmonary (5), renal (4), CVA (1), infection (3), wound dehiscence (9) Minor: 8% LSC: NR
Gehrig et al 2005–2007 BMI ≥30 UNC	49 vs 32		✓	HC	NR	189 vs 215	50 vs 150	1.0 vs 1.3	31 vs 24	DRS: 0 LSC: 3	NR	DRS: enterotomy (1) LSC: none	DRS: Major: 8% Port-site hernia (3), cuff complicaiton (1) Minor 2% LSC: Major 6% Port-site hernia (1), cuff complicaiton (1) Minor 3%

Study				n				Mortality	Complication rate	Complications	Details
Boggess et al 2005–2007 UNC	103 vs 138 103 vs 81	✓ ✓	HC HC	DS SS	191 vs 146 191 vs 213	75 vs 266 75 vs 146	1 vs 4.4 1 vs 1.2	33 vs 15 33 vs 23	DRS: 2.8% LSC: 3.7%	DRS: 1% OS: 1.4% LSC: 2.5%	DRS: bowel injury (1) OS: enterotomy (1) LSC: caval injury (1), bowel injury (1)	DRS: Major: 2% Port-site hernia (1), PE (1) Minor: 3% OS: Major 8% CVA (1), ileus + readmission (7), DVT (2), PE (1), respiratory failure (1) Minor: 21% LSC: Major: 5% port-site hernia (1), ileus readmission (1), vaginal dehiscence (1), abscess (1) Minor: 5%
Bell et al 2005–2007 Sanford Clinic, Sioux Falls, SD	40 vs 40 40 vs 30	✓ ✓	HC + CC retro- spective HC + CC	SS SS	184 vs 209 184 vs 171	166 vs 316 166 vs 253	2.3 vs 4.0 2.3 vs 4.0	17 vs 14 17 vs 17	NR	DRS: 5% OS: 15% LSC: 10%	DRS: None OS: genital femoral n, damage (1) LSC: cava; injury (1)	DRS: 8% Port-site hernia (1), re-operation for bleeding (1), delayed void (1) OS: 25% Ileus (5), wound infection (2), lymphedema (1), cuff hematoma (1), incisional hernia (1) LSC: 23%

(continued on next page)

Table 1
(Continued)

Surgery	N	DRS vs OS	DRS vs LSC	Control	Surgeon	OR Time (min)	EBL (mL)	Hospital Stay (days)	Lymph Node Count	Conversions	Bld Tx	Intraoperative Complications	Postoperative Complications
													Wound infection (3), DVT (1), cuff dehiscence (1), superficial phlebitis (1), A-fib (1)
DeNardis et al 2006–2007 Florida Hospital Cancer Institute	56 vs 106	✓		HC retrospective	DS	177 vs 79	105 vs 241	1.0 vs 3.2	19 vs 18	DRS: 5.4%	0% vs 9%	None	**DRS: 20%** Respiratory failure (1), ileus (1), fever 92), atelectasis (1), wound complication (1), cuff hematoma/separation (4), UTI (1)

Seamon et al 2006–2008 OU	✓	HC pro-spective	SS	105 vs 76	242 vs 287	100 vs 250	1 vs 2 (med)	31 vs 33	DRS: 12% LSC: 26%	3% vs 13%	3 vs 2 DRS: vessel injury (1), GI injury (2) vs OS: nerve injury (1), urinary tract injury (1)	DRS: 9% Port-site herniation (1), cardiac (1), pulmonary (1), other (5) LSC: 10% LSC: 10% DVT (1), cardiac (1), neurologic (1), other (3)
Seamon et al 2006–2008 BMI ≥30	✓	HC retro-spective	SS	228 vs 143	109 vs 394		1 vs 3	25 vs 24	DRS: 15.6%	2% vs 9%	1 vs 2 DRS: GI injury (1) vs OS: vessel injury (1), GI injury (1)	DRS: 10% Cardic (1), pulmonary (2), GI (2), urologic (1), fever (1), fistula (1), bleeding (1), other (3)

OS: 61%
Fever (17), anemia (13), Ileus (4), ARF (2), PE (1), colitis (1), urinary retention (2), thrush (1), UTI (4), atelectasis (4), wound complicaiton (13), lymphocele (1), cuff hematoma/ seperation (2)

(continued on next page)

Table 1
(Continued)

Surgery	N	DRS vs OS	DRS vs LSC	Control	Surgeon	OR Time (min)	EBL (mL)	Hospital Stay (days)	Lymph Node Count	Conversions	Bld Tx	Intraoperative Complications	Postoperative Complications
OU + UAB Matched: BMI + surgeon 1:2													OS: 26% DVT (1), cardiac (2), pulmonary (2), GI (19), urologic (2), (neurologic (1), fever (4), ARF (3), opiated OD (1), parasthesia (2), arrest (1), death (1) Wound complicaitons: **11% vs 27%**
Jung et al 2006–2009 Korea	28 vs 56, 28 vs 25	✓	✓	CC, CC pro-septive	SS, SS	193 vs 187, 193 vs 165	NR	7.9 vs 10.8, 7.9 vs 7.7	21 vs 24, 21 vs 18	none	DRS: 14% OS: 43% LSC: 16%	DRS: none OS: 1 vessel injury LSC: none	**DRS: 7%** pelvic infection (2) **OS: 23%** uretral stricture (1), pelvic infection (2), ileus (1), incisional hernia (1), wound dehiscence (6), lymphocele (1), lymphedema (1)

Cardenas-Goicoechea et al 2007–2010 U Penn	✓	HC retrospective SS	237 vs 178	109 vs 187	1.9 vs 2.3	22 vs 23	DRS: 1% LSC: 5.2%	2.9% vs 1.7%	DRS: 2GI injury (2) LSC: 6 Urinary tract injury (6) Higher rates of uretral injury in LSC	LSC: 8% Pelvic infection (2) DRS: Major (2) PE (1), enterocutaneous fistula (1) DRS: Minor 8%: lymphocele (1), UTI (2), cuff dehiscence (1), abscess (2), incsional hernia (1), ileus (1) LSC: Major (0%) Minor 8%: lymphocele (3), UTI (1), Pna (2), wound seroma (2), cuff cellulitis (2), SBO (1), hematoma (1), port-site abscess (1)

(continued on next page)

Table 1
(Continued)

Surgery	N	DRS vs OS	DRS vs LSC	Control	Surgeon	OR Time (min)	EBL (mL)	Hospital Stay (days)	Lymph Node Count	Conversions	Bld Tx	Intraoperative Complications	Postoperative Complications
Lim et al 2008–2009 Center of Hope-Reno, Nevada	56 vs 36 56 vs 56	✓	✓	HC HC prospective	SS initial exp SS initial exp	163 vs 137 163 vs 192	89 vs 266 89 vs 209	1.6 vs 4.9 1.6 vs 2.6	27 vs 56 27 vs 45	DRS: 1.8% LSC: 7.1%	DRS: 0% OS: 3% LSC: 0%	DRS: 0 OS:0 LSC: 13% (7) obturator n. injury (3), cystotomy (2), entertomy (1), vessel injury (1)	DRS: Major: 5% PE (1), abscess (1), perforated gastric ulcer (1) Minor: 9% OS: Major: 14% Abscess/sepsis (1), fistula (1), pna (1), PE (1), hypertensive crisis (1) Minor: 3% LSC: Major: 11% Fistula (1), obturatory pasly (3), bacteremia (1), DVT (1) Minor: 4%

				SS Initial ex	147 vs 187	81 vs 207	1.5 vs 3.2	25 vs 43	DRS: 0.8% LSC: 6.6%	DRS: 0% LSC: 2.5%	DRS: 0.8% enterotomy (1) LSC: 6% Obturator n. injury (3), cystotomy (2), enterotomy (1), vessel injury (1)	DRS: Major: 4% PE (1), abscess (1), perforated gastric ulcer (1), bowel perforation (1) Minor: 6% LSC: Major: 10% Fistula (1), obturatior palsy (3), bacteremia (1), DVT (1), richter hernia (1), CVA (1) Minor: 2%
Lim et al 2008–2010 Center of Hope Reno, Nevada	122 vs 122	✓	HC prospective									

(continued on next page)

Table 1
(Continued)

Surgery	N	DRS vs OS	DRS vs LSC	Control	Surg-eon	OR Time (min)	EBL (mL)	Hospital Stay (days)	Lymph Node Count	Conver-sions	Bld Tx	Intraoperative Complications	Postoperative Complications
Paley et al 2006–2009 Swedish Medical Center-Seattle, WA	377 vs 131	✓		HC Pro-spective	DS	**184 vs 139**	**47 vs 198**	**1.4 vs 5.3**	**16 vs 13**	DRS: 3.5%	DRS: 0.5% OS: 0.8%	**DRS: 0.5%** Vessel injury (1), cystotomy (1) **OS: 3%** Uretral injury/ARF	**DRS: 5%** cardiac (1), pulmonary (3), DVT/PE (3), infection (4), labile bld sugar (2), ileus/SBO (2), chylous ascites (1), cuff dehiscence (4) **OS: 17%** Cardiac (5), pulmonary (1), DVT/PE (1), infection (6), wound dehiscence (9)

Abbreviations: ARF, acute renal failure; CC, concurrent controls; CVA, cerebrovascular accident; DRS, da vinci robotic system; DS, different surgeon(s); DVT, deep venous thrombosis; EBL, estimated blood loss; HC, historic controls; LSC, laparoscopy; n, sample size; NR, not reported; OR, operating room; OS, open surgery; PE, pulmonary embolism; SBO, small bowel obstruction; SS, same surgeon(s).

When not specified, DRS outcomes are reported first. Items in **bold** are **significantly** different determined by a two-sided alpha <0.05. Outcomes are reported as means unless otherwise noted.

From Weinberg L, Rao S, Escobar PF. Robotic surgery in gynecology: an updated systematic review. Obstet Gynecol Int 2011;2011:852061.

CERVICAL CANCER
Role of Minimally Invasive Surgery

Minimally invasive surgical techniques are commonly used in the treatment of cervical carcinoma. Many gynecologic oncologists began using the technology to perform laparoscopic radical hysterectomies. Many studies have shown decreased blood loss, hospital stay, recovery times, and increased quality of life by performing radical hysterectomy with laparoscopy compared with traditional abdominal approach.[12,13] Despite these advantages, the laparoscopic approach presented technical challenges that prevented it from becoming widely accepted. Radical hysterectomy is a challenging surgery independent of the approach because of the extensive dissection required around the ureter, bladder, and rectum. Robotic-assisted radical hysterectomy is becoming more common because it offers improved dexterity and visualization for this complex procedure. Recently, many investigators have reported on comparison studies between abdominal versus laparoscopic versus robotic approaches for radical hysterectomy. Next we review some of the key comparative studies in the literature today.

Magrina and colleageus[14] published their experience with 27 robotic radical hysterectomies compared with laparoscopic and abdominal cases. The robotic cases were matched with laparoscopic and abdominal cases for age, BMI, type of malignancy, stage, and type of radical hysterectomy. Blood loss for the robotic and laparoscopic groups was lower compared with the abdominal group. Operative times were longest with the laparoscopic technique and equivalent for robotic and abdominal cases. They reported no conversion to open technique and the complication rates were equivalent across all modalities. No recurrences were reported in the 18 cervical cancer patients with an average follow-up of 31 months. The authors concluded that robotic and laparoscopic radical hysterectomy were safe and often the preferred surgical approach.

Boggess and co-workers[15] reported their experience with the first 51 consecutive cases of type III robotic radical hysterectomy compared with 49 cases of type III abdominal radical hysterectomy. The groups had comparable stage, BMI, and uterine size. The robotic group was more likely to have had prior abdominal surgery (51% vs 18%). The robotic group had significantly shorter operative times, lower blood loss, shorter hospital stays, and higher node counts compared with the abdominal radical hysterectomy group. This study again supported the role of robotic radical hysterectomy approach over abdominal approach. This group of investigators recently published survival outcomes for women undergoing robotic radical hysterectomy.[16] The majority of patients included in the study had stage IBI cervical carcinoma. The survival analysis demonstrated 94% progression-free survival and overall survival at 36 months owing to the recurrence and death in 1 patient. When compared with the institutional historical cohort, there was no difference in progression-free ($P = .27$) or overall survivals ($P = .47$). The authors conclude that there data are supportive of acceptable oncologic outcomes at 3 years, although longer follow-up is required.

The studies comparing robotic radical hysterectomy with abdominal radical hysterectomy suggest that the robotic approach is preferable owing to decreases in blood loss, hospital stay, recovery time, and complications. Longer follow-up is needed to evaluate the oncologic outcomes, but early data support similar outcomes for the 3 approaches. The recent Society of Gynecologic Oncology consensus statement stresses the importance of interpreting the data with caution since all studies to date are retrospective and often represent a sequential time comparison or single surgeon experience. Long-term survival outcomes and cost effective analyses are needed to further the acceptance of robotic radical hysterectomy into common practice for the treatment of early stage cervical cancer.[17]

OVARIAN CANCER
Role of Minimally Invasive Surgery

Similar to uterine and cervical cancers, there has been increasing interest in applying minimally invasive surgical techniques for the staging of presumed early stage ovarian cancer. Historically, ovarian cancer staging has been performed through a vertical midline abdominal incision that provides excellent exposure, but is also associated with increased blood loss, increased postoperative pain, and longer recovery time. For these reasons, some gynecologic oncologists have begun to explore the feasibility and safety of utilizing minimally invasive surgery in this setting.

Early stage epithelial ovarian cancer is uncommon, accounting for only 15% of all cases at diagnosis. However, presumed early stage ovarian cancer patients require comprehensive staging to determine prognosis and to plan treatment options. Often these cancers are identified incidentally during laparoscopic oophorectomy for presumed benign adnexal masses and the issue of proceeding with a second surgery for staging is considered. Many critics have argued that adequate staging requires detailed exploration of the peritoneal cavity is neither safe nor feasible with minimally invasive techniques. A few recent studies have attempted to address this issue.[18]

Tozzi and co-workers[19] reported on 24 patients with FIGO stage IA or IB ovarian or fallopian tube cancer who underwent comprehensive laparoscopic staging over 7-year period. Thirteen patients were undergoing primary staging, whereas 11 were undergoing completion staging. The average operative time was 176 minutes. No intraoperative complications were reported. The mean number of pelvic lymph nodes was 19 and the mean number of para-aortic lymph nodes was 19. At a median follow-up of 46 months, the progression-free survival was 92% and the overall survival was 100%. This small study does demonstrates support for the safety and feasibility of minimally invasive approach to primary and completion staging for patients with presumed early stage ovarian cancer.[19]

Another report published by Spirtos and associates[20] addressed the issue of completion staging for women with incompletely staged ovarian, fallopian tube, peritoneal cancers. Seventy-three patients were evaluated in the report. The conversion rate was high compared with previous reports, with 17 patients (23%) requiring conversion to laparotomy to complete the staging procedure. The most common reason cited for conversion was adhesions preventing adequate visualization.[20] Nezhat and colleagues[21] conducted a retrospective review of 36 patients who underwent laparoscopic staging for presumed early stage ovarian cancer. Eleven of the patients were ultimately diagnosed with borderline ovarian tumors. The complication rate was acceptable. Seven (19%) patients had their disease upstaged. With a 4-year median follow-up, there were 3 recurrences in patients (92% progression-free survival) and no patient deaths (100% overall survival).[21]

Several case series, retrospective reviews, and case-control studies have demonstrated that minimally invasive surgery is both safe and effective for the staging of presumed early stage ovarian cancer when performed by a gynecologic oncologist. On the other hand, there are few data regarding the use of minimally invasive techniques for advanced stage ovarian cancer and its use in this setting cannot be recommended.

ROBOTIC-ASSISTED SURGERY IN GYNECOLOGIC ONCOLOGY

In recent years, robotic-assisted surgery has had a significant impact on the operative treatment of gynecologic malignancies. The robotic system was approved by the US Food and Drug Administration in 2005 for gynecologic surgery. The robotic technology offers many advantages over traditional laparoscopic surgery, including 3-dimensional vision, wristed instrumentation for improved dexterity, and ergonomic console systems. The introduction of the robotic systems has had a dramatic change in the pattern of clinical practice for the gynecologic oncology field. A recent Society of Gynecologic Oncology consensus statement reported that currently there are 1400 robotic systems installed in 950 hospitals.[17] Most surgeons report the greatest benefit of robotic surgery is its ease of use and improvement in patient quality of life. Gynecologic oncologists are most commonly applying the technology to surgical staging of uterine cancer and radical pelvic surgery for cervical cancer.[22] In this section, we review the issue of costs associated with robotic technology and the role of robotics in the obese patient.

Cost Analysis

Increased cost is among the most commonly cited concerns regarding adoption of robotic technology. As more and more data accumulate that demonstrate comparable surgical outcomes between laparoscopic and open approaches, it is only appropriate to consider the cost of treatment in the decision regarding surgical approach. Three groups have reported on costs of robotics and other surgical approaches in the management of endometrial cancer. Bell and associates[23] compared cost for endometrial cancer staging via laparotomy versus laparoscopy versus robotic techniques. The average cost for hysterectomy and staging was greatest for laparotomy, followed by robotic, and lowest for laparoscopy. The cost reduction for the minimally invasive approaches was related to shorter length of hospital stay and reduced postoperative morbidity.[23] Another group found that robotic assisted procedures were associated with higher total hospital costs and mean operative costs than laparoscopic procedures.[24] The cost differences were driven by use of disposable instruments and longer operating room times. A third group used a decision model analysis to compare costs of the 3 different surgical approaches in endometrial cancer. The decision model included a societal perspective model which included costs associated with surgery, acquisition and maintenance of the robot, hospitalization, lost wages, and caregiver costs. In the societal perspective model, laparoscopy was the least costly approach with an average cost of $10,128 per case compared with robotic ($11,476) and open hysterectomy ($12,847). The cost difference was most dependent on the use of disposable robotic equipment and the total recovery time from robotic surgery. The authors concluded that robotic assisted surgery is less costly than abdominal hysterectomy when the societal costs associated with recovery time are accounted for and can be more economical if disposable equipment use is minimized.[25] As robotic technology gains popularity, cost analysis and strategies to reduce cost will be needed to improve the economic advantage of this approach.

Optimizing the Surgical Approach in the Obese Patient

Obesity has reached epidemic status in the United States. One of the most common risk factors for endometrial cancer is obesity. Obesity has been associated with greater surgical risks; there is more difficulty with exposure, longer operative times, increased blood loss, and a greater number of comorbidities that complicate the perioperative and postoperative course. For these reasons, gynecologic surgeons are commonly challenged to operate on obese if not morbidly obese patients and achieve similar oncologic outcomes in a safe setting. We know from LAP2 that the feasibility of laparoscopic surgical staging for endometrial cancer is affected by the patient's weight. The conversion from laparoscopy to laparotomy was drastically increased for increasing BMI.[8] Scribner and co-workers[26] reported similar difficulties when comparing laparoscopic with open staging in the obese with a 64% success rate in nodal dissection in obese patients dropped to 44% in the morbidly obese patient. However, for women who were able to undergo laparoscopic staging, they required less postoperative IV pain medication, shorter hospitalizations, fewer wound infections, and fewer postoperative fevers.[26] The introduction of the robotic surgical platform has seemingly improved the technical aspects of surgery in the obese while maintaining all the minimally invasive advantages. The feasibility and advantages of robotic surgery in patients with high BMIs has recently become a common topic in the gynecologic oncology literature.

There are no prospective, randomized trials evaluating the robotic surgical platform as the preferred surgical approach in women with obesity (BMI >30) or morbid obesity (BMI >40). However, more and more experience is being reported with favorable outcomes in this difficult patient population. One of the earliest reports was from Gehrig and associates,[27] reporting on consecutive robotic endometrial cancer staging procedures from 2005 to 2007 compared with consecutive laparoscopic cases (2000–2004). There were 36 obese and 13 morbidly obese women who underwent surgery with the robotic platform and 25 obese and 7 morbidly obese women who underwent traditional laparoscopy. For both the obese and morbidly obese patients, robotic surgery was associated with shorter operative times, less blood loss, increased lymph node counts, and shorter hospital stays.[27] Similarly, in a retrospective cohort study comparing 73 obese patients with endometrial cancer who underwent robotic surgery with 104 obese patients who underwent laparotomy, Subramaniam and colleagues[28] reported longer operative times; however, estimated blood loss, the percentage of patients receiving transfusion, hospital length of stay, wound complications (4% vs 20%; $P = .002$) and other complications (10% vs 30%; $P = .001$) were improved in the robotic cohort.[28]

VULVAR CANCER
Sentinel Lymph Node Biopsy

Surgery for vulvar cancer surgery has undergone many advances. Historically, these women were treated with radical vulvectomy and en bloc inguinofemoral lymph node dissection, a procedure with high survival rates as well as morbidity. This radical approach moved to a triple incision technique and has maintained optimal survival while decreasing morbidity. The next surgical advance being evaluated in vulvar cancer is the role of sentinel lymph node biopsy. Inguinofemoral lymphadenectomy has relatively high rates of perioperative complications, with as many as two thirds of patients experiencing wound breakdown, lymphocyst formation, and/or lymphedema. For these reasons, and based on our understanding of the anatomic drainage patterns, lymphatic mapping and sentinel node dissection in vulvar cancer have been explored.

The largest study evaluating the sensitivity and false negative rate of patients with vulvar cancer undergoing sentinel lymph node biopsy is the GROINSS-V study.[29] This observational study evaluated 403 patients. The trial was conducted at 15 sites with surgical skill verification procedures required.[29] Patients with less than a 4-cm squamous cell cancer of the vulva were studied using radioactive tracer and blue dye for sentinel node dissection. If the sentinel node was negative at pathologic ultrastaging, inguinofemoral lymphadenectomy was omitted and the patient was observed. A group of 276 patients with a negative sentinel lymph node biopsy were observed for a median of 35 months. Six groin recurrences were diagnosed (2.3%) and the 3-year survival rate was 97%. Short-term morbidity was decreased in patients after sentinel node dissection only when compared with patients with a positive sentinel who underwent inguinofemoral lymphadenectomy (wound breakdown in groin, 12% vs 34%; cellulitis, 5% vs 21%). Long-term morbidity was also decreased in the sentinel lymph node biopsy only group specifically lymphedema of the legs: 2% versus 25% (P<.0001). The authors concluded that sentinel lymph node biopsy was safe in appropriate patients and quality-controlled multidisciplinary teams.

In addition to the large observational study discussed, the Gynecologic Oncology Group is conducting a large validation study prospectively evaluating the sensitivity, false-negative rate, and negative predictive value of sentinel lymph node dissection. This study did not require skill verification and was conducted at many more hospitals, perhaps simulating a more community-based practice approach. The study has met the accrual goal and the final results should be available soon.

Common Questions

Despite these promising results, many questions and safety issues remain with introducing this surgical technique into routine clinical practice.

What is the best technique for sentinel lymph node detection?
A meta-analysis recently compared the following approaches of detecting lymph node metastases in women with vulvar cancer: Blue dye (isosulfan blue, patent blue, or methylene blue), technetium-99m-labelled nanocolliod, groin ultrasonography with or without fine needle aspiration, computed tomography, magnetic resonance imaging, and positron emission tomography. The most accurate tests were sentinel lymph node biopsy with either technetium (sensitivity, 97% [95% confidence interval (CI), 91–100]; negative likelihood ratio, 0.12 [95% CI, 0.053–0.28]) or blue dye (sensitivity, 95% [95% CI, 82–99]; negative likelihood ratio, 0.18 [95% CI, 0.07–0.32]). Sensitivities for the other tests ranged from 45% to 86%.[30] In an expert panel statement, most panelists recommended the combined approach (blue dye and radiocolliod) allowed surgeons to become more comfortable with sentinel lymph node biopsy.[31]

Is the false-negative rate acceptable?
The validation trials for sentinel lymph node biopsy in breast cancer and melanoma reported false-negative rates of 4% to 5%. In patients with early stage breast cancer, investigators have reported false-negative rates as high as 10%; however, the majority of sentinel node–negative patients in this disease site are still receiving adjuvant treatment. The status of the groin nodes in vulvar cancer is the most important prognostic factor and their status is often what dictates the need for adjuvant therapy. There is little margin for error in detecting groin node metastasis because groin recurrence is usually fatal.

Tips for Successful Use of Sentinel Lymph Node Biopsy

The gynecologic oncologist should demonstrate competence in their ability to identify the sentinel lymph node. Most experts recommended performing 10 sentinel lymph node biopsies followed by lymphadenectomy to provide for adequate learning of the procedure. Patient selection is critical; one should exclude multifocal disease or large tumors. Preoperative imaging is also helpful to exclude patients with gross nodal involvement in whom mapping procedures may be inaccurate. Nuclear medicine specialists trained to perform intradermal injections for vulvar tumors and a surgical pathologist familiar with ultra-staging techniques should be included. Given our current level of data, sentinel lymph node biopsy is a reasonable alternative to full inguinal lymphadenectomy when the procedure is performed by a skilled multidisciplinary team in well-selected patients.[32]

SUMMARY

The numerous advances in the surgical care of gynecologic oncology patients are allowing clinicians to offer improved quality of life while maintaining excellent cancer outcomes. Advances in technology and disease understanding will only enhance our surgical abilities beyond what can be imagined today. Surgeons have a responsibility to evaluate new technology critically and incorporate the technology into patient care safely and efficiently.

REFERENCES

1. Baskett TF. Hysterectomy: evolution and trends. Best Pract Res Clin Obstet Gynaecol 2005;19:295–305.
2. Querleu D, Leblanc E, Castelain B. Laparoscopic pelvic lymphadenectomy in the staging of early carcinoma of the cervix. Am J Obstet Gynecol 1991;164:79–81.
3. Childers JM, Spirtos NM, Brainard P, et al. Laparoscopic staging of the patient with incompletely staged early adenocarcinoma of the endometrium. Obstet Gynecol 1994;83:597–600.
4. Spirtos NM, Schlaerth JB, Spirtos TW, et al. Laparoscopic bilateral pelvic and paraaortic lymph node sampling: an evolving technique. Am J Obstet Gynecol 1995;173:105–11.
5. Childers JM, Brzechffa PR, Hatch KD, et al. Laparoscopically assisted surgical staging (LASS) of endometrial cancer. Gynecol Oncol 1993;51:33–8.
6. Tozzi R, Malur S, Koehler C, et al. Laparoscopy versus laparotomy in endometrial cancer: first analysis of survival of a randomized prospective study. J Minim Invasive Gynecol 2005;12:130–6.
7. Malzoni M, Tinelli R, Cosentino F, et al. Total laparoscopic hysterectomy versus abdominal hysterectomy with lymphadenectomy for early-stage endometrial cancer: a prospective randomized study. Gynecol Oncol 2009;112:126–33.
8. Walker JL, Peidmonte MR, Spirtos NM, et al. Laparoscopy compared with laparotomy for comprehensive surgical staging of uterine cancer: Gynecologic Oncology Group Study LAP2. J Clin Oncol 2009;27:5331–6.
9. Weinberg L, Rao S, Escobar PF. Robotic surgery in gynecology: an updated systematic review. Obstet Gynecol Int 2011;2011:852061.
10. Kornblith AB, Huang HQ, Walker JL, et al. Quality of life of patients with endometrial cancer undergoing laparoscopic international federation of gynecology and obstetrics staging compared with laparotomy: a Gynecologic Oncology Group study. J Clin Oncol 2009;27:5337–42.
11. Janda M, Gebski V, Brand A, et al. Quality of life after total laparoscopic hysterectomy versus total abdominal hysterectomy for stage I endometrial cancer (LACE): a randomised trial. Lancet Oncol 2010;11:772–80.
12. Frumovitz M, dos Reis R, Sun CC, et al. Comparison of total laparoscopic and abdominal radical hysterectomy for patients with early-stage cervical cancer. Obstet Gynecol 2007;110:96–102.
13. Ramirez PT, Slomovitz BM, Soliman PT, et al. Total laparoscopic radical hysterectomy and lymphadenectomy: the M. D. Anderson Cancer Center experience. Gynecol Oncol 2006;102:252–5.

14. Magrina JF, Kho RM, Weaver AL, et al. Robotic radical hysterectomy: comparison with laparoscopy and laparotomy. Gynecol Oncol 2008;109:86–91.
15. Boggess JF, Gehrig PA, Cantrell L, et al. A case-control study of robot-assisted type III radical hysterectomy with pelvic lymph node dissection compared with open radical hysterectomy. Am J Obstet Gynecol 2008;199:357 e1–7.
16. Cantrell LA, Mendivil A, Gehrig PA, et al. Survival outcomes for women undergoing type III robotic radical hysterectomy for cervical cancer: a 3-year experience. Gynecol Oncol 2010;117:260–5.
17. Ramirez PT, Adams S, Boggess JF, et al. Robotic-assisted surgery in gynecologic oncology: A Society of Gynecologic Oncology consensus statement Developed by the Society of Gynecologic Oncology's Clinical Practice Robotics Task Force. Gynecol Oncol 2012;124:180–4.
18. Iglesias DA, Ramirez PT. Role of minimally invasive surgery in staging of ovarian cancer. Curr Treat Options Oncol 2011;12:217–29.
19. Tozzi R, Kohler C, Ferrara A, et al. Laparoscopic treatment of early ovarian cancer: surgical and survival outcomes. Gynecol Oncol 2004;93:199–203.
20. Spirtos NM, Eisekop SM, Boike G, et al. Laparoscopic staging in patients with incompletely staged cancers of the uterus, ovary, fallopian tube, and primary peritoneum: a Gynecologic Oncology Group (GOG) study. Am J Obstet Gynecol 2005;193:1645–9.
21. Nezhat FR, Ezzati M, Chuang L, et al. Laparoscopic management of early ovarian and fallopian tube cancers: surgical and survival outcome. Am J Obstet Gynecol 2009;200:83 e1–6.
22. duPont NC, Chanfrasekhar R, Wilding G, et al. Current trends in robot assisted surgery: a survey of gynecologic oncologists. Int J Med Robot 2010;6:468–72.
23. Bell MC, Torgerson J, Seshadri-Kreaden U, et al. Comparison of outcomes and cost for endometrial cancer staging via traditional laparotomy, standard laparoscopy and robotic techniques. Gynecol Oncol 2008;111:407–11.
24. Holtz DO, Miroshnichenko G, Finnegan MO, et al. Endometrial cancer surgery costs: robot vs laparoscopy. J Minim Invasive Gynecol 2010;17:500–3.
25. Barnett JC, Judd JP, Wu JM, et al. Cost comparison among robotic, laparoscopic, and open hysterectomy for endometrial cancer. Obstet Gynecol 2010;116:685–93.
26. Scribner DR Jr, Walker JL, Johnson GA, et al. Laparoscopic pelvic and paraaortic lymph node dissection in the obese. Gynecol Oncol 2002;84:426–30.
27. Gehrig PA, Cantrell LA, Shafer A, et al. What is the optimal minimally invasive surgical procedure for endometrial cancer staging in the obese and morbidly obese woman? Gynecol Oncol 2008;111:41–5.
28. Subramaniam A, Kim KH, Bryant SA, et al. A cohort study evaluating robotic versus laparotomy surgical outcomes of obese women with endometrial carcinoma. Gynecol Oncol 2011;122:604–7.
29. Van der Zee AG, Oonk MH, De Hulliu JA, et al. Sentinel node dissection is safe in the treatment of early-stage vulvar cancer. J Clin Oncol 2008;26:884–9.
30. Selman TJ, Luesley DM, Acheson N, et al. A systematic review of the accuracy of diagnostic tests for inguinal lymph node status in vulvar cancer. Gynecol Oncol 2005;99:206–14.
31. Levenback CF, van der See AG, Rob L, et al. Sentinel lymph node biopsy in patients with gynecologic cancers Expert panel statement from the International Sentinel Node Society Meeting, February 21, 2008. Gynecol Oncol 2009;114:151–6.
32. Levenback CF. How safe is sentinel lymph node biopsy in patients with vulvar cancer? J Clin Oncol 2008;26:828–9.

Hereditary Gynecologic Cancers
Risk Assessment, Counseling, Testing and Management

Lori L. Ballinger, MS

KEYWORDS

- Genetic counseling • Genetic testing • Gynecologic cancer • Hereditary cancers

KEY POINTS

- Identification of patients at risk for hereditary cancer syndromes is critical for early diagnosis or prevention of cancers.
- Many cancer genetic syndromes present with specific clinical or pathological features, or specific family history patterns.
- Genetic risk assessment and counseling is integral to the process of genetic testing for hereditary cancer syndromes.

Recognition of women and families at risk for inherited cancer syndromes is critical for both management and prevention of gynecologic cancers as well as other syndrome-associated malignancies. Most hereditary cancer syndromes have risks for multiple cancers, and surveillance for affected women is radically different than for those with sporadic disease. High-penetrance hereditary cancer syndromes account for 5% to 10% of all cancers, including those of the female reproductive organs. In this article, inherited syndromes that involve tumors and malignancies of the uterus and ovaries are discussed.

OVARIAN CANCER

Every year, approximately 22,000 women are diagnosed with an ovarian malignancy in the United States. The population lifetime risk is 1.4% (1/71). Risk factors for ovarian cancer include advancing age and nulliparity; other possible risk factors include early age of menarche and infertility. Family history also plays a role, with a 4.6 relative risk of ovarian cancer in the mother of an affected patient, and 1.6 relative risk in a sister (7.0% and 2.5%, respectively).[1] However, women with inherited cancer

The author has nothing to disclose.
Hereditary Cancer Assessment Program, University of New Mexico, Cancer Research and Treatment Center, MSC 07 4025, 1 University of New Mexico, Albuquerque, NM 87131, USA
E-mail address: lballinger@salud.unm.edu

Obstet Gynecol Clin N Am 39 (2012) 165–181
doi:10.1016/j.ogc.2012.02.006
0889-8545/12/$ – see front matter © 2012 Elsevier Inc. All rights reserved.

syndromes have a lifetime risk as high as 12% to 50% for ovarian malignancy. Hereditary ovarian cancers also often present at an earlier age than those in the general population. Inherited ovarian neoplasms are associated with several genetic cancer syndromes, including hereditary breast/ovarian cancer syndrome, the Lynch syndrome also known as hereditary nonpolyposis colon cancer, and other, rare syndromes, such as Peutz–Jeghers syndrome.

ENDOMETRIAL CANCER

Based on rates from 2006 through 2008, approximately 2.5% (1/40) of women born today will be diagnosed with cancer of the endometrium, most between ages 50 and 70.[2] In the United States, more than 46,000 cases are diagnosed each year. Risk factors for endometrial cancer include nulliparity, infertility, exposure to unopposed estrogens, anovulation, obesity, and type 2 diabetes. The incidence of endometrial carcinoma is higher in Caucasians than Blacks.[2] The most common genetic risk factor for development of endometrial cancer is the Lynch syndrome. The risk of endometrial cancer is also increased in other hereditary cancer syndromes, such as PTEN Hamartoma Tumor syndrome (Cowden syndrome) and Peutz-Jeghers syndrome.

HEREDITARY BREAST/OVARIAN CANCER SYNDROME

The large majority of patients with hereditary breast/ovarian syndrome have mutations in BRCA1 or BRCA2, and these genes account for the major proportion of inherited ovarian cancers.[3–5] Both are tumor suppressor genes that function in the DNA damage response pathway. The greatest risk for women who have BRCA mutations is breast cancer; mutations confer a lifetime risk of 50% to 85%, but ovarian cancer risk is also significantly increased.

Risks

The risk of ovarian cancer is higher in women with BRCA1 mutations, and 80% of families with both breast and ovarian cancer have mutations in this gene. In women from families with a high incidence of breast and/or ovarian cancer, mutations in BRCA1 confer a lifetime risk of epithelial ovarian cancer of 20% to 60%.[6,7] The lifetime risk of epithelial ovarian cancer associated with BRCA2 mutations in these families has been estimated between 10% and 20%.[7–9] Mutations in the ovarian cancer cluster region of exon 11 in the BRCA2 gene also confer higher risks of ovarian malignancies (relative risk, 1.88). There is also a higher ratio of ovarian to breast cancer than in families with mutations elsewhere in the BRCA2 gene.[10,11] Antoniou and associates[12] estimated the risks to be lower for family members of unselected cases of BRCA-positive ovarian cancer (39% for BRCA1 and 11% for BRCA2).

Epidemiology

The frequency of BRCA1 or BRCA2 mutations in the general population is estimated to be 1 in 300 to 1 in 800[13]; however, the frequency of founder mutations in some populations is much higher. In individuals of eastern European Jewish (Ashkenazi) ancestry, 3 founder mutations (187delAG and 5382insC in BRCA1 and 6174delT in BRCA2) account for more than 90% of mutations detected. In the United States, 1 in 40 of such individuals carries 1 of these 3 mutations.[14] High frequencies of founder mutations have been described in several other populations and ethnic groups.[15]

Approximately 6% to 13% of unselected ovarian cancers are due to mutations in BRCA genes.[16,17] The risk of BRCA-related ovarian cancer rises significantly after the age of 35 to 40 in BRCA1 mutation carriers and age 40 to 45 in BRCA2 mutation carriers, whereas the risk of breast cancer in these women levels off after age 60.[12,18,19]

Pathology

BRCA-related ovarian cancers are exclusively epithelial, and most are of high-grade serous or undifferentiated histology,[20,21] although and endometrioid type has been described.[22] Borderline and mucinous tumors have not been observed in most studies.[4,16,23–25] Fallopian tube neoplasms seem to play an important role in the molecular pathogenesis of BRCA-related ovarian cancers.[26,27] More than half of all occult carcinomas found in women who undergo risk-reducing salpingo-oophorectomy (RRSO) are found in the distal fallopian tube.[28–30]

Ovarian Cancer Risk Reduction in BRCA1 and BRCA2

Chemoprevention

Oral contraceptive use by women with BRCA mutations has been shown to be associated with a lower risk of ovarian cancer.[31,32] An estimated 50% reduction has been observed in multiple studies, with greater reduction observed in women who used oral contraceptives for longer than 3 years.[33,34] In some studies, the risk of breast cancer in BRCA mutation carriers was slightly increased for those who used pre-1975 formulations, or in those who used oral contraceptives before age 30[35]; however, a meta-analysis of the impact of oral contraceptive use on breast cancer risk in mutation carriers did not show any increase in breast cancer risk.[36]

Risk-reducing bilateral salpingo-oophorectomy

Several studies have demonstrated that ovarian cancer screening using transvaginal ultrasonography and serum CA-125 levels in women at high risk results in both a high prevalence of false positive results, in addition to late-stage presentation for the majority of the affected women.[37–41] Nonetheless, for women who decline surgical prophylaxis, current guidelines include both examinations, starting at age 35 or earlier, depending on the earliest age of onset of ovarian cancer in the family.[42,43]

Multiple studies have demonstrated a greatly reduced risk of ovarian cancer and subsequent mortality risk in BRCA mutation carries who undergo bilateral RRSO.[41,43,44] Risk reduction is estimated to be 85% to 95%,[44,45] especially if performed by the age of 40.[42,46,47] Domchek and colleagues[48] found that among a cohort of women with BRCA mutations, RRSO was associated with a lower risk of not only ovarian cancer, but also breast cancer, all-cause mortality, breast cancer–specific mortality, and ovarian cancer–specific mortality.[48]

Several studies have shown that short-term hormone replacement therapy after RRSO has little, if any effect on breast cancer risk[49,50] in BRCA-positive women who have not previously been diagnosed with breast cancer, and can be considered for quality-of-life issues. The recommended duration of HRT from time of RRSO is to around age 50 years.[51]

The risk of occult ovarian or fallopian tube malignancy at the time of RRSO has been estimated to be between 2% and 11%, depending on the gene involved and the age at the time of surgery.[41,52,53] Therefore, special consideration for both the procedure and pathologic examination of RRSO specimens is recommended.[42,54–56] It is essential that as much as possible of the tissue at risk be removed, although the majority of the fallopian tube cancers occur in the distal or mid portion, and no cancers have been reported in the interstitial fallopian tube in the cornua of the uterus.[57–59] Adequate pathologic examination of the ovaries and fallopian tubes requires serial sectioning (2–3 mm) to detect small cancers.[41,60] The risk of primary

- *Early onset breast cancer (<45y)*
- *Two breast primaries in a single individual*
- *Breast and ovarian cancer in the same individual*
- *Breast cancer **and** ≥1 close blood relative with breast cancer ≤age 50 years **or** ≥1 close relative with ovarian cancer at any age **or** ≥2 close relatives with breast cancer at any age*
- *Breast or ovarian cancer at any age and Ashkenazi Jewish ancestry*
- *Male breast cancer*
- *Ovarian cancer and family history of breast or ovarian cancer*
- *Women from families that meet the above criteria*

Fig. 1. Criteria for risk evaluation in women from families with breast/ovarian cancer.

peritoneal carcinoma is low, but exact estimates vary, and are hampered by different surgical and pathologic procedures in the studies. Chapman and associates[61] recommend that follow-up of women post RRSO be standardized to include dual-energy x-ray absorptiometry bone scanning 1 to 2 years after RRSO, as well as exercise, calcium, and vitamin D supplementation. Data supporting or refuting biannual serum CA-125 screening do not yet exist. The Gynecologic Oncology Group 199 protocol has completed a 5-year follow-up of a large cohort of high-risk women, and it is hoped that this study will improve the evidence for CA-125 serum screening post-RRSO.

Although current guidelines do not recommend hysterectomy at the time of RRSO, some controversy remains about the risk of uterine serous carcinoma in germline BRCA mutation carriers[62,63]; however, all published series regarding this are limited to Ashkenazi or other Jewish populations.

Survival in BRCA-Related Ovarian Cancers

Some studies report improved survival in ovarian cancer patients with BRCA mutations over that in noncarriers.[64–66] BRCA gene products play a vital role in DNA repair mechanisms.[67,68] It has been demonstrated that the deficiency of the BRCA proteins confers cellular sensitivity to the inhibition of poly (ADP-ribose) polymerase enzyme. As this polymerase is a key enzyme in the repair of single strand DNA damage, the loss of poly (ADP-ribose) polymerase enzyme activity in BRCA mutant tumors is thought to lead to increased chromosome instability and programmed cell death.[69,70] Because there is no functional protein within the tumor cells, the capacity to repair DNA damage is lost. Cisplatin, used in first-line treatment of ovarian malignancy, also acts through the induction of DNA damage by causing double-strand breaks in DNA, leading to cell death and better therapeutic response.[69,71]

Identification of Those at Risk

Standard guidelines exist for identifying women with BRCA mutations (**Fig. 1**). Clinicians should be aware of the need for eliciting extended family history for affected patients as well as those with significant family histories. Maternal and paternal sides of the family should be considered independently for patterns of cancer. A 3-generational history, including siblings, children, parents, aunts, uncles, cousins, and grandparents is the standard for determining risk.

Close attention to the type of cancer, bilaterality, age of diagnosis, and history of chemoprevention or risk-reducing surgeries is required. Documentation, particularly pathology reports of primary cancers diagnosed in affected family members, should be obtained when possible. Distinction should be made between primary and

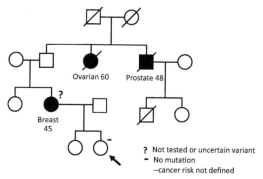

Fig. 2. Patient who is negative for mutations and no mutation identified in affected family member. Cancer risks are not defined for this patient.

metastatic sites. Identification of the ancestry/ethnicity of the individual is important for reasons discussed below.

Testing Considerations

Whenever possible, testing of an affected family member with early onset disease, bilateral disease, or multiple primaries is preferred, because that individual has the highest likelihood of having a mutation. Because negative test results in an unaffected family member are considered to be less informative in the absence of a known mutation in the family, before such testing is performed, a woman should be fully informed of the limitations (**Fig. 2**). If a mutation is identified in a family member, unless there is history of early onset breast or ovarian cancer on both the maternal and paternal sides, single-site testing for the identified mutation is adequate for affected as well as unaffected patients. If an affected individual with a family history of an identified mutation is negative for that mutation, further testing by sequence analysis should also be considered (eg, a woman with ovarian cancer at age 50 who is negative for a known familial mutation). Women who test negative for a known familial mutation are considered to be "true negatives" and are not at increased risk for breast or ovarian cancers (**Fig. 3**).

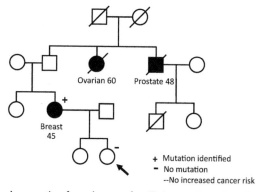

Fig. 3. Patient who is negative for a known familial mutation identified in affected family member. Cancer risks are not increased for this patient.

Women of Ashkenazi Jewish ancestry should be tested first for the 3 founder mutations in BRCA1 and BRCA2, and in those families with a known founder mutation, testing for all 3 mutations is recommended, based on the high prevalence of these mutations in this population. A woman who meets criteria for testing in non-Ashkenazi populations should undergo further testing by sequence analysis if she is negative for the founder mutations.[12]

Variants of uncertain significance pose a significant dilemma for interpretation, especially in unaffected women with a concerning family history. These variants may be benign polymorphisms unrelated to increased cancer risk, or may be deleterious mutations that cause a significant increase in risk. This illustrates the importance of testing an affected relative, and patients with variants of uncertain significance should be encouraged to participate in research aimed at defining the clinical impact of the gene variant.

Certain mutations (some large rearrangements and deletions) are not detectible by sequence analysis and should be considered in mutation-negative families with high-suspicion for hereditary breast/ovarian cancer.[72,73] There are tests that detect the large rearrangements that account for 7.5% of all mutations in BRCA1 and BRCA2.[74] These rearrangements are rare in Ashkenazi Jewish families with hereditary breast/ovarian cancer.[75]

As discussed in detail at the end of this paper, appropriate genetic counseling is integral to the process of evaluation and testing of individual or families suspected of having inherited cancer syndromes.

THE LYNCH SYNDROME

The Lynch syndrome is a multiple cancer disorder that carries greatly increased risks of colon and other gastrointestinal tumors, and endometrial, ovarian, hepatobiliary tract, and uroepithelial tract neoplasms. Originally called hereditary nonpolyposis colon cancer syndrome (because colorectal cancers seemed to be the defining feature), endometrial and ovarian malignancies, among other cancers, have now been recognized as part of the spectrum of this disorder. The Lynch syndrome accounts for 2% to 3% of all endometrial cancers.[76,77] The Lynch syndrome is associated with mutations in 1 of 4 genes (MLH1, MSH2, MSH6, or PMS2). These genes function as DNA mismatch repair (MMR) genes, excising errors that occur during DNA replication.

Epidemiology

The prevalence of the Lynch syndrome varies from 0.3% to 5.8%; early on, population incidence was estimated at 1/600 to 1/2000[78]; however, because of the complexities of identifying families and affected individuals by clinical criteria alone, this is certainly an underestimate.[79] The Lynch syndrome accounts for 2.2% of colon cancers and 2% of ovarian cancers unselected for age.[80,81] The prevalence of the Lynch syndrome mutations in women with endometrial cancer who are under age 50 is approximately 9% to 20%[82,83]; the prevalence is even higher for nonobese women diagnosed with endometrial cancer in this age group.[84,85]

Cancer Risks

Genotype–phenotype correlations have emerged in the Lynch syndrome. Individuals with mutations in MLH1 and MSH2 have higher cancer risks, with a lifetime risk of colon cancer of approximately 50% to 82%, and a risk of endometrial cancer of 21% to 57%.[86–88] The risk for colon cancer in MSH6 and PMS2 are approximately 18% and 15%, respectively; the risk of endometrial cancer in mutation carriers of MSH6 is

---

Box 1
Revised Bethesda guidelines for testing colorectal tumors for microsatellite instability

- Colorectal cancer diagnosed in a patient less than 50 years of age.

- Presence of synchronous metachronous colorectal or other hereditry non-polyposis colorectal (HNPCC) related tumorsa, regardless of age.

- Colorectal cancer with MSI-H histologyb diagnosed in a patient who is less than 60 years of age.

- Colorectal cancer diagnosed in one or more first degree relatives with an HNPCC-related tumor, with one of the cancers being diagnosed under age 50 years.

- Colorectal cancer diagnosed in two or more first- or second-degree relatives with HNPCC- related tumors, regardless of age.

aHNPCC-related tumors include colorectal, endometrial, stomach, ovarian, pancreas, ureter and renal pelvis, biliary tract, brain and small bowel.

bPresence of tumor infiltrating lymphocytes, Crohn's-like lymphocytic reaction, mucinous/sign-etring differentiation, or medullary growth pattern.

(Adapted from Umar A, Boland DR, Terdiman JP, et al. Revised Bethesda guidelines for hereditary nonpolyposis colorectal cancer (Lynch syndrome) and microsatellite instability. J Natl Cancer Inst 2004;96:261–8;with permission).

17% to 26% and approximately 15% in PMS2 mutation carriers.[87,89,90] The ratio of endometrial to colon cancer is greater for women with MSH6 mutations[77,89] than with the other genes. The risk of ovarian cancer in Lynch syndrome is 4% to 12%. Risks of other cancers are increased over the population, including gastric (6%–13%), urothelial (1%–4%), small bowel, (3%–6%), and biliary tract (1.4%–4%).[86,91–95]

Identification of the Lynch Syndrome in Women with Endometrial or Ovarian Cancer

Guidelines for identifying the Lynch syndrome in women gynecologic cancers is less well-defined than for those with colorectal cancer.[96] Because women with mutations can present with endometrial cancer as the first or sentinel malignancy, identification is important, given the personal and family risk for other malignancies. The revised Bethesda guidelines for identifying patients focus almost exclusively on colorectal cancers, although in patients with colon and another Lynch syndrome cancer (endometrial and ovarian included) consideration of testing is recommended (**Box 1**).[97] Screening based on patient age and family history has been proposed,[82,98] but it has been shown that women with the Lynch syndrome, especially those with mutations in MSH6 and PMS2, often present with age of onset of less than 50 years.[99] Resnick and co-workers[100] have advocated for universal screening for Lynch syndrome in all endometrial cancers as the most cost-efficient way of diagnosing the greatest number of patients.[100]

   Multiple tumor testing modalities exist to identify women who should be offered definitive germline genetic testing. These include microsatellite instability, immuno-histochemistry for MMR gene expression, and MLH1 promotor hypermethylation studies. Because most microsatellite instability–high and MLH1-absent endometrial tumors have MLH1 promotor hypermethylation, testing of endometrial tumors for MMR gene expression, followed by MLH1 hypermethylation studies in those tumors with absent MLH1 staining, is the most efficient way to identify those who need germline testing. **Fig. 4** illustrates an algorithm adapted from Garg and Soslow,[96] using this approach. Because a MLH1 dimerizes with PMS2 and MSH2 dimerizes MSH6, germline testing for the dominant protein (MLH1 or MSH2) should be

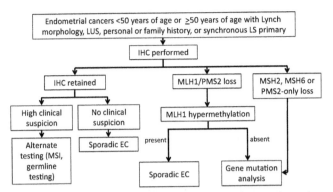

Fig. 4. Proposed algorithm for testing endometrial cancers for Lynch syndrome. *(Adapted from* Garg K, Soslow RA. Lynch syndrome (hereditary non-polyposis colorectal cancer) and endometrial carcinoma. J Clin Pathol 2009;62:679–84;with permission).

performed when both are absent in tumor tissue. In cases of MSH6- or PMS2-only absent staining, germline testing should be performed first for gene with absent staining. Because there are a few case reports in the literature where MLH1 mutations in patients were identified with PMS2-only absent in colon cancers,[97] it may be appropriate to further investigate those who are negative for PMS2 mutations. Additionally, because not all mutations are identified by current technology, patients whose tumors have confirmed absence of immunohistochemistry staining and nonmethylation should be assumed to have the Lynch syndrome and should be followed accordingly, even if a mutation is not identified.

Gynecologic Cancer

Endometrial cancer can often be the sentinel cancer in women with the Lynch syndrome, especially in women with MSH2 mutations,[86,101,102] emphasizing the need to identify these patients to prevent or provide increased surveillance for other Lynch syndrome cancers. Women who present with synchronous endometrial and nonserous ovarian cancers are more likely to have the Lynch syndrome, especially those with family history of a Lynch syndrome malignancy.[103]

In a large study, Broaddus and associates[104] examined the histopathologic features of 50 women with Lynch syndrome-associated endometrial cancer and compared them with 2 groups of women with sporadic endometrial cancer (42 women <50 years and 50 women of all ages with tumors demonstrating microsatellite instability secondary to MLH1 promotor methylation). No difference in myometrial invasion, lymphovascular invasion, or stage was found; however, there were striking differences in the histologic subtype of the Lynch syndrome cancers. Whereas sporadic tumors were almost all (96%–97%) of endometrioid histology, 24% of Lynch tumors were of papillary serous, clear cell, or mixed Müllerian histology. The mean age of diagnosis of non-endometrioid tumors was 46.4 years, younger than the general population age of less than 65 years for these histologic subtypes. Another study by Walsh and co-workers[83] identified 26 microsatellite high, non–MLH1-hypermethylated endometrial tumors in a series of 148 early onset endometrial cancers (≤50 years). In this study, the Lynch syndrome tumors were more likely to be poorly differentiated, FIGO II or above, and have tumor-infiltrating lymphocytes, a higher mitotic rate, and deeper myometrial invasion than patients with microsatellite stable or MLH1 hypermethylation of their tumors.

Two recent papers have described an association of carcinoma of the lower uterine segment and the Lynch syndrome. Westin and colleagues[105] found 29% of 1009 endometrial cancers of the lower uterine segment to be Lynch syndrome related. Compared with patients with endometrial carcinoma of the corpus, these women were more likely to be younger, have higher stage tumors, and deeper myometrial invasion. Garg and co-workers[106] describes absent MMR gene staining in 5 of 6 lower uterine segment tumors from 71 cases meeting selection criteria for Lynch syndrome tumor testing.

Ovarian cancer in Lynch syndrome presents with a younger age of onset (average, 45–50 years) and is more likely to be of endometrioid or clear cell histology.[98,107] The lifetime risk of ovarian cancer is estimated to be between 6% and 12%.[82,91,93,102]

Surveillance and Risk Reduction

In addition to colon cancer surveillance, women with the Lynch syndrome can benefit from surveillance for endometrial cancers. Although somewhat controversial, most authors feel that transvaginal ultrasonography plus endometrial sampling in women over the age of 30 is appropriate.[108–111] Because many endometrial cancers can often be diagnosed at early stages on the basis of symptoms, women should be educated about the signs of endometrial cancers. Surveillance for ovarian cancer has not been proven to be effective. Most sources recommend hysterectomy and bilateral salpingo-oophorectomy for women with the Lynch syndrome after childbearing is complete.[112–114] Occult endometrial and fallopian tube cancer at the time of risk reducing surgery has been reported,[115] emphasizing the need for complete removal to the tubes, ovary, and uterus, as well as careful pathologic examination.

RARE SYNDROMES THAT INCREASE THE RISK OF GYNECOLOGIC MALIGNANCY

Peutz-Jeghers syndrome is an autosomal-dominant disease characterized by hamartomatous polyps of the gastrointestinal tract and mucocutaneous melanin pigmentation (freckling). There is a greatly increased risk of multiple types of cancers in patients with Peutz-Jeghers syndrome. Cancers of the small intestine, stomach, colon, and pancreas predominate. The majority of ovarian neoplasms are sex cord tumors with annular tubules and granulosa cell tumors,[116,117] with a mean age of onset of 28 years. Patients with Peutz-Jeghers syndrome also have a 10% risk of adenoma malignum of the cervix, with the mean age of diagnosis at 28 years[116–118]; the lifetime risk of uterine cancer is 9% by age 65.[116]

PTEN Hamartoma Tumor syndrome (Cowden syndrome) is a multiple cancer syndrome that involves hamartomatous overgrowth in multiple organs. It is characterized by multiple hamartomas of the skin, mucous membranes, breast, thyroid, and endometrium. Breast and thyroid cancers are the most common malignancies (25%–50% and 3%–10%, respectively). The lifetime risk of endometrial cancer has been estimated to be between 5% and 19%.[119,120] Endometrial leiomyomas are also common and usually multiple. In a series of cases, Rustad and associates[120] found no mutations patients with endometrial cancer who did not have personal history otherwise suggestive of Cowden syndrome.

GENETIC RISK EVALUATION AND COUNSELING IN HEREDITARY GYNECOLOGIC CANCERS

A genetic counselor, medical geneticist, or other health professional with expertise and experience in cancer genetics should be involved in counseling patients regarding inherited cancer syndromes. Genetic counseling is recommended both when genetic testing is offered and after results are disclosed. Multiple organizations and professional societies emphasize the importance of cancer risk assessment and genetic counseling with genetic testing.[121]

Genetic risk assessment uses pedigree analysis and available risk assessment tools[122] to determine whether a family history is suggestive of a known inherited cancer syndrome. These tools are useful for families with adequate numbers of gender-appropriate members, but can underestimate risk in women with small families or few female relatives.[123]

Appropriate genetic counseling includes the assessment of patient knowledge of genetic testing for cancer risk, including risks, benefits, and limitations. Pretest counseling should include an evaluation of the extended family history and explanation of the sensitivity of the testing, as well as the recommended follow-up for those with and those without identified mutations. The patient's perception of her risks and risks to her relatives should be assessed, and an understanding of how the testing could influence management or prevention of disease is vital for informed decision making.

Genetic counseling for hereditary cancers should be customized to the experiences of each individual, thereby placing genetic risk in the context of other related risk factors. The purpose of genetic counseling is to educate the individual about the biological, genetic, and environmental risk factors related to the diagnosis or risk of cancer development. Risks to other relatives should be discussed. Patient understanding of this information should be assessed and misunderstandings addressed so that patients can make independent, informed decisions regarding their desire to undergo genetic testing, cancer screening, and prevention.

SUMMARY

Gynecologists and gynecologic oncologists have a major role in identifying patients at increased risk of inherited cancer syndromes. Awareness of the biological and familial risk factors is useful in this practice, and can assist patients and families in navigating the follow-up for these complex disorders. Large national and international cohorts of women with known BRCA1/2 mutations or high risk continue to collect data in an attempt to better understand genetic risk, risk modifiers, and quality-of-life impact or screening, testing and risk reduction strategies. The Consortium of Investigators of Modifiers of BRCA1/2 is beginning to identify other genetic modifiers of BRCA1/2 risk and cancer cluster regions in an attempt to better individualize site specific cancer risk and prevention strategies. The Gynecologic Oncology Group has initiated a long-term follow-up study to the Gynecologic Oncology Group 199 protocol, which will continue to advance understanding of patient decisions, quality-of-life impact, and other genetic factors responsible for cancer initiation and progression. These and other large consortia are invaluable resources with massive datasets requiring herculean analyses that will continue to rapidly advance our present knowledge and management of women with hereditary cancer syndromes.

REFERENCES

1. Ziogas A, Gildea, M, Cohen P, et al. Cancer risk estimates for family members of a population-based family registry for breast and ovarian cancer. Cancer Epidemiol Biomarkers Prev 2000;9:103–11.
2. SEER Cancer Statistics Review, 1975-2008, National Cancer Institute, Bethesda, Available at: http://seer.cancer.gov/statfacts/. Accessed November 10, 2011.

3. Gayther SA, Russell P, Harrington P, et al. The contribution of germline BRCA1 and BRCA2 mutations to familial ovarian cancer: no evidence for other ovarian cancer-susceptibility genes. Am J Hum Genet 1999;65:1021–9.

4. Pal T, Permuth-Wey J, Betts JA, et al. BRCA1 and BRCA2 mutations account for a large proportion of ovarian carcinoma cases. Cancer 2005;104:2807–16.

5. Rasmus SJ, Gather SA. The contribution of BRCA1 and BRCA2 to ovarian cancer. Molec Oncol 2009;3:138–50.

6. Brose MS, Rebbeck TR, Calzone, KA, et al. Cancer risk estimates for BRCA1 mutation carriers identified in a risk evaluation program. J Natl Cancer Inst 2002;94:1365–72.

7. Struewing JP, Hartge P, Wacholder S, et al. The risk of cancer associated with specific mutations of BRCA1 and BRCA2 among Ashkenazi Jews. J Natl Cancer Inst Monogr 1995;17:33–5.

8. King MC, Marks JH, Mandell JB. New York Breast Cancer Study Group. Breast and ovarian cancer risks due to inherited mutations in BRCA1 and BRCA2. Science 2003;302:643–6.

9. Satagopan JM, Boyd J, Kauff ND, et al. Ovarian cancer risk in Ashkenazi Jewish carriers of BRCA1 and BRCA2. Clin Cancer Res 2002;8:3776–81.

10. Thompson D, Easton D. Variation in cancer risks, by mutation position, in BRCA2 mutation carriers Am J Hum Genet 2001;68:410–9.

11. Lubinski J, Phelan CM, Ghadirian P, et al. Cancer variation associated with the position of the mutation in the BRCA2 gene. Fam Cancer 2004;3:1–10.

12. Antoniou AC, Pharoah PD, Narod S, et al. Breast and ovarian cancer risks to carriers of the BRCA1 5382insC and 185delAG and BRCA2 6174delT mutations: a combined analysis of 22 population based studies. J Med Genet 2005;42:602–3.

13. Whittemore AS, Gong G, Imyre J. Prevalence and contribution of BRCA1 mutations in breast cancer and ovarian cancer: results form 3 US population-based case-control studies of ovarian cancer. Am J Hum Genet 1997;60:496–504.

14. Antoniou A, Pharoah PD, Narod S, et al. Average risks of breast and ovarian cancer associated with BRCA1 and BRCA2 mutations detected in a case series unselected for family history: a combined analysis of 22 studies. Am J Hum Genet 2003;72:117–30.

15. Ferla R, Calo V, Cascio S, et al. Founder mutations in BRCA1 and BRCA2 genes. Ann Oncol 2007;18(Suppl 6):vi93–8.

16. Risch HA, McLaughlin JR, Cole DE, et al. Prevalence and penetrance of germline BRCA1 and BRCA2 mutations in a population series of 649 women with ovarian cancer. Am J Hum Genet 2001;68:700–10.

17. Lu KH, Cramer DW, Muto MG, et al. A population-based study of BRCA1 and BRCA2 mutations in Jewish women with epithelial ovarian cancer. Obstet Gynecol 1999;94:34–7.

18. Suthers G. Cancer risks for Australian women with a BRCA1 or BRCA2 mutation. Aust N Z J Surg 2007;77:314–9.

19. van der Kolk DM, de Bock GH, Leegte BK, et al. Penetrance of breast cancer, ovarian cancer and contralateral breast cancer in BRCA1 and BRCA2 families; high cancer incidence at older age. Breast Can Res Treat 2010;124:643–51.

20. Evans DGR, Young K, Bulman M, et al. Probability of BRCA1/2 mutation varies with ovarian histology: results from screening 442 ovarian cancer families. Clin Genet 2008;73:338–45.

21. Press JZ, De Luca A, Boyd N, et al. Ovarian carcinomas with genetic and epigenetic BRCA1 loss have distinct molecular abnormalities. BMC Cancer 22;8:17–29–28.

22. Lakhani SR, Manek S, Penault-Llorca F, et al. Pathology of ovarian cancers in BRCA1 and BRCA2 carriers. Clin Cancer Res 2004;10:2473–81.

23. Shaw PA, McLaughlin JR, Zweemer RP, et al. Histopathologic features of genetically determined ovarian cancer. Int J Gynecol Pathol 2002;21:407–11.

24. Werness BA, Ramus S, DiCioccio RA, et al. Histopathology, FIGO stage, and BRCA mutation status of ovarian cancers from the Gilda Radner Familial Ovarian Cancer Registry. Int J Gynecol Pathol 2004;23:29–34.

25. Stratton JF, Gayther SA, Russell P, et al. Contribution of BRCA1 mutations to ovarian cancer. N Engl J Med 1997;336:1125–30.

26. Vicus D, Finch A, Cass I, et al. Prevalence of BRCA1 and BRCA2 germ line mutations among women with carcinoma of the fallopian tube. Gynecol Oncol 2010;118:299–302.

27. Norquist B, Garcia R, Allison K, et al. The molecular pathogenesis of hereditary ovarian carcinoma. Cancer 2010;116:5261–71.

28. Callahan MJ, Crum CP, Mederios F, et al. Primary fallopian tube malignancies in BRCA-positive women undergoing surgery for ovarian cancer risk reduction. J Clin Oncol 2007;25:3985–90.

29. Finch A, Shaw P, Rosen B, et al. Clinical and pathologic findings of prophylactic salpingo-oophorectomies in 159 BRCA1 and BRCA2 carriers. Gynecol Oncol 2006;100:58–64.

30. Hermsen BB, vanDiest PJ, Berkhof J, et al. Low prevalence of (pre) malignant lesions in the breast and high prevalence in the ovary and Fallopian tube in women at hereditary high risk of breast and ovarian cancer. Int J Cancer 2006;119:1412–8.

31. Narod SA, Risch H, Moslehi R, et al. Hereditary Ovarian Cancer Clinical Study Group. Oral contraceptives and the risk of hereditary ovarian cancer. N Engl J Med 1998;339:424–8.

32. Whittemore AS, Balise RR, Pharoah PDP, et al. Oral contraceptive use and ovarian cancer risk among carries of BRCA1 or BRCA2 mutations. Br. J Cancer 2004;91:1911–5.

33. McGuire V, Felberg A, Mills M, et al. Relation of contraceptive and reproductive history to ovarian cancer risk in carriers and noncarriers of BRCA1 gene mutations. Am J Epidemiol 2004;160:613–8.

34. McLaughlin JR, Risch HA, Lubinski J, et al. Hereditary Ovarian Cancer Clinical Study Group. Reproductive risk factors for ovarian cancer in carriers of BRCA1 or BRCA2 mutations: a case-control study. Lancet Oncol 2007;8:26–34.

35. Narod SA, Dubé MP, Kiljn J, et al. Oral contraceptives and the risk of breast cancer in BRCA1 and BRCA2 mutation carriers. J Natl Cancer Inst 2002;94:1773–9.

36. Iodice S, Barile M, Rotmensz N, et al. Oral contraceptive use and breast or ovarian cancer risk in BRCA1/2 carriers: a meta-analysis. Eur J Cancer 2010;46:2275–84.

37. Gaarenstrom KN, van der Hiel B, Tollenaar R, et al. Efficacy of screening women at high risk of hereditary ovarian cancer: results of an 11-year cohort study. Int J Cancer 2006;16(Suppl 1):54–9.

38. Oei AL, Massuger LF, Bulten J, et al. Surveillance of women at high risk for hereditary ovarian cancer is inefficient. Br J Cancer 2006;94:814–9.

39. Olivier RI, Lubsen-Brandsma MA, Berhoef S, et al. CA125 and transvaginal ultrasound monitoring in high-risk women cannot prevent the diagnosis of advanced ovarian cancer. Gynecol Oncol 2006;100:20–6.

40. Rebbeck TR, Lynch HT, Neuhausen SL, et al. Prophylactic oophorectomy in carriers of BRCA1 or BRCA2 mutations. N Engl J Med 2002;346:1616–22.

41. Finch A, Beiner M, Lubinski J, et al. Hereditary Ovarian Cancer Clinical Study Group. Salpingo-oophorectomy and the risk of ovarian, fallopian tube, and peritoneal cancers in women with a BRCA1 or BRCA2 mutation. JAMA 2006;296:185–92.
42. National Comprehensive Cancer Network Guidelines. Hereditary Breast and Ovarian Cancer Syndrome. Version 1.2011. Available at: www.nccn.org. Accessed November 25, 2011, with permission.
43. Kauff ND, Barakat RR. Risk-reducing salpingo-oophorectomy in patients with germline mutations in BRCA1 or BRCA2. J Clin Oncol 2007;25:2921–6.
44. Kauff ND, Satagopan JM, Robson ME, et al. Risk-reducing salpingo-oophorectomy in women with a BRCA1 or BRCA2 mutation. N Engl J Med 2002;346:1609–15.
45. Rebbeck TR, Lynch HT, Neuhausen SL, et al. Prophylactic oophorectomy in carriers of BRCA1 or BRCA2 mutations. N Engl J Med 2002;346:1616–22.
46. Clark AS, Domchek SM. Clinical management of hereditary breast cancer syndromes. J Mammary Gland Biol Neoplasia 2011;16:17–25.
47. ACOG Practice Bulletin. Hereditary breast and ovarian cancer syndrome. Obstet Gynecol 2009;113:957–66.
48. Domchek SM, Friebel TM, Singer CF, et al. Association of risk-reducing surgery in BRCA1 or BRCA2 mutation carriers with cancer risk and mortality. JAMA 2010;304: 967–75.
49. Rebbeck TR, Friebel T, Wagner T, et al. Effect of short-term hormone replacement therapy on breast cancer risk reduction after bilateral prophylactic oophorectomy in BRCA1 and BRCA2 mutation carriers: the PROSE Study Group. J Clin Oncol 2005;23:7804–10.
50. Eisen A, Lubinski J, Gronwald J, et al. Hormone therapy and the risk of breast cancer in BRCA1 mutation carriers. J Natl Cancer Inst 2008;100:1361–7.
51. Armstrong K, Schwartz JS, Randall T, et al. Hormone replacement therapy and life expectancy after prophylactic oophorectomy in women with BRCA1/2 mutations: a decision analysis. J Clin Oncol 2004;22:1045–54.
52. Carcangiu ML, Peissel B, Pasini B, et al. Incidental carcinomas in prophylactic specimens in BRCA1 and BRCA2 germ-line mutation carriers, with emphasis on fallopian tube lesions: report of 6 cases and review of the literature. Am J Surg Pathol 2006;30:1222–30.
53. Powell BC. Occult ovarian cancer at the time of risk-reducing salpingo-oophorectomy. Gynecol Oncol 2006;100:1–2.
54. Powell BC, Chen LM, McLennan J, et al. Risk-reducing salpingo-oophorectomy (RRSO) in BRCA mutation carriers: experience with a consecutive series of 111 patients using a standardized surgical-pathological protocol. Intl J Gynecol Cancer 2011;21:846–51.
55. Rhiem K, Foth D, Wappenschmidt B, et al. Risk-reducing salpingo-oophorectomy in BRCA1 and BRCA2 mutation carriers. Arch Gynecol Obstet 2011;283:623–7.
56. Hirst JE, Gard, GB, McIllroy K, et al. High rates of occult fallopian tube cancer diagnosed at prophylactic bilateral salpingo-oophorectomy. Intl J Gynecol Cancer 2009;19:826–9.
57. Rabban JT, Crawford B, Chen LM, et al. Transitional cell metaplasia of fallopian tube fimbriae: a potential mimic of early tubal carcinoma in risk reduction salpingo-oophorectomies from women with BRCA mutations. Am J Surg Pathol 2009;33: 111–9.
58. Medeiros F, Muto MG, Lee Y, et al. The tubal fimbria is a preferred site for early adenocarcinoma in women with familial ovarian cancer syndrome. Am J Surg Pathol 2006;30:3230–6.

59. Narod SA, Sun P, Ghadirian P, et al. Tubal ligation and risk of ovarian cancer in carriers of BRCA1 or BRCA2 mutations: a case-control study. Lancet 2001;357: 1467–70.

60. Powell BC, Kenley E, Chen LM, et al. Risk-reducing salpingo-oophorectomy in BRCA mutation carriers: role of serial sectioning in the detection of occult malignancy. J Clin Oncol 2005;23:127–32.

61. Chapman JS, Powell CB, McLennan J, et al. Surveillance of survivors: follow-up after risk-reducing salpingo-oophorectomy in BRCA1/2 mutation carriers. Gynecol Oncol 2011;122:339–43.

62. Lavie O, Ben-Arie A, Segev Y, et al. BRCA germline mutations in women with uterine serous carcinoma–still a debate. Int J Gynecol Cancer 2010;20:1531–4.

63. Bruchim I, Amichay K, Kidron D, et al. BRCA 1/2 germline mutations in Jewish patients with uterine serous carcinoma. Int J Gynecol Cancer 2010;20:1148–53.

64. Lacour RA, Westin SN, Meyer LA, et al. Improved survival in non-Ashkenazi Jewish ovarian cancer patients with BRCA1 and BRCA2 gene mutations. Gynecol Oncol 2011;121:358–63.

65. Chetrit A, Hirsh-Yechezkel G, Ben-David Y, et al. Effect of BRCA1/2 mutations on long-term survival of patients with invasive ovarian cancer: the national Israeli study of ovarian cancer. J Clin Oncol 2008;26:20–5.

66. Ramus SJ, Fishman A, Pharoah PDP, et al. Ovarian cancer survival in Ashkenazi Jewish patients with BRCA1 and BRCA2 mutations. EJSO 2001;27:278–328.

67. Boyd J, Sonoda Y, Federici MG, et al. Clinicopathologic features of BRCA-linked and sporadic ovarian cancer. JAMA 2000;283:2260–5.

68. Foulkes WD. BRCA1 and BRCA2: chemosensitivity, treatment outcomes and prognosis. Fam Cancer 2006;5:135–42.

69. McCabe N, Lord CJ, Tutt AN, et al. BRCA2-deficient CAPAN-1 cells are extremely sensitive to the inhibition of Poly (ADP-Ribose) polymerase: an issue of potency. Cancer Biol Ther 2005;4:934–6.

70. Farmer H, McCabe N, Lord CJ, et al. Targeting the DNA repair defect in BRCA mutant cells as a therapeutic strategy. Nature 2005;434:917–21.

71. Kennedy RD, Quinn JE, Mullan PB, et al. The role of BRCA1 in the cellular response to chemotherapy. J Natl Cancer Inst 2004;96:1659–68.

72. Weitzel JN, Lagos VI, Herzog JS, et al. Evidence for common ancestral origin of a recurring BRCA1 genomic rearrangement identified in high-risk Hispanic families. Cancer Epidemiol Biomarkers Prev 2007;16:1615–20.

73. Palma MD, Domchek SM, Stopfer J, et al. The relative contribution of point mutations and genomic rearrangements in BRCA1 and BRCA2 in high-risk breast cancer families. Cancer Res 2008;68:7006–14.

74. Myriad Genetic Laboratories. Available at: http://www.myriad.com/lib/brac/BART-table-faq.pdf. Accessed November 28, 2011.

75. Stadler ZK, Saloustros E, Hansen NA, et al. Absence of genomic BRCA1 and BRCA2 rearrangements in Ashkenazi breast and ovarian cancer families. Br Cancer Res Treat 2010;123:581–5.

76. Hampel H, Frankel W, Panescu J, et al. Screening for Lynch syndrome (hereditary nonpolyposis colorectal cancer) among endometrial cancer patients. Cancer Res 2006;66:7810–7.

77. Wijnen J, deLeeuw W, Vasen H, et al. Familial endometrial cancer in female carriers of MSH6 germline mutations. Nat Genet 1999;23:142–4.

78. de la Chapelle A. The incidence of Lynch syndrome. Fam Cancer 2005;4:233–7.

79. Hampel H, Frankel WL, Martin E, et al. Feasibility of screening for Lynch syndrome among patients with colorectal cancer. J Clin Oncol 2008;26:5783–8.

80. Malander S, Rambech E, Kristoffersson U, et al. The contribution of the hereditary nonpolyposis colorectal cancer syndrome to the development of ovarian cancer. Gynecol Oncol 2006;101:238–43.

81. Rubin SC, Blackwood MA, Bandera C, et al. BRCA1, BRCA2, and hereditary nonpolyposis colorectal cancer gene mutations in an unselected ovarian cancer population: relationship to family history and implications for genetic testing. Am J Obstet Gynecol 2006;178:670–7.

82. Lu KH, Schorge JO, Rodabaugh KJ, et al. Prospective determination of prevalence of Lynch syndrome in young women with endometrial cancer. J Clin Oncol 2007;25: 5158–64.

83. Walsh MD, Cummings MC, Buchanan DD, et al. Molecular pathologic, and clinical features of early-onset endometrial cancer: identifying presumptive Lynch syndrome patients. Clin Cancer Res 2008;14:1692–700.

84. Lu, KH. Hereditary gynecologic cancers: differential diagnosis, surveillance, management and surgical prophylaxis. Fam Cancer 2008;7:53–8.

85. Matthews KS, Estes JM, Conner MG, et al. Lynch syndrome in women less than 50 years of age with endometrial cancer. Obstet Gynecol 2008;111:1161–6.

86. Aarnio M, Sankila T, Pukkala E, et al. Cancer risk in mutation carriers of DNA mismatch repair genes. Intl J Cancer 1999;81:214–8.

87. Bonadona V, Bonaiti B, Olschwang S, et al. Cancer risks associated with germline mutations in MLH1, MSH2, and MSH6 genes in Lynch syndrome. JAMA 2011;305: 2304–10.

88. Quehenberger F, Vasen HF, van Houwelingen HC. Risk of colorectal and endometrial cancer for carriers of mutations of the hMLH1 and hMSH2 gene: correction for ascertainment. J Med Genet 2005;42:491–6.

89. Baglietto L, Lindor NM, Dowty JG, et al. Dutch Lynch Syndrome Study Group. Risks of Lynch syndrome cancers for MSH6 mutation carriers. J Natl Cancer Inst 2010; 102:193–201.

90. Senter L, Clendenning M, Sotamaa K, et al. The clinical phenotype of Lynch syndrome due to germ-line PMS2 mutations. Gastroenterology 2008;135:419–28.

91. Vasen HF, Stormorken A, Menko FH, et al. MSH2 mutation carriers are at higher risk for cancer than MLH1 mutation carriers: a study of hereditary nonpolyposis colorectal cancer families. J Clin Oncol 2001;19:4074–80.

92. Hampel H, Stephens JA, Pukkala E, et al. Cancer risk in hereditary nonpolyposis colorectal cancer syndrome: later age of onset. Gastroenterology 2005;129: 415–21.

93. Watson P, Butzow R, Lynch HT, et al. The clinical features of ovarian cancer in hereditary nonpolyposis colorectal cancer. Gynecol Oncol 2001;82:223–8.

94. Barrow E, Robinson L, Alduaij W, et al. Cumulative lifetime incidence of extracolonic cancers in Lynch syndrome: a report of 121 families with proven mutations. Clin Genet 2009;75:141–9.

95. Stoffel E, Mukherjee B, Raymond VM, et al. Calculation of risk of colorectal and endometrial cancer among patients with Lynch syndrome. Gastroenterology 2009; 137:1621–7.

96. Garg K, Soslow RA. Lynch syndrome (hereditary non-polyposis colorectal cancer) and endometrial carcinoma. J Clin Pathol 2009;62:679–84.

97. Umar A, Boland DR, Terdiman JP, et al. Revised Bethesda guidelines for hereditary nonpolyposis colorectal cancer (Lynch syndrome) and microsatellite instability. J Natl Cancer Inst 2004;96:261–8.

98. Ketabi Z, Bartuma K, Bernstein I, et al. Ovarian cancer linked to Lynch syndrome typically presents as early-onset, non-serous epithelial tumors. Gynecol Oncol 2011;121:462–5.

99. Hampel H, Stephens JA, Pukkala E, et al. Cancer risk in hereditary nonpolyposis colorectal cancer syndrome: later age of onset. Gastroenterology 2005;129: 415–21.

100. Resnick K, Straughn JM Jr, Backes F, et al. Lynch syndrome screening strategies among newly diagnosed endometrial cancer patients. Obstet Gynecol 2009;114: 530–6.

101. Hendriks YM, Wagner A, Morreau H, et al. Cancer risk in hereditary non-polyposis colorectal cancer due to MSH6 mutations: impact on counseling and surveillance. Gastroenterology 2004;127:17–25.

102. Dunlop MG, Farrington SM, Carothers AD, et al. Cancer risk associated with germline DNA mismatch repair gene mutations. Hum Mol Genet 1997;6:105–10.

103. Soliman PT, Broaddus RR, Schmeler KM, et al. Women with synchronous primary cancers of the endometrium and ovary: do they have Lynch syndrome? J Clin Oncol 2005;23: 9344–50.

104. Broaddus RR, Lynch HT, Chen L, et al. Pathologic features of endometrial carcinoma associated with HNPCC. Cancer 2006;106:87–94.

105. Westin SN, Lacour RA, Urbauer DL, et al. Carcinoma of the lower uterine segment: a newly described association with Lynch syndrome. J Clin Oncol 2008;26:5965–71.

106. Garg K, Leitao M, Kauff N, et al. Selection of endometrial carcinomas for DNA mismatch repair protein immunohistochemistry using patient age and tumor morphology enhances detection of mismatch repair abnormalities. Am J Surg Pathol 2009;33:925–33.

107. DeLair D, Oliva E, Köbel M, et al. Morphologic spectrum of immunohistochemically characterized clear cell carcinoma of the ovary: a study of 155 cases. Am J Surg Pathol 2011;35:36–44.

108. Lu KH. Hereditary gynecologic cancers: differential diagnosis, surveillance, management and surgical prophylaxis. Fam Cancer 2008;7:53–8.

109. Renkonen-Sinisalo L, Butzow R, Leminen A, et al. Surveillance for endometrial cancer in hereditary nonpolyposis colorectal cancer syndrome. Int J Cancer 2006; 120:821–4.

110. Auranen A, Joutsiniemi T. A systematic review of gynecological cancer surveillance in women belonging to hereditary nonpolyposis colorectal cancer (Lynch syndrome) families. Acta Obstet Gynecol Scand 2011;90:437–4.

111. Gerritzen LH, Hoogerbrugge N, Oei AL, et al. Improvement of endometrial biopsy over transvaginal ultrasound alone for endometrial surveillance in women with Lynch syndrome. Fam Cancer 2009;8:391–7.

112. Lynch HT, Casey MJ. Prophylactic surgery prevents endometrial and ovarian cancer in Lynch syndrome. Nat Clin Pract Oncol 2007;4:672–3.

113. Chen LM, Yang KY, Little SE, et al. Gynecologic cancer prevention in Lynch syndrome/hereditary nonpolyposis colorectal cancer families. Obstet Gynecol 2007; 110:18–25.

114. Kwon JS, Sun CC, Peterson SK, et al. Cost-effectiveness analysis of prevention strategies for gynecologic cancers in Lynch syndrome. Cancer 2008;113:326–35.

115. Palma L, Marcus V, Gilbert L, et al. Synchronous occult cancers of the endometrium and fallopian tube in an MSH2 mutation carrier at time of prophylactic surgery. Gynecol Oncol 2008;111:575–8.

116. Giardiello FM, Brensinger JD, Tersmette AC, et al. Very high risk of cancer in familial Peutz-Jeghers syndrome. Gastroenterology 2000;119:447–53.
117. Chen KT. Female genital tract tumors in Peutz-Jeghers syndrome. Hum Pathol 1986;17:858–61.
118. Fujiwaki R, Takahashi K, Kitao M. Adenoma malignum of the uterine cervix associated with Peutz-Jeghers syndrome. Int J Gynaecol Obstet 1996;53:171–2.
119. Pilarski R. Cowden syndrome: a critical review of the literature. J Genet Counsel 2009;18:13–27.
120. Rustad CF, Bjørnslett M, Heimdal KR, et al. Germline PTEN mutations are rare and highly penetrant. Hered Can Clin Pract 2006;4:177–85.
121. Genetic counseling is endorsed by the following. American College of Medical Genetics, American College of Obstetrics and Gynecology, American Gastroenterology Association, American Society of Clinical Oncology, American Society of Breast Surgeons, American Society of Colon and Rectal Surgeons, International Society of Nurses in Genetics, National Comprehensive Cancer Network, National Society of Genetic Counselors, Oncology Nursing Society, Society of Gynecologic Oncology, Society of Surgical Oncology and US Preventative Services Task Force.
122. Parmigiani G, Chen S, Iversen ES Jr, et al. Validity of models for predicting BRCA1 and BRCA2 mutations. Ann Intern Med 2007;147:441–50.
123. Weitzel JN, Lagos VI, Cullinane CA, et al. Limited family structure and BRCA gene mutation status in single cases of breast cancer. JAMA 2007;297:2587–95.

Ovarian Cancer
Screening and Early Detection

Barbara A. Goff, MD

KEYWORDS

- Diagnosis • Early detection • Screening • Symptoms

KEY POINTS

- Screening for ovarian cancer is not recommended for women of average risk.
- Using biomarkers with secondary screening by transvaginal ultrasound show the most promise for effective screening in research studies.
- Most women with ovarian cancer will have symptoms and this disease should no longer be considered "silent".
- Currently the best method for early diagnosis is for both patients and practitioners to have a high index of suspicion when symptoms are present.
- The most common symptoms of ovarian cancer include bloating, abdominal or pelvic pain, feeling full quickly or difficulty eating and urinary symptoms. Symptoms that are relatively new to a patient and occur about 50% of the month are the symptoms to be most concerned about.

SCREENING

In 1994 the US National Institutes of Health convened a consensus conference for the management of ovarian cancer.[1] At that time, the recommendation was to obtain a family history and offer screening to those who had 2 or more affected family members (ovarian cancer or premenopausal breast cancer). However, no guidance was given as to what screening modality should be used or how frequently. Screening women without a significant family history was not recommended.[1] Unfortunately, almost 20 years later, there still are no recommended screening tests for average risk women. For women at elevated risk secondary to family history consistent with BRCA1, BRCA2, or the Lynch syndrome, genetic testing is recommended because screening has not been shown to reduce the morbidity or mortality of ovarian cancer in these patients.[2] Identifying women with deleterious mutations allows practitioners

Disclosure: The author is a consultant for Fujirebio.
Division of Gynecologic Oncology, Department of Obstetrics and Gynecology, University of Washington School of Medicine, Box 356460, 1950 NE Pacific, Seattle, WA 98195–6460, USA
E-mail address: bgoff@uw.edu

Obstet Gynecol Clin N Am 39 (2012) 183–194
doi:10.1016/j.ogc.2012.02.007
obgyn.theclinics.com
0889-8545/12/$ – see front matter © 2012 Elsevier Inc. All rights reserved.

to offer counseling and possible interventions to those at elevated risk of developing ovarian cancer.[3]

In 2012, no organization recommends screening average risk women. The American Congress of Obstetricians and Gynecologists recommends against screening for ovarian cancer in the general population.[4] The US Preventative Services Task Force gives ovarian cancer screening a grade "D" recommendation, which indicates this should be eliminated from a periodic health examination because more women are harmed by the false–positive results than helped by early detection.[5] The Society of Gynecologic Oncologists also does not advocate screening for ovarian cancer outside of clinical trials.[2] The US Preventative Services Task Force does give a grade "B" recommendation for genetic counseling and testing of women with a pedigree consistent with a familial mutation that would increase the risk of ovarian and other malignancies.[3] Those found to have mutations can be offered risk-reducing surgery, which dramatically lowers the risk of developing ovarian, fallopian tube, or primary peritoneal cancers.

There are several challenges in developing screening strategies in ovarian cancer.[6] First, unlike breast cancer or cervical cancer, there is no defined in situ lesion. Some recent evidence suggests that, for high-grade serous tumors associated with BRCA1 or BRCA2 mutations, the fallopian tube may be the initial site of a precursor lesion.[7] These results are preliminary and it is unclear if the same association between in situ lesions in fallopian tube and ovarian cancer will be found in women without these mutations. Another challenge is that a major operative procedure (laparotomy or laparoscopy) is usually required for diagnosis.[6,8] Given that there is a low, but definite risk, of morbidity from these types of surgical procedures, any screening strategy for ovarian cancer needs to ensure that the morbidity and possible mortality from false-positive screens will not outweigh the possible benefits of early detection.

The risk of false-positive screens with ovarian cancer screening is a significant concern. This is a major challenge to overcome in the effort to design effective screening programs. The main issue is that the incidence of ovarian cancer in women over age 50 is only 40/100,000.[9] That means even with a perfect screening test, 2500 screens are needed to detect 1 case of ovarian cancer. It also means that if a screening test has only a 1% false-positive rate (sensitivity of 99%), then of every 2500 women screened 25 would have false-positive tests yielding a positive predictive value (PPV) of 4%. In general, it has been accepted that a screening test that results in a major surgical procedure should have a PPV of at least 10%. That means for every case of cancer detected there would be no more than 10 "unnecessary" surgeries (false positives). With an incidence of 40 in 100,000, a screening test would need a specificity of 99.6% or a false-positive rate of less than 0.4% to have a PPV of 10% or higher. The final challenge with ovarian cancer screening is developing a screening test that is not only effective, but also reasonably inexpensive. Because 2500 women need to be screened to detect a single ovarian cancer, the cost must be affordable, and the test readily available and acceptable to patients.

Two large, prospective, randomized screening trials for ovarian cancer have recently been conducted in average-risk women.[10,11] The results of the Prostate Lung Colorectal and Ovarian Cancer screening trial have been reported over the last decade.[10,12] There were 78,232 women between the ages of 55 and 74 who were enrolled between 1993 and 2001. Women randomly assigned to screening underwent annual transvaginal ultrasonography (TVS) for 4 years and annual CA125 for 6 years. Controls consisted of women who were assigned to receive routine care. For the group randomized to screening, any abnormalities and decisions about surgery were managed by the patient's physician according to standard of care. In the initial

Table 1
Pathologic results from the United Kingdom collaborative trial of ovarian cancer screening prevalence screen

Participants Undergoing Surgery	MMS	TVS
n (%)	97 (0.2)	845 (1.8)
Pathology		
Benign	40	732
LMP*	8	20
Primary ovary/fallopian tube	34	5
Metastatic	3	5
Early stage disease	47.1%	50.0%

Abbreviation: LMP, low malignant potential tumor.
Data from Menon U, Gentry-Maharaj A, Hallett R, et al. Sensitivity and specificity of multimodal and ultrasound screening for ovarian cancer, and stage distribution of detected cancers: results of the prevalence screen of the UK Collaborative Trial of Ovarian Cancer Screening (UKCTOCS). Lancet Oncol 2009;10:327–40.

prevalence screen, the investigators found that CA125 was elevated in 1.5% of the population and TVS was abnormal in 4.7% of the population. The PPV of the screening tests was 3.7% and 1%, respectively. Over a 4-year period, compliance with screening dropped to 77.6%. The overall ratio of surgeries to screen detected cancers was 19.5:1 and 72% of the screen detected cancers were late stage.[12]

In June 2011, the final results of the effect of screening on ovarian cancer mortality were reported for the Prostate Lung Colorectal and Ovarian Cancer trial.[10] The median follow-up of participants was 12.4 years. Ovarian cancer was diagnosed in 212 women in the screened group and 176 in the control group. There were 118 deaths caused by ovarian cancer in the screened group compared with 100 deaths among the controls. Screening with an annual TVS and CA125 did not reduce ovarian cancer mortality. In addition, of the 3285 women with a false-positive result, 1080 underwent surgery and 163 (15%) experienced at least 1 serious complication. This confirms that cancer screening can lead to unintended harm.

More encouraging results have been found in the United Kingdom Collaborative Trial of Ovarian Cancer Screening.[11] Results from the prevalence screen were reported in 2009. Between 2001 and 2005, a total of 202,632 postmenopausal women aged 50 to 74 years were randomly assigned to no screening (control; n = 101,359), annual CA125 screening (interpreted using an unpublished risk of ovarian cancer algorithm) with TVS as a secondary screen for those with abnormal CA125s (multimodality screening [MMS]; n = 50,640) or annual screening with TVS (TVS; n = 50,639). Of those in the MMS group, 97 (0.2%) underwent surgery owing to the screening process compared with 845 (1.8%) in the TVS group. Pathologic evaluation is shown in **Table 1**. In both screening groups, approximately 50% of ovarian cancers were diagnosed in the early stage. In the group screened with TVS there were 732 surgical procedures performed for benign conditions, indicating a relatively high false-positive rate of TVS compared with the MMS. For primary invasive epithelial and tubal cancers the sensitivity, specificity and PPVs were 89.5%, 99.8%, and 35.1% for MMS and 75.0%, 98.2%, and 2.8% for TVS, respectively. There was a significant difference in specificity (*P*<.0001), but not sensitivity between the 2 groups. Because a PPV of 10% is considered the minimal acceptable value for a screening test that would lead to an invasive surgical procedure, then a huge advantage of the MMS

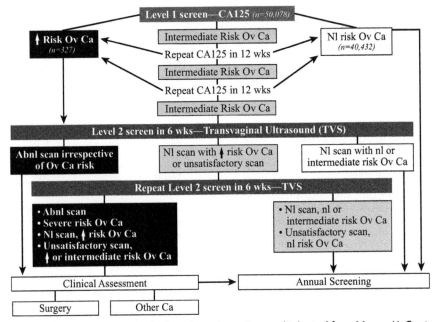

Fig. 1. UKCTOS Pathologic Results from Prevalence Screen. (*Adapted from* Menon U, Gentry-Maharaj A, Hallett R, et al. Sensitivity and specificity of multimodal and ultrasound screening for ovarian cancer, and stage distribution of detected cancers: results of the prevalence screen of the UK Collaborative Trial of Ovarian Cancer Screening (UKCTOCS). Lancet Oncol 2009;10:327–40; with permission.)

process is that with a PPV of 35.1, only 2.8 surgeries would be performed for each case of ovarian cancer detected. In contrast, for the TVS group, a PPV of 2.8% means that 35.2 surgeries would be performed for each case of cancer. Although the preliminary results are encouraging, final analysis comparing cancer mortality between screened and controls will need to be performed to assess efficacy. In addition, the screening algorithm for the MMS arm is quite complex and may be difficult to replicate outside a clinical trial (**Fig. 1**).

A screening algorithm similar to the UK MMS group was evaluated by researchers at the M.D. Anderson Cancer Center.[13] In a single-arm study, investigators screened women for ovarian cancer using CA125 levels with a Risk of Ovarian Cancer Algorithm (ROCA) followed by secondary screening with additional CA125 or TVS if patients were intermediate or high risk. There were 3238 postmenopausal women who participated over 8 years. After each CA125 level drawn, women were triaged based on risk into these categories: Annual CA125 (low risk), repeat CA125 in 3 months (intermediate risk), or TVS and referred to a gynecologic oncologist (high risk). Surgery was performed at the discretion of the gynecologic oncologist. Eight women underwent surgery as a result of screening, with 3 invasive ovarian cancers, 2 borderline ovarian cancers, and 3 benign ovarian tumors. All 3 ovarian cancers were early stage. The specificity of the ROCA was 99.7% and PPV was 37.5%.

It is clear from these studies that using TVS as a secondary screening tool significantly improved both the specificity as well as PPV when detecting ovarian cancer.[14] There has been 1 large study of TVS as a primary screen in over 25,000 women from the University of Kentucky. Over an 18-year period, asymptomatic women over age 50 and women over age 25 with a significant family history were offered TVS for screening. In this study, 364 women underwent surgery (1.4%). TVS had a sensitivity of 85%, specificity of 98.7%, and a PPV of 14.0%. However, this center has special expertise in TVS and screening for ovarian cancer; therefore, these results have not been replicated by other investigators. Specifically, in the Prostate Lung Colorectal and Ovarian Cancer trial, where TVS was performed at multiple centers in over 39,000 women, the PPV was only 1.0%.[12] For a screening regimen to have adequate specificity to prevent potential harm form unnecessary surgery, TVS will most likely need to be utilized as a secondary screen after biomarker evaluation.

Given that the prevalence of ovarian cancer is significantly higher among women with a strong family history or know genetic mutation (BRCA1, BRCA2, mismatch repair genes), hopes were that screening strategies may be more successful in this high-risk group than in the general population. Unfortunately, this hope has not been realized.[15] One of the initial large studies came from the National Ovarian Cancer Early Detection Program.[16] Women at elevated risk of ovarian cancer based on family history, but not genetic testing, were screened every 6 months with TVS. Women had to have a normal TVS to enter the trial. There were 4526 women enrolled in the study. A total of 49 women underwent invasive operative procedures and 12 gynecologic malignancies were diagnosed in women with a normal TVS 12 and 6 months before their diagnosis. All 10 ovarian and fallopian tube cancers were detected in advanced stages. The authors concluded that TVS, even every 6 months, had limited value as a screening test in women at increased risk for disease.

Other studies have focused specifically on women with BRCA1 and BRCA2 mutations. Annual surveillance using both CA125 and TVS has not been associated with earlier stage diagnosis.[17–19] The vast majority of women with mutations who are screening are diagnosed in advanced stages. All of these studies have concluded that annual screening with TVS and CA125 for mutation cancers is ineffective because cancer is not detected at an early enough stage to influence survival. This is why risk-reducing surgery is recommended when child bearing is complete for those with known mutations.[20]

In 2010 and 2011, the US Food and Drug Administration approved the OVA1 test[21] and ROCA with CA125 and HE4.[22] Both tests have the same indications: To be used in women with a pelvic mass to determine the likelihood of malignancy and allow appropriate triage of these women to a gynecologic oncologist. Neither test is approved, or should be used, as a screening test.

DIAGNOSIS

Currently, ACOG recommends that the best way to detect ovarian cancer is for both the patient and her clinician to have a high index of suspicion of the diagnosis in symptomatic women.[4] The Society of Gynecologic Oncologists also recognizes that most women with ovarian cancer are symptomatic, yet go undiagnosed for many months.[2] Unfortunately, no currently available test has been shown to reliably detect ovarian cancer in its earliest and most curable stages, and so educating women and practitioners about symptoms and promptly initiating a diagnostic workup in these women is currently the best method for timely diagnosis.[4]

Historically, ovarian cancer was thought to be a "silent killer" because symptoms were not thought to develop until advanced stages when chances of cure were poor. In the 1980s and 1990s, there were several retrospective studies that evaluated symptoms in ovarian cancer patients.[23–25] All of these studies concluded that women with ovarian cancer frequently have symptoms before diagnosis, although the symptoms were often vague and not necessarily gynecologic in nature. Although

Table 2
Frequency of symptoms in ovarian cancer

Symptom	Frequency (%)
Increased abdominal size	61
Bloating	57
Fatigue	47
Abdominal pain	36
Indigestion	31
Urinary frequency	27
Pelvic pain	26
Constipation	25
Back pain	23
Pain with intercourse	17
Unable to eat normally	16
Palpable mass	14
Vaginal bleeding	13
Weight loss	11
Nausea	9
Bleeding with intercourse	3
Diarrhea	1
Deep venous thrombosis	1
None	5

Data from Goff BA, Mandel L, Muntz HG, et al. Ovarian carcinoma diagnosis. Cancer 2000;89: 2068–75.

there was significant agreement across these studies, they were criticized because of small numbers and data collection from retrospective chart analysis.

In 2000, a survey of 1725 women with ovarian cancer from the United States and Canada was published evaluating the type of symptoms, if any, that women experienced before diagnosis.[26] The findings were significant in that 95% of women with ovarian cancer recalled developing symptoms an average of 3 to 6 months before seeing a physician. The most common symptoms (**Table 2**) were abdominal (77%), gastrointestinal (70%), pain (58%), constitutional (50%), urinary (34%), and pelvic (26%). Ovarian cancer patients often had multiple symptoms; interestingly, gynecologic symptoms were the least common. In women with early stage disease, 89% had symptoms before diagnosis, and symptoms were not different for women with early stage disease compared with those with advanced stages.

This survey also evaluated delays in diagnosis.[26] Physicians and patients both contributed to delays in diagnosis. Physicians commonly misdiagnosed women with irritable bowel syndrome, stress, gastritis, or depression months before the diagnosis of ovarian cancer. In this study, 30% of women were actually treated with a prescription medication for another condition within the 3 to 6 months preceding their ovarian cancer diagnosis. Physician misdiagnosis was associated with more advanced stage of disease. In addition, patients themselves frequently did not recognize their symptoms could be due to a serious diagnosis. Women who said they ignored their symptoms were significantly more likely to be diagnosed with advanced stage disease compared with those who felt they did not ignore their symptoms.

Table 3			
Comparison of symptoms between ovarian cancer cases and controls			
Symptom	Olson et al,[27] All Stages	Olsen et al,[27] Early Stages	Goff et al,[28] All Stages
Bloating	25.3 (15.5–40.9)	19.2 (9.4–37.5)	3.6 (1.8–2.0)
Difficulty eating/lack of appetite	8.8 (4.3–18.2)	—	2.5 (1.3–5.0)
Abdominal pain	6.2 (4.0–9.6)	5.5 (2.8–10.8)	2.3 (1.2–4.4)
Urinary symptoms	3.5 (2.2–5.7)	—	2.5 (1.3–4.8)
Constipation	3.5 (2.0–6.3)	5.5 (2.5–12.0)	1.6 (0.7–1.4)
Fatigue	2.9 (2.5–6.1)	—	1.4 (0.7–2.7)

Data from Olson SH, Mignone L, Nakraseive C, et al. Symptoms of ovarian cancer. Obstet Gynecol 2001;98:212–7 and Goff BA, Mandel LS, Melancon CH, et al. Frequency of symptoms of ovarian cancer in women presenting to primary care clinics. JAMA 2004;291:2705–12.
Values are presented as odds ratios (95% confidence interval).

In 2001, investigators from Memorial Sloan-Kettering Cancer Center published a case-control study evaluating symptoms before diagnosis.[27] Women with ovarian cancer (n = 168) and controls (n = 251) were interviewed about symptoms experienced during the preceding 6 months. The authors found that ovarian cancer patients were significantly more likely to complain of bloating, lack of appetite, abdominal pain, fatigue, urinary frequency, and constipation than controls. In this study, 89% of women with early stage disease also complained of symptoms before diagnosis, and there was no significant difference in the symptoms reported between those with early versus late stage disease. When the authors compared symptoms in women with early stage disease with controls assessed by telephone using random-digit dialing (**Table 3**), the odds ratios (OR) were still significant: Bloating (odds ratio [OR], 19.2; 95% confidence interval [CI], 9.9–37.5); abdominal pain (OR, 5.5; 95%, CI, 2.8–10.8); constipation (OR, 5.5; 95% CI, 2.5–12.0). Although these results suggested very significant differences between cases and controls, the controls were not women visiting a physician's office, and therefore may not represent the typical patient, with a variety of complaints, seen in clinical practice.

To address the concerns raised about the control group in the Memorial study, researchers at the University of Washington evaluated symptoms typical of ovarian cancer in 1709 women presenting to a primary care clinic. Women were surveyed about the types of symptoms they had experienced over the prior year as well as the frequency, severity, and duration of symptoms.[28] The primary care clinic patients were then compared as controls with a group of 128 women with pelvic masses who filled out an identical survey about symptoms before surgery and before they knew whether or not their mass was malignant. Symptoms such as bloating, increased abdominal size, urinary symptoms, and pelvic and abdominal pain were found significantly more frequently in women with ovarian cancer than in those presenting to primary care clinics, although the OR of symptoms for cases as compared with controls were quite a bit lower than was seen in the Memorial study. One of the potential reasons that the OR are so much lower in the study from Goff and associates is that the control group used were actual patients visiting their primary care physician for a problem visit (see **Table 3**), in contrast with people reached in their home by telephone.

The study from the University of Washington also evaluated the characteristic of symptoms in cancer versus clinic patients.[28] Cancer patients typically reported that their symptoms occurred 20 to 30 times per month compared with 2 to 3 times per month for the clinic patients. The symptoms in cancer patients were significantly of more recent onset. For instance, the duration of symptoms was usually less than 3 to 6 months for cancer patients compared with a year or longer for the clinic controls. The authors found that although the types of symptoms that women with ovarian cancer experience are vague and frequently reported by women presenting to primary care clinics, the important distinction between cases and controls seems to be the frequency and duration of the symptoms. Researchers from other institutions across the United States and in other countries have found remarkably similar findings.[29-36] In addition, large, population-based studies have identified the majority of ovarian cancer patients as experiencing symptoms before diagnosis.[34,36,37]

A follow-up, case-control study was conducted by Goff and colleagues[38] to establish a symptom index that might be useful in the early diagnosis of ovarian cancer. In this study, 149 women with ovarian cancer were surveyed about symptoms before surgical exploration; controls consisted of 255 women in an ovarian cancer screening program and 233 women who were referred for pelvic ultrasonography. Logistical regression was used to determine which factors independently predicted ovarian cancer in an exploratory group and then sensitivity and specificity were tested in a confirmatory group. The symptom index that was most sensitive for detecting ovarian cancer was a woman having any 1 of 6 symptoms (bloating, increased abdominal size, difficulty eating, feeling full quickly, and abdominal or pelvic pain), which occurred more than 12 times per month and were present for less than 1 year. The overall sensitivity and specificity for detecting ovarian cancer were 70% and 86%, respectively. The sensitivity for detecting early stage disease was 57% and 80% for advanced stage disease. These investigators are currently conducting a clinical trial using symptom triggered screening for ovarian cancer.[39] Women who screen positive on a symptom index (**Fig. 2**) are referred for testing with CA125 and TVS. Critics have raised concerns that evaluation of symptoms will lead to unnecessary operations.[40-43] However, a recent clinical trial of more than 2000 women evaluated with symptom screening followed by symptom-triggered TVS and CA125 found that none of the screened patients underwent a laparotomy or laparoscopy because of enrollment in a symptom screening program.[39] Although the sensitivity of the symptom index is likely to be a significant weakness, symptom identification may be a low-cost method to improve rates of early detection in the general population, because this is a group for which a screening test neither exists nor is recommended.

One of the main concerns about symptom reporting is the potential of recall bias. However, there have been several case-control studies evaluating symptoms from claims data and chart notes of ovarian cancer patients before their diagnosis.[34,36,37,44] These studies also confirm that women with ovarian cancer are significantly more likely than controls to have specific symptoms 3 to 6 months before diagnosis. Smith and co-workers[37] evaluated the Surveillance, Epidemiology, and End Results Medicare database for 1985 ovarian cancer patients, 6024 breast cancer patients, and 10,941 noncancer patients. ICD-9 diagnosis codes were compared before the ovarian cancer diagnosis date or reference date for noncancer patients. Ovarian cancer patients were significantly more likely to have visits for target symptoms, including abdominal pain, abdominal swelling, and gastrointestinal complaints within 6 months before diagnosis. Hamilton and colleagues[44] performed a chart review of 212 ovarian cancer patients and 1060 controls and found that 85% of cases had 1 of 7 ovarian cancer symptoms documented in the medical records before diagnosis, compared with 15% of controls. Abdominal distension, urinary frequency,

Symptom Index

Are you currently experiencing any of the following symptoms frequently? Check the box Yes or No. If yes, also check the box for number of days per month and the box for the number of months you experience each symptom.

1. Pain: Abdominal/Pelvic Pain
   ☐ No
   ☐ Yes⟶**1a.**   **If yes,** how many **days** per month do you experience this symptom?

		More than 13
0-5 days	6–12 days	days
☐	☐	☐

     1b.   **If yes,** how **long** have you had this symptom?

Less than 1 month	1–6 months	7-12 months	More than 1 year
☐	☐	☐	☐

2. Eating: Feeling full quickly or unable to eat normally
   ☐ No
   ☐ Yes⟶**2a.**   **If yes,** how many **days** per month do you experience this symptom?

		More than 13
0-5 days	6–12 days	days
☐	☐	☐

     2b.   **If yes,** how **long** have you had this symptom?

Less than 1 month	1–6 months	7-12 months	More than 1 year
☐	☐	☐	☐

3. Abdomen: Abdominal bloating or increased abdomen size
   ☐ No
   ☐ Yes⟶**3a.**   **If yes,** how many **days** per month do you experience this symptom?

		More than 13
0-5 days	6–12 days	days
☐	☐	☐

     3b.   **If yes,** how **long** have you had this symptom?

Less than 1 month	1–6 months	7-12 months	More than 1 year
☐	☐	☐	☐

Fig. 2. Symptom Index screening tool. (*Adapted from* Goff BA, Lowe KA, Kane JC, et al. Symptom triggered screening for ovarian cancer: a pilot study of feasibility and acceptability. Gynecol Oncol 2012;124:230–5; with permission.)

and abdominal pain were significantly associated with ovarian cancer even at 6 months before diagnosis.

Other investigators have evaluated the University of Washington symptom index retrospectively and have found limited utility.[40,41] In a study by Pavlik and associates,[41] only 6 of 30 patients (20%) who had undergone surgery for ovarian cancer had a positive symptom index. The authors did not provide information as to how long after surgery symptom information was collected. Rossing and co-workers[40] also retrospectively surveyed women about symptoms before diagnosis and compare this with age-matched controls. In this study, women were surveyed on average of 9 months after diagnosis. The symptom index was positive in 62.3% of women with early stage disease and 70.7% of those with advanced stage disease, but only 30% of women with a positive symptom index became positive more than 5 months before their diagnosis. In addition, the authors retrospectively calculated PPV and found it to be low, approximately 1%. Because of the low PPV the authors argue for a cautious approach to the use of symptoms to trigger an extensive medical evaluation for ovarian cancer. The low estimates of PPV are not surprising given the frequency of these symptoms in the general population and the low incidence of ovarian cancer, but it does not mean that these symptoms should be ignored.

SUMMARY

Ultimately, the timely diagnosis of ovarian cancer will rely on clinical judgment and careful analysis of presenting symptoms within the context of a thoughtful dialogue between the patient and her physician. Symptoms most typical of ovarian cancer include bloating, abdominal or pelvic pain, and difficulty eating. In some studies, urinary symptoms are also a common presenting symptom. When these symptoms occur more than 12 times per month and are of recent onset, then ovarian cancer should be considered as a possibility. Although most women who have these symptoms do not have ovarian cancer, it is important that providers include ovarian cancer in their differential diagnosis. Through research from the past decade, we now understand that there are patterns of symptoms associated with ovarian cancer. Importantly, we now know that ovarian cancer is not a "silent disease." Finally, clinicians must always listen carefully to their patients avoid potentially harmful delays in diagnosis. Until there is a screening test, awareness is best.

REFERENCES

1. National Institutes of Health Consensus Development Conference Statement. Ovarian cancer: screening, treatment, and follow-up. Gynecol Oncol 1994;55:S4–14.
2. Schorge JO, Modesitt SC, Coleman RL, et al. SGO White paper on ovarian cancer: etiology, screening and surveillance. Gynecol Oncol 2010;119:7–17.
3. US Preventive Services Task Force. Genetic risk assessment and BRCA mutation testing for breast and ovarian cancer susceptibility. Ann Intern Med 2005;143: 355–61.
4. The American College of Obstetricians and Gynecologists Committee Opinion. The role of the obstetrician-gynecologist in the early detection of epithelial ovarian cancer. Obstet Gynecol 2011;117:742–6.
5. US Preventive Services Task Force Agency for Healthcare Research and Quality. Screening for ovarian cancer. Rockville (MD): US Department of Health and Human Services; 2004.
6. Menon U, Jacobs IJ. Ovarian cancer screening in the general population. Curr Opin Obstet Gynecol 2001;13:61–4.
7. Crum CP. Intercepting pelvic cancer in the distal fallopian tube: theories and realities. Mol Oncol 2009;3:165–70.
8. Jacobs IJ, Menon U. Progress and challenges in screening for ovarian cancer. Mol Cell Proteomics 2004;3:355–66.
9. Bast RC Jr, Brewer M, Zou C, Hernandez MA, et al. Prevention and early detection of ovarian cancer: mission impossible? Recent Results Cancer Res 2007;174:91–100.
10. Buys SS, Partridge E, Black A, et al. Effect of screening on ovarian cancer mortality. The Prostate, Lung, Colorectal and Ovarian (PLCO) Cancer Screening Randomized Controlled Trial. JAMA 2011;305: 2295–303.

11. Menon U, Gentry-Maharaj A, Hallett R, et al. Sensitivity and specificity of multimodal and ultrasound screening for ovarian cancer, and stage distribution of detected cancers: results of the prevalence screen of the UK Collaborative Trial of Ovarian Cancer Screening (UKCTOCS). Lancet Oncol 2009;10:327–40.

12. Partridge E, Kreimer AR, Greenlee RT, et al. Results from four rounds of ovarian cancer screening in a randomized trial. Obstet Gynecol 2009;114:775–82.

13. Lu KH, Skates S, Bevers TB, et al. A prospective U.S. ovarian cancer screening study using the risk of ovarian cancer algorithm (ROCA). J Clin Oncol 2010;28:15s.

14. van Nagell JR Jr, DePriest PD, Ueland FR, et al. Ovarian cancer screening with annual transvaginal sonography. Cancer 2007;109:1887–96.

15. Hogg R, Friedlander M. Biology of epithelial ovarian cancer: implications for screening women at high genetic risk. J Clin Oncol 2004;22:1315–27.

16. Fishman DA, Cohen L, Bland SV, et al. The role of ultrasound evaluation in the detection of early-stage epithelial ovarian cancer. Am J Obstet Gynecol 2005;192: 1214–22.

17. van der Velde NM, Mourits MJE, Arts HJG, et al. Time to stop ovarian cancer screening in BRCA1/2 mutation carriers? Int J Cancer 2009;1214:919–23.

18. Hermsen BB, Olivier RI, Verheijen RH, et al. No efficacy of annual gynaecological screening in BRCA 1/2 mutation carriers: observational follow-up study. Br J Cancer 2007;96:1335–42.

19. Evans DG, Gaarenstroom KN, Stirling D, et al. Screening for familial ovarian cancer: poor survival of BRCA1/2 related cancer. J Med Genet 2009;46:593–7.

20. Pruthi S, Gostout BS, Lindor NM. Identification and management of women with BRCA mutations or hereditary predisposition for breast and ovarian cancer. May Clin Proc 2010;85:1111–20.

21. Ueland FR, Desimone CP, Seamon LG, et al. Effectiveness of a multivariate index assay in the preoperative assessment of ovarian tumors. Obstet Gynecol 2011;117: 1289–97.

22. Moore RG, Miller MC, Disilvestro P, et al. Evaluation of the diagnostic accuracy of the risk of ovarian malignancy algorithm in women with a Pelvic Mass. Obstet Gynecol 2011;118:280–8.

23. Smith EM, Anderson B. The effects of symptoms and delay in seeking diagnosis among women with cancers of the ovary. Cancer 1985;56:2727–32.

24. Flam F, Einhorn N, Sjovall K. Symptomatology of ovarian cancer. Eur J Obstet Gynecol Reprod Biol 1988;27:53–7.

25. Eltabbakh GH, Yadav PR, Morgan A. Clinical picture of women with early stage ovarian cancer. Gynecol Oncol 1999;75:476–9.

26. Goff BA, Mandel L, Muntz HG, et al. Ovarian carcinoma diagnosis. Cancer 2000;89: 2068–75.

27. Olson SH, Mignone L, Nakraseive C, et al. Symptoms of ovarian cancer. Obstet Gynecol 2001;98:212–7.

28. Goff BA, Mandel LS, Melancon CH, et al. Frequency of symptoms of ovarian cancer in women presenting to primary care clinics. JAMA 2004;291:2705–12.

29. Vine MF, Calingaert B, Berchuck A, et al. Characterization of prediagnostic symptoms among primary epithelial ovarian cancer cases and controls. Gynecol Oncol 2003;90: 75–82.

30. Yawn PB, Barrette BA, Wollan PC. Ovarian cancer: the neglected diagnosis. Mayo Clin Proc 2004;79:1277–82.

31. Freidman GD, Skilling JS, Udaltsove NV, et al. Early symptoms of ovarian cancer: a case-control study without recall bias. Fam Pract 2005;22:548–53.

32. Kim MK, Kim K, Kim SM, et al. A hospital-based case control study of identifying ovarian cancer using a symptom index. J Gynecol Oncol 2009;20:238–42.

33. Devlin SM, Diehr PH, Andersen MR, et al. Identification of ovarian cancer symptoms in health insurance claims data. J Womens Health 2010;19:381–9.

34. Ryerson AB, Eheman C, Burton J, et al. Symptoms, diagnoses, and time to key diagnostic procedures among older U.S. women with ovarian cancer. Obstet Gynecol 2007;109:1053–61.

35. Wynn ML, Chang S, Peipins LA. Temporal patterns of conditions and symptoms potentially associated with ovarian cancer. J Women Health (Larchmt) 2007;16: 971–86.

36. Laurie G, Thompson PJ, McDuffie KE, et al. Prediagnostic symptoms of ovarian carcinoma: a case-control study. Gynecol Oncol 2009;114:231–6.

37. Smith LH, Morris CR, Yasmeen S, et al. Ovarian cancer: can we make the clinical diagnosis earlier? Cancer 2005;104:1398–407.

38. Goff BA, Mandel LS, Drescher CW, et al. Development of an ovarian cancer symptom index: possibilities for earlier detection. Cancer 2007;109221–7.

39. Goff BA, Lowe KA, Kane JC, et al. Symptom triggered screening for ovarian cancer: a pilot study of feasibility and acceptability. Gynecol Oncol 2012;124:230–5.

40. Rossing MA, Wicklund KG, Cushing-Haugen KL, et al. Predictive value of symptoms for early detection of ovarian cancer. J Natl Cancer Inst 2010;102:222–9.

41. Pavlik EJ, Saunders BA, Doran S, et al. The search for meaning – symptoms and transvaginal sonography screening for ovarian cancer: predicting malignancy. Cancer 2009;115:3689–98.

42. Daly MB, Ozols RF. Symptoms of ovarian cancer – where to set the bar? JAMA 2004;291:2755–6.

43. Cass I. The search for meaning – symptoms and transvaginal sonography screening for ovarian cancer. Cancer 2009;115:3606–9.

44. Hamilton W, Peters TJ, Bankhead C, et al. Risk of ovarian cancer in women with symptoms in primary care: population based case-control study. BMJ 2009;339: b2998.

Gestational Trophoblastic Neoplasia

R. Osborne, MD, FRCSC, MBA[a],*, J. Dodge, MD, FRCSC, MEd[b]

KEYWORDS

- Trophoblastic disease • Neoplasm • Gestational • Choriocarcinoma

KEY POINTS

- Origin
  Trophoblastic disease is an allograft of fetal tissue consisting of paternally-derived tissue that invades the maternal decidual plate in an uncontrolled manner.
- GTN
  Trophoblastic neoplasia is defined by the F.I.G.O. (2002) definition of persistent disease (a rise or plateau in the quantitative β-hCG titer).
- Treatment
  The type of treatment is determined by the W.H.O. risk score (low risk 0-6 and high risk >6). Patients with the former receive single-agent, and the latter, combination chemotherapy.
- Prognosis
  Low risk disease is almost universally curable and most high risk disease is also successfully treated unless there are liver (and brain) metastases.
- Regionalization
  Since this is a very rare but potentially curable disease, treatment should be centralized in tertiary centers, by oncologists with particular knowledge and expertise in the management of trophoblastic neoplasia.

Trophoblastic neoplasms are a truly fascinating set of diseases that arise from a failed gestation. A molar pregnancy is an allograft of fetal tissue typically containing only paternal chromosomes that may invade the maternal decidua following a failed gestation that may have arisen up to decades earlier. Choriocarcinoma (CCA), the most common malignant form of trophoblastic disease, represented the very first

The authors have nothing to disclose.
[a] Division of Gynecologic Oncology, Odette Cancer Centre, 2075 Bayview Avenue, Toronto, Ontario M4N 3M5, Canada; [b] Division of Gynecologic Oncology, Princess Margaret Hospital, Toronto, Ontario, Canada
* Corresponding author.
E-mail address: ray.osborne@sunnybrook.ca

Obstet Gynecol Clin N Am 39 (2012) 195–212
http://dx.doi.org/10.1016/j.ogc.2012.03.002
0889-8545/12/$ – see front matter © 2012 Elsevier Inc. All rights reserved.

medical cure of a solid cancer in 1956[1–3] following an observation by pathologist M.C. Li in 1954 that the urine human chorionic gonadotropin (hCG) level declined in a woman undergoing treatment for melanoma. Dr Roy Hertz then used this anecdotal information to successfully treat trophoblastic disease using a drug called amethopterin, a less toxic form of the drug aminopterin first used by Lucy Willis in 1930 to treat pernicious anemia of pregnancy.[4,5]

PATHOLOGY

These tumors are derived from the fetus/conceptus and not from the mother. With the single exception of partial mole (PHM), all of these lesions will be composed, in whole or in part, of paternal genetic material, a process called androgenesis.

Trophoblastic Function and Differentiation

Human trophoblast is derived from trophectoderm, the outermost layer of the blastocyst. The earliest cell layer of the trophectoderm, cytotrophoblast, lines the blastocyst and serves as the stem cell for the other layers of the developing trophoblast. Cytotrophoblast also makes a primitive hCG molecule called hyperglycosylated hCG (H-hCG; ITA or invasive trophoblast antigen) for the first 14 days after conception that seems to promote blastocyst adhesion and the earliest invasion by the syncytiotrophoblastic mass beneath the blastocyst at the implantation site. Immediately after implantation (day 7), cytotrophoblast, in its function as the trophoblast stem cell, differentiates into a syncytial mass (previllous trophoblast).[6]

Early cytotrophoblast, also referred to as the Langhans cell layer, is the germinative layer that proliferates and differentiates along two distinct pathways. First, on the incipient villus surface it fuses into syncytiotrophoblast cells (ST), a terminally differentiated cell line that loses its proliferative capability but secretes hormones/proteins including human placental lactogen (hPL), hCG, and other paracrine proteins. These proteins regulate the microenvironment of the implantation site and establish the villus interface with maternal blood permitting fetomaternal oxygen/carbon dioxide transfer as well as nutrition and metabolic product exchange.[6]

Second, the extravillus trophoblast, cytotrophoblast, differentiates into intermediate trophoblast (IT). IT is a heterogenous cell population that can be subcategorized based on its anatomic location. In the intravillus mesenchyme, the so-called anchoring columns, cytotrophoblast evolves imperceptibly into implantation site IT (ISIT). ISIT loses its proliferative ability (low Ki-67 assay) but is now able to invade the maternal decidua and myometrium, dissecting between the smooth muscle fibers. By tropism, ISIT migrates to and invades the maternal spiral arteries (high MelCAM assay) leaving their overall structure intact. ISIT coats the vascular endothelial surface with extracellular matrix resulting in incompetence of the arterial valves that in turn results in a very low resistance environment that facilitates oxygen and waste transfer between mother and fetus. ISIT makes hPL, whereas chorion-type IT (CTIT) does not. ISIT also loses its proliferative capability and does not invade the decidua parietalis. In normal early pregnancy, the ISIT invades the maternal decidual plate but is tightly controlled both spatially and temporally, involving only the decidua and, at most, the inner 30% of the myometrium solely beneath the implantation site. Later, in normal pregnancy, the ISIT cells fuse into multinucleated cells with accompanying loss of both their migratory and invasive characteristics.[6]

Gestational Trophoblastic Diseases

The gestational trophoblastic diseases (GTDs) include all molar gestations, both complete and partial, even though over 90% will resolve without treatment following uterine evacuation. The term *GTD* also includes persistent moles that are not completely expelled after curettage and go on to require active management, and its malignant analogue, CCA. The definition also includes the malignant variant of exaggerated placental site reaction (EPS), placental site trophoblastic tumor (PSTT) that arises from the ISIT, and the malignant variant of benign placental nodule (PN), and epithelioid trophoblastic tumor (ETT) that arises from CTIT of the chorion laeve. As would be expected from its pathologic characteristics, PSTT extensively invades myometrium and its vascular structures. CCA, ETT, PSTT, and persistent mole all require active management and are referred to collectively as gestational trophoblastic neoplasia (GTN).[6]

The several forms of GTD are related to discrete pathologic errors that occur at different stages of differentiation of the trophoblast. Some of these lesions are neoplasms (CCA, ETT, PSTT), whereas their benign counterparts (EPS, PN, and molar pregnancy, respectively) are best described as abnormal placentas with the potential to develop malignant placental lesions. The cytogenetics of molar pregnancy are well-understood, but the pathogenesis of these other trophoblast lesions is not, in part because of the rarity of these abnormalities and the absence of an experimental model.

CCA arises from a prior molar pregnancy in 50% of cases as evidenced by the fact that most are homozygous (85% of complete moles have an XX karyotype) because they have arisen through diandry; duplication of a single X sperm in an empty ovum. Approximately 95% of PSTT and ETT lesions arise after a term pregnancy or a nonmolar abortion. Based on histopathologic studies, PSTT and ETT are believed to arise from distinct subpopulations of extravillous IT (ISIT and CTIT, respectively). Recent molecular evidence confirms both their fetal (trophoblastic) origin and the presence of paternal genes.[7]

Partial moles are nonrecurring and have a very low risk of persistence (.5%–2%). Partial moles are typically, but not invariably, triploid. Triploid gestations only demonstrate trophoblastic proliferation (GTD) when there are at least two paternal haploid chromosome sets arising either by dispermy (fertilization by two sperm) or diandry (one sperm that duplicates through a meiosis-1 error), plus a maternal haploid set. When the extra haploid set is maternal the gestational villi are hydropic but there is no trophoblastic proliferation, the hallmark of trophoblastic disease. Such gestations are not a GTD but usually consist of a nonviable fetus and a hydropic but nonproliferative placenta.

Complete moles have a 10-fold risk of recurrence in the next gestation and a further 10-fold risk with a third pregnancy. Partial moles have no increased risk of persistence in follow-on gestations because they are due to nonrecurring errors of fertilization. A very few families seem to have a predisposition to repeated GTD. The defect is thought to be on chromosome 7 at the NLRP locus. In one recent report, the NLRP7 mutation was present in 60% of patients with two hydatidiform moles (HMs), 13% with one HM, and 8% of patients with three or more spontaneous abortions. If the patient had two defective alleles, reproductive wastage was even higher.[8]

The diagnosis of a complete mole is sometimes difficult, particularly in very early pregnancy. Classically the diagnosis is based on histologic and genetic criteria, but the former, based on morphology, is highly subjective and prone to significant interobserver variability.[9] The unique genetic features of CHM (androgenetic diploidy), PHM (diandritic triploidy), and hydropic abortus (biparental diploidy) permit the use of certain molecular discriminators. The immunohistochemical expression of the p57[kip2] gene, a cell cycle inhibitor and tumor suppressor that is strongly paternally imprinted and maternally expressed, has been shown to reliably differentiate CHM from PHM and hydropic abortus. The villous cytotrophoblast cells of CHM lack the maternal genome and stain negatively for the gene, whereas PHM and hydropic abortus stain strongly positive for the gene regardless of gestational age.[10,11] Recent evidence suggests that a second marker gene PHLDA2 may also accurately differentiate CHM from PHM and other gestational mimics.[12] Whereas p57 expression can identify CHM, because of the absence of maternal DNA, fluorescence in situ hybridization can determine the genetic identity of PHM and abortus by determining their ploidy status. By allowing accurate subclassification of moles and unusual products of conception, more accurate prognostic information can be obtained.[13,14]

TUMOR BIOMARKERS
Human Chorionic Gonadotropin

HCG is a near-perfect biomarker. Each trophoblastic cell makes a relatively finite amount of hCG per day (10^{-5} mIU/mL), and the assay result provides an accurate indication of the trophoblastic cell burden. The most primitive trophoblast cell, cytotrophoblast, makes hyperglycosylated hCG for only the first few weeks of the gestation. This autocrine hormone likely plays an active role in establishment of both the implantation site and the fetomaternal circulation and also evolves into syncytiotrophoblast that makes regular hCG of normal pregnancy. Production of hCG increases logarithmically from implantation (day 7) and peaks at 10 weeks at a median level of about 60,000 mIU/mL, then declines between the 10th and 20th weeks and remains stable at around 12,000 mIU/mL until term.[15,16]

The hCG molecule is not a single biological molecule. Regular hCG is produced by differentiated syncytiotrophoblast cells and consists of a common 92 amino acid glycopeptide chain, with asparagine-linked mono- and biantennary sugar moieties and a unique 145 amino acid beta (β) chain with both asparagine and serine linked disaccharide moieties, the latter attached to the C-terminal peptide of the chain. The hCG molecule acts to maintain the vascular supply of the placenta in normal gestation by stabilizing the myometrial and decidual spiral arteries.[17] The molecule, particularly the β chain, often becomes fragmented, particularly when malignant transformation occurs. In normal pregnancy, the free β fragment comprises less than 1% of the total hCG assay, the nicked β fragment less than 10%, and there may be a very small amount of H-hCG. The β core fragment, a terminal degradation product of β chain metabolism, is only detectable in the urine. The more common fragments, β core, nicked β, and hyperglycosylated free β, are produced in varying amounts. Hyperglycosylated free β also functions as an autocrine hormone (acts on its tissue of origin) by independently promoting growth and invasion in GTN.[18]

Hyperglycosylated hCG

H-hCG, also called ITA or invasive trophoblast antigen, is regular hCG with double-sized, tri- and tetrasaccharide O-linked sugars and is made by undifferentiated extravillous cytotrophoblast. H-hCG functions as an autocrine hormone by facilitating ordered trophoblast invasion at the implantation site in normal gestation and supporting disordered malignant invasion in GTN.[16] A hyperglycosylated free β subunit is produced by a high proportion of GTN and other malignancies.[17] H-hCG functions as an autocrine and has the ability to signal normal placental cytotrophoblast to grow and invade, whereas hCG promotes uterine vascularization. Insufficient H-hCG levels are associated with pregnancy loss and preeclampsia.[18]

It is very important to use an assay that can detect not only the intact hCG molecule but also H-hCG and H-free β, as well as all their degradation products (hCG β radioimmunoassay and the Siemens Immulite assay), because most automated commercial laboratory tests (12 are currently on the market) detect only regular hCG with accuracy.[19] In the same study, when the same sera were tested against other hCG assays, there was as much as a 58-fold variation in the assay titer results. When the same assay was retested with the same sera there was a 1.4-fold difference using pregnancy sera and a 2.2-fold difference with GTN sera. This discordance was related to differences in assay recognition of nicked hCG, free β, and other hCG variants.[20] H-hCG and its degradation fragments may be significantly overproduced, particularly in early pregnancy, CCA, and germ cell malignancies. A nonquantitative hCG assay therefore may not accurately reflect the true disease burden.[18]

Free β and the β Core Fragment

The free β assay is the biomarker of choice for detecting/following PSTT, a neoplasm characterized by intermediate cell invasion of the myometrium. Because there is very little syncytiotrophoblast present, the amount of hCG present is very low and is not a useful marker of response for PSTT. The free β assay is also part of early pregnancy serum screening for Downs syndrome (2 fold increase in free b and 9 fold increase in H-hCG). ETT tumors make low level hCG and are best monitored with the urinary β core fragment assay.[6,17]

Clinical syndromes involving hCG assay

Quiescent hCG syndrome. Some patients continue to make small amounts of real hCG in the absence of any radiologic evidence of GTN. Typically the titer is only double-digit and remains stable for months or up to 16 years.[21,22,23] It seems that a small focus of, or perhaps individual, dispersed, differentiated syncytiotrophoblast cells are present, sometimes after prior chemotherapy. These slow growing cells make small static amounts of hCG and do not have invasive potential so long as there is no cytotrophoblast or IT present. These syncytiotrophoblast cells do not respond to chemotherapy, and hysterectomy does not normalize the hCG titer. H-hCG is usually absent but may constitute no more than 6% of the total hCG assay result. Cole and Khanian[22] have reported that 7% of these patients will begin to secrete increased H-hCG within 5 years, weeks to months before the hCG titer begins to rise and before there is clinically detectable GTN.

Phantom hCG. About 2% of reproductive aged women will have a low level positive conventional hCG test without trophoblast seemingly present (< 300 mIU/mL). This is a false-positive test result due to the presence of nonspecific heterophile antibody in the patient's serum usually due to childhood (smallpox) immunization. The term *heterophile antibody* implies the presence of a cross-species antibody. HCG tests involve two animal antibodies, one that is specific for binding one molecular site on hCG and one specific for binding a distant site on hCG. This second site has a dye, enzyme, chemoluminescence, or tracer attached that will identify the amount of hCG present. The hCG molecule is sandwiched between the immobilized antibody and the tracer antibody. Antibodies are always bivalent and, when heterophile antibody (human antianimal antibody) is present, it binds the animal antibodies used in the hCG assay and causes a false-positive or "phantom" result.[24,25] The large heterophile molecule does not enter the urine because of its size. True elevated hCG will produce a positive serum and urine assay for hCG, but in this syndrome the urine hCG assay is usually nondetectable (and never >50 mIU/mL). The diagnosis can also be made with serial dilution of the sample (false titers are not affected by dilution) or use of a second commercial assay that will often result in a marked fluctuation in the titer (most will be negative). Occasionally the false report is related to the reagent, so repeating the assay with an assay from a different species (sheep vs rabbit) will strip off the heterophile antibody. No treatment is required if the hCG result is a false-positive, because no abnormal trophoblast is present.[22]

Menopausal elevation of the hCG assay. A small number of perimenopausal and postmenopausal women will be found to have a low level positive hCG test result. One percent of perimenopausal and 7% of postmenopausal women have a serum hCG concentration above the conventional cutoff level of 4 to 5 mIU/mL. Both serum follicle-stimulating hormone (FSH) and hCG are known to increase with age. In one study it was suggested that women over 55 years of age should have a reset hCG cutoff value of 14 mIU/mL to minimize the possibility of such a false-positive assay result. These false results are due to elevated pituitary FSH and luteinizing hormone and/or benign low level pituitary hCG production.[26] If truly pituitary in origin, the hCG titer can be suppressed with a small dose of an oral contraceptive tablet over as few as 7 days.[27]

Posttreatment low level hCG elevation. In a report from Sheffield, a small percentage of women (.05%) had a low level persistent hCG assay following apparent successful treatment of GTN where the titer either reached normal then rose slightly or plateaued at a very low level. The hCG titer did not respond to a change in treatment, or remained static for a protracted period, without any clinical sign or disease. The test result was rarely higher than 40 mIU/mL. The presumed cause was either a small residual focus of syncytiotrophoblast or a false-positive assay due to elevated gonadotropin or heterophile antibody.[28]

DIAGNOSIS AND STAGING
Tumors of Cytotrophoblasts and Syncytiotrophoblasts

When a molar pregnancy is first detected, the following basic investigations are indicated: pelvic ultrasound (if not already performed), quantitative hCG, complete blood count (CBC), creatinine, thyroid function tests, and a chest radiograph. The diagnosis of GTD is typically made by pelvic ultrasound that demonstrates a snowstorm-like appearance within the uterine cavity. Current ultrasound can resolve down to hydropic placental vesicles as small as 2 mm. A partial mole usually is found with an accompanying nonviable gestation present in addition to an enlarged hydropic placenta. Most molar gestations are nowadays identified at the time of the early pregnancy screening sonogram in the absence of symptoms. Previously, patients usually presented with vaginal bleeding, an enlarged uterus, or occasionally signs of hyperthyroidism or early toxemia. Surprisingly, the incidence of persistent disease has not changed despite earlier diagnosis, suggesting that the likelihood of developing neoplasia is determined at a very early developmental stage. Complete moles may also occasionally be found as the second gestation in a twin pregnancy where the other fetus is normal and potentially viable. Other diagnoses to consider based on a hydropic uterine mass are Beckwith-Wiedemann syndrome, viral placentitis, and syphilis or Rh isoimmunization.

Ultrasound will provide information on the type of molar gestation, whether the disease involves the endometrial cavity or if it is partial or wholly intramyometrial (suggesting that second curettage may not be useful), the potential risk of uterine perforation, and the presence of theca lutein cysts or adnexal/vaginal metastases. There is also recent information that a uterine artery pulsatility quotient may be able to differentiate patients at higher risk of developing persistent and resistant disease at an earlier time point.[29]

A simple chest radiograph is obtained when persistence is diagnosed, but imaging of the brain or abdomen is not performed unless the chest film demonstrates pulmonary disease. The chest radiograph will resolve disease of at least 10^9 cells, whereas a computed tomographic or magnetic resonance (MR) scan will detect 10^7 cells and a positron emission tomography scan as few as 10^6 cells. However, a computed tomographic lung scan is the dose equivalent of 100 chest films (roughly the equivalent of a single long-haul air flight).[30] The value of a computed tomographic lung scan for disease staging remains controversial.

Once a molar pregnancy is found, the uterus is emptied. The mode of uterine emptying is important. Typically patients undergo a suction curettage, but medical methods of evacuation are sometimes used. The evidence suggests that the latter results in a higher likelihood of incomplete emptying and a higher rate of persistence and subsequent chemotherapy. As a result, medical evacuation should be discouraged.[31]

Following evacuation of a molar gestation, the hCG titer is monitored weekly until it either returns to normal (80%–95%) or persists (a rise or plateau as defined by the World Health Organization [WHO] and International Federation of Gynecology and Obstetrics [FIGO] criteria) requiring active management. The diagnosis of persistent disease GTN is also made if there is extrauterine disease not including vagina, adnexa, or lung if no single pulmonary lesion exceeds 2 cm. The definitions of a rise or plateau are contained in the WHO and FIGO guidelines for GTN but are purposely imprecise. These definitions are, at best, surrogate measures of GTN. This imprecision is a major reason why it is very difficult to compare results from different trophoblastic disease units (TDUs), given the differing institution-specific diagnostic criteria, risk scoring differences, and different regimens and reporting criteria.

Some patients may be falsely labeled as having GTN when in fact, the titer would return to normal with further observation alone. Historically, centers in the United Kingdom and Europe have tended to observe these patients for a longer period (up to 6 months as long as the titer continues to decline) than have most North American centers, accounting for the geographic discrepancy in persistence rates (5%–7% vs 15%–30%).[32]

Rarely, abnormal trophoblast may be found in the fallopian tube, where it usually presents as a typical ectopic gestation with abdominal pain and/or vaginal bleeding, or it may be diagnosed on an early pregnancy ultrasound. The abnormality may equally be PHM, CHM, or CCA. Treatment is usually removal of the abnormal tissue, but only 25% persisted and required chemotherapy in a series from Sheffield.[33]

Tumors of Intermediate Trophoblast

Tumors of IT have only recently been identified and described, so long-term clinical data are lacking. These tumors include EPS and PSTT and PN and ETT.

PSTT typically presents with abnormal vaginal bleeding. The tumor invades and destroys myometrial smooth muscle. As a result, the mass is poorly defined both clinically and radiologically. The assay for free β is the best biomarker for following PSTT.

ETT is typically a disease of reproductive aged women that follows a term pregnancy in 70% of patients (15% after either molar pregnancy or spontaneous abortion). The interval from the index gestation to diagnosis is an average of 6.2 years (range 1 to 18). It is typically a discrete nodule composed of hyalinized extracellular matrix and necrosis measuring as much as 5 cm in size. Blood vessel structure within the tumor is preserved, and intratumor hemorrhage is atypical. Patients usually present with abnormal vaginal bleeding. Metastases are unusual (<25%) but typically involve lung. The serum hCG level is elevated but usually remains below 2500 mIU/mL. This lesion is best followed with the β core fragment assay.[17]

The best treatment for both PSTT and ETT is hysterectomy. However, in young reproductive aged women, these lesions are occasionally managed by localized, hysteroscopic resection.

PRIMARY TREATMENT

When GTD persists, or if the curettings contain CCA (or PSTT or ETT), the patient's disease is staged (FIGO criteria) and a risk score (WHO criteria) assigned that determines the primary treatment regimen. The FIGO stage is an anatomic staging that has no bearing on the clinical management of disease. The risk score is composed of eight distinct criteria that are each assigned a score from 0 to 4. Initial disease staging includes CBC, creatinine, liver and thyroid function tests, pelvic ultrasound, and chest radiograph. There is little likelihood that a patient will have metastatic disease (brain, liver, or gastrointestinal tract) if the chest radiograph is negative (no lung lesion $\geq$ 1 cm); therefore, further investigation of the brain or liver is not indicated at that point.

The hCG titer, an excellent measure of the burden of disease, independently predicts for the failure of low-risk regimens. The hCG titer is assigned a risk score value of between 0 and 4 but, in the absence of other risk factors, even patients with a titer greater than 10^6 can have a low-risk score. In a report from the United Kingdom, if the initial titer exceeds 400,000 mIU/mL most patients will eventually require combination therapy that should be commenced at the outset of treatment. If the titer is between 100,000 and 400,000 mIU/mL, 30% of patients will be cured with a low-risk dose regimen. The remaining 70% will require a change in regimen, but with no loss of curability, and with only an additional 2 weeks of treatment.[34]

Chemotherapy for Low-Risk Disease

WHO determined "low-risk" disease (risk score 0–6) is treated with single agent chemotherapy using one of several published methotrexate regimens, with or without folinic acid rescue, or using dactinomycin, usually as a biweekly parenteral injection. Both drugs have relatively low side effect profiles; methotrexate produced mucositis and marrow depression in multiple single-institution reports, whereas dactinomycin resulted in grade 1 alopecia in 15% and grade 1 nausea in 40% in the phase III Gynecologic Oncology Group (GOG) study.[35]

The specific single drug regimen chosen is unfortunately both institution- and/or continent-specific. Europeans generally prefer an 8-day methotrexate regimen (Charing Cross TDU) that includes alternate-day folinic acid. North Americans typically prefer either a 5-day methotrexate regimen without folinic acid rescue or biweekly "pulse" dactinomycin. These regimens are very difficult to compare because of the paucity of prospective randomized studies.

The very large Charing Cross TDU data set, and collaborative single-institution results, have all reported an approximately 78% likelihood of cure using the 8-day methotrexate regimen, and a 2% to 26% chance that the patient will require a change in protocol because of toxicity (mucositis or marrow depression).[36]

The other commonly used methotrexate treatment is the 5-day methotrexate regimen (without folinic acid rescue) developed by the Brewer TDU at Northwestern University, Chicago. The Brewer regimen recently reported an 81% primary response rate and a 6% incidence of regimen change due to toxicity.[37]

There are two randomized trials comparing pulse dactinomycin and methotrexate at 30 mg/m^2 that included randomized data on response and toxicity.[35,38] In the GOG study, biweekly dactinomycin was 71% effective using strict definitions and failure criteria, rising to 75% if the "failure" was statistically correct but clinically trivial (and had gone unrecognized by the treating physician). Furthermore, in the GOG study, if only patients with a risk score of 0 to 4 were counted (all previous studies excluded harder-to-cure patients with risk scores of 5 or 6) the outcome was 79%.[35]

Gleeson and colleagues[39] published a phase III study that compared weekly methotrexate at 40 mg/m^2 and 8-day methotrexate/folinic acid. His group found no difference in response rate between the regimens, although the former was better tolerated and was preferred by patients.[39] Two other large TDUs have reported nonrandomized comparisons of low-risk treatment options. Kang and colleagues[40] compared weekly methotrexate at 50 mg/m^2 and 8-day methotrexate and folinic acid. Each regimen was approximately 70% effective as first line treatment. Mousavi and colleagues[41] compared biweekly dactinomycin and 5-day methotrexate and found the former to be 90% effective and the latter only 68% effective ($P = 0.018$). Both reports favored dactinomycin based on treatment outcome, toxicity, and ease of use.

We know from several large data sets, and from the GOG study, that a risk score of 5 or 6 confers a much lower chance of primary response/cure. Some investigators now question whether the inclusion of risk score 5 and 6 patients and the collapsing of the separate intermediate risk category into the low-risk group were in error.[42]

Several other regimens have been tested on patients with low-risk disease, all in nonrandomized, single-institution studies. Ng and colleagues and others have reported on the effectiveness of methotrexate infusion at 150 mg/m^2, and a dose of 1000 mg/cycle has also been studied.[43,44] Single agent etoposide has been used for low-risk disease at 100 mg/m^2.[45] It is a very effective regimen, but the alopecia, nausea, and risk of second malignancy have prevented its use as a primary treatment for all but high-risk patients. Methotrexate and dactinomycin in tandem have also been reported for low-risk disease. The investigators reported a 98% primary response rate, but there was a 10% likelihood of grade 3 or 4 toxicity.[46] The question arises whether so-called low-risk disease should be treated with two of the three most active agents and whether the toxicity of this regimen is acceptable for so-called low-risk patients.

Finally, there are reports from China and the Peking Union Hospital (Song) stretching back several decades on the use of high dose 5-fluoruracil for these patients. This regimen, although quite cost-effective, is toxic (nausea and gastrointestinal symptoms) and has not found favor in Western countries to date.

Single agent methotrexate and dactinomycin have both been used as prophylactic single dose treatment for low-risk patients and, whereas the likelihood of a patient requiring full treatment is decreased, this approach does result in unnecessary treatment for a very many patients whose disease would likely have resolved spontaneously.[47,48,49]

Low-risk metastatic disease, as defined by the older National Cancer Institution criteria for low-risk disease, has been successfully treated with sequential 5-day methotrexate and dactinomycin. The success rate in this harder-to-treat low-risk group in the Brewer series was 67%, but drug resistance was reported in 22% and drug toxicity in another 11%, suggesting that, although effective, this regimen is likely too toxic for general use.[50]

It is very difficult to compare the available regimens on outcome and toxicity because of the differences in patient selection, risk scoring criteria, and rigid institutional preference for specific regimens. Therefore, there is no international consensus about a" best" primary regimen for low-risk disease.[51–53]

Follow-Up

Given the significant loss-to-follow-up rates in the United States where 3% to 13% of patients do not complete treatment and 40% are lost before follow-up is completed, Goldstein and colleagues[54] have suggested that prompt introduction of single agent chemotherapy for persistent disease may be prudent in some circumstances.[54,55]

In the United Kingdom, if the titer normalizes with 50 days (7 weeks), there is scant chance of recurrence. This finding was confirmed by a report from the Dutch Central Registry of Hydatidiform Mole where only 1 out of 265 patients developed recurrence after as few as two normal titers.[56]

Management of Low-risk Primary Treatment Failure

Early diagnosis of resistance to low-dose single agent chemotherapy is highly desirable in order to limit the number of ineffective treatment cycles before a switch is made to a curative regimen. Several investigators have used a regression graph to predict need for treatment. These investigators have graphed the slope of normal postevacuation hCG regression and applied 95% confidence limits to the curves. If the patient's titer falls outside the confidence intervals, the patient is deemed to have persistent disease requiring active management. Rotmensch and colleagues[57] designed a 90th percentile log-exponential regression curve based on a small number of patients successfully treated with methotrexate. Shigematsu and colleagues[58] developed a receiver operating characteristic curve with an hCG cutoff value that identifies refractory patients at an earlier point in their treatment. More recently, von Trommel and Kerkmeijer[59] collaborated to develop a cutoff value (737 mIU/mL) that predicted resistance to 8-day methotrexate in 50% of patients who eventually did not respond to methotrexate a full 2.5 cycles earlier than with conventional definitions. A very high test specificity is essential so that very few patients are switched unnecessarily to combination chemotherapy, and in this study, a 97.5% level of specificity was obtained.[59]

Between 17% and 36% of patients initially treated with low-dose methotrexate regimens will require a change in treatment because of drug resistance. When this requirement occurs, the patient's disease is restaged and the risk score is recalculated. If the score is still low-risk (0–6), patients may be retreated with 5-day methotrexate or dactinomycin. The Sheffield group has also reported that a combination of etoposide and dactinomycin (EA regimen) has a very high (97%) chance of cure in these patients without significant toxicity and no observed second malignancy risk.[60] If the hCG titer is less than 150 mIU/mL, the two UK sites would offer 5-day or biweekly dactinomycin. This has proven to be an excellent regimen in this circumstance (cure rate of 94% and no observed grade 3–4 toxicity). Given the success of the regimen, the Sheffield and Charing Cross groups have recently increased the hCG assay threshold to 300 mIU/mL.[61]

If the recalculated risk score exceeds 6, the EMACO regimen is used. If the chest radiograph is now positive, the liver (computed tomography of abdomen) and brain should be imaged (MR brain) to rule out metastatic disease.

Chemotherapy for High-risk Disease

If the curettings contain CCA, the patient may be treated with a single agent regimen if the risk score is 0 to 6, but if it is 7 or higher, the patient should receive a first line multiagent regimen, usually EMACO. This protocol contains not only methotrexate and dactinomycin but, in addition, etoposide, vincristine and cyclophosphamide. The regimen is repeated every 14 days and is more emetogenic and marrow-toxic than the single agent protocols. In addition, use of etoposide confers a small (2%) but dose-dependent lifetime risk of late-developing acute myelogenous leukemia.[62]

The Sheffield group has studied treating these women with methotrexate, etoposide, and dactinomycin (MEA) and omitting the much less active CO part of EMACO with good effect (75%).[60]

Patients with a primary diagnosis of PSTT should be treated with a different regimen, the EPEMA regimen, which contains biweekly platinum and weekly etoposide. Some investigators would also use this regimen as primary treatment for "very high-risk" CCA (risk score $\geq$12). This regimen is quite marrow-toxic and typically requires granulocyte-stimulating factor support by the third cycle. Other possible first line options are MEA[60] that contains a higher dose of etoposide (300 vs 200 mg/m^2) or methotrexate, actinomycin, cyclophosphamide, which was an effective regimen in the 1980s but one that was associated with potentially life-threatening myelosuppression.[32]

Management of High-risk Primary Treatment Failure

If treatment with EPEMA fails, the treatment options are quite limited. Taxol may have a role to play at this stage. Several centers have successfully used a doublet containing etoposide/Taxol and etoposide/platinum, and there is evidence that this regimen may be less toxic than EPEMA as second line therapy.[63]

Other regimens are largely salvage treatments that are unlikely to result in cure and are typically marrow-suppressive and toxic. These additional protocols include cis-platin, etoposide, bleomycin, ifosfamide, cis-platin, etopiside, high dose 5-flurorouracil, gemcitabine, and ultra high dose etoposide with autologous bone marrow transplantation.

PSTT and ETT are easily cured by hysterectomy when the disease is confined to the uterus. However, metastatic PSTT and ETT are relatively chemotherapy-insensitive, and cure when the disease is extrauterine is problematic.

Postchemotherapy Fertility

Once cured, regardless of regimen, chemotherapy patients are normally fertile, although after chemotherapy, menopause typically occurs about 3 years earlier than normal.[64]

METASTATIC DISEASE
Pulmonary Disease

Approximately 10% of patients will have a positive chest radiograph at presentation. Unless individual lesions are greater than 2 cm they can be observed as long as there is no other sign of metastatic disease and the hCG titer continues to decline appropriately. Patients with lesions larger than 2 cm are unlikely to spontaneously resolve and therefore should be treated. The chest film may remain radiologically positive for as long as several years after the hCG titer has normalized. If the chest film is normal, there is very little likelihood that there is disease elsewhere, specifically brain or liver. Therefore, in the absence of specific symptoms to suggest metastatic disease, imaging of brain or abdomen is not indicated when the chest radiograph is normal.

A computed tomographic scan of the lung is positive in 10% to 25% of asymptomatic patients who have a negative chest film. Several studies have suggested that these micrometastatic lesions do not confer a higher risk of distant disease, presumably because this small-volume disease can still be cleared by maternal immune surveillance mechanisms.[65] On the other hand, a recent report from Sheffield revealed that, of 192 patients with GTN, 52 had a normal chest radiograph and a positive computed tomographic scan. Of those whose risk score remained low-risk, even when the computed tomographic scan result was incorporated into the risk score, 27% failed first line treatment. Additionally, of 20 patients whose disease became high-risk when the computed tomography findings were incorporated into the risk score, 70% needed a regimen change, suggesting that computed tomographic lung scanning may indeed predict outcome. If this finding is confirmed, computed tomographic scanning of the lung may need to replace simple chest radiograph in the scoring system in the future.[66]

Central Nervous System Disease

Most patients who develop brain metastases had an antecedent term pregnancy or a long interval after the last pregnancy. Patients who present with evidence of intracranial disease and an elevated hCG titer (typically headache, nausea, or visual disturbance) need to be managed aggressively. Most of the deaths from central nervous system metastases occur in the first 14 days after presentation.[67,68] A neurosurgeon should assess the patient as soon as an MR brain scan is completed because some isolated superficial lesions can be effectively treated by surgical resection.[69] Patients need to receive immediate parenteral steroids to minimize cerebral edema that might result in coning if there is bleeding from the lesion(s). Chemotherapy is begun as soon as possible, usually with single agent etoposide at 100 mg/m^2. Seven days later full dose EMACO can be started.[68]

Radiotherapy for acute intracranial disease is controversial. Some TDUs treat these women with 24 to 30 cGy to the whole brain with or without stereotactic boost.[70] However, there is theoretic concern about the long-term neurologic effects.[71] Furthermore, radiation-induced tumor vessel sterilization usually requires up to 14 days to be effective, so rapid control of potential intracranial bleeding is problematic. Stereotactic radiotherapy has been successfully used to treat brain metastases, particularly when the disease is in areas of the brain that cannot be accessed neurosurgically. There was longstanding concern that the blood-brain barrier was relatively impervious to chemotherapeutic drugs, but that may not entirely be the case.[72] Charing Cross, in particular, has used prophylactic intrathecal methotrexate in patients who have a positive chest film on the assumption that these women are most at risk of developing intracranial disease. At Charing Cross, cranial irradiation is not used for patients with brain metastases. Instead, intrathecal methotrexate is given in addition to systemic multiagent chemotherapy for patients with documented brain disease. Based on data from Charing Cross, it seems that if patients survive the initial 14 days after diagnosis, their outlook is substantially better with cure rates in the order of 80%.[68]

Liver/Gastrointestinal Disease

Liver metastases are very uncommon (2.7%). Two-thirds of liver lesions follow a term pregnancy, often over 12 months earlier. Synchronous lung metastases are very common (93%), and concomitant brain metastases are found in 33% of the women. Almost all patients fall into the high-risk category based on the WHO criteria. Liver disease often presents as right upper quadrant pain due to bleeding into the liver parenchyma and distention of the hepatic capsule. These areas cannot be safely treated with radiotherapy, so chemotherapy is the preferred treatment. Regional chemotherapy of the liver and occasionally selective resection have been used but with little success. The curability of patients with liver metastases is approximately

30% but falls to 10% if there are synchronous cerebral metastases. None of the various high-risk chemotherapy regimens seem to offer a significant outcome advantage.[73]

SURGERY FOR GTN

Initial management of GTD should always include uterine curettage rather than medical evacuation (prostaglandin, an antiprogestin, or oxytocin), regardless of the size of the uterus. There is a higher likelihood of incomplete emptying with a nonsurgical approach and an associated 1.7- to 1.9-fold increased risk of persistence requiring chemotherapy.[31] In a small percentage of perimenopausal and postmenopausal women, hysterectomy may be curative and/or may decrease the likelihood that the patient will need chemotherapy, or it may reduce the number of chemotherapy cycles needed to achieve cure.[74]

Reports from the Netherlands, Charing Cross, and the Sheffield TDU suggest that a second therapeutic uterine curettage is of as yet undetermined value. The report from van Trommel and colleagues[75] concluded that 9.4% of women were saved chemotherapy but with an accompanying 2.5% likelihood of uterine perforation. The investigators concluded that second curettage was not useful.[75] In contrast, the Sheffield group determined that, for persistent low-risk disease, patients with an hCG titer between 1500 to 5000 mIU/mL, second curettage rather than immediate chemotherapy was curative for 60% of women. The Sheffield group used a much less rigid definition of persistence that might explain their higher observed cure rate.[76] In another study, the Charing Cross group observed that, if the preevacuation titer exceeded 5000 mIU/mL, 70% of patients went on to require chemotherapy. If the titer exceeded 100,000 mIU/mL the potential benefit was quite small, whereas the risk of uterine perforation and hemorrhage was significant.[34] A phase II trial has been mounted by the GOG to prospectively study the utility of second curettage and the significance of the depth of uterine infiltration.[77]

Selected patients with drug-resistant foci of disease in the uterus, lung, brain, or liver may be cured by hysterectomy or by partial lung, liver, or brain resection.

A small number of women will experience significant vaginal bleeding either during or after treatment. If the blood loss originates from a vaginal or uterine mass, hysterectomy may be required. Selective arterial embolization of a symptomatic residual arteriovenous malformation after normalization of the hCG assay is often curative.[78,79,80,81] This minimally invasive approach preserves fertility in younger aged women and should be offered whenever possible.

DISCUSSION

This disease is very uncommon and is often highly complicated, particularly if the disease is high-risk with or without extrapelvic metastases. In addition, the incidence of the disease is declining, presumably as the nutrition of women in underdeveloped countries improves. It seems that the mortality rate from this disease is greatly improved if the disease is treated in regional TDUs where experience and expertise can be centralized. Such an arrangement also fosters better research, because the number of cases seen in noncentralized areas can be very low. The United Kingdom has had a centralized system for both hCG testing and treatment for 30 years, and they remain the world leaders in clinical and basic science research in this disease. The Netherlands has mandated the "rule of 20," implying that if a clinician manages fewer than 20 cases of a given condition per year they may not have the required expertise to manage specific diseases, and as a result there is regionalization of GTN management.[82] Several European centers have recently formed a collaborative group to standardize data collection, clinical expertise, and research into one common entity, European Trophoblastic Diseases Group. In North America, there are three well-known regional centers: the Brewer TDU at Northwestern University, New England Trophoblastic Disease Center at Brigham and Women's in Boston, and the South East Trophoblastic Disease Center at Duke University, North Carolina, but the clinical material in most centers is declining as more gynecologic oncologists are trained and enter community-based practice. Trophoblastic disease is a very interesting disease and is typically both low-risk and easily cured, so many of these community-based oncologists will treat GTN without registration or referral to a regional center. As a result, there is evidence that high-risk patients are referred regionally later than should be the case and, as a result, outcomes may be less than optimal.

There are incipient efforts to foster international cooperation to ask relevant clinical questions about this rare disease. Particularly for high-risk and recurrent disease, few centers, if any, have the necessary patient volumes to ask important clinical questions in a prospective and randomized setting. So much of the existing literature on the management of GTN is based on single-institution reports that are nonrandomized and therefore open to a variety of potential methodologic biases. What is needed is prospective unbiased data on the effectiveness of the various regimens, particularly for low-risk disease, and randomized information on toxicity and side effects. The term *low-risk* implies easy to cure, cost-efficient, and safe. Several of the current low-risk regimens are both toxic and resource-intense, and their place in the GTN armamentarium needs to be reexamined in prospective, multiinstitution studies.

Another area where progress may occur is in the field of biomarkers. What is the clinical value of hyperglycosylated hCG testing (H-hCG or ITA)? Does an increase in this marker above a threshold value represent impending invasive disease? Can a simple, reliable assay be developed to test for this biomarker? Is hyperglycosylated hCG, with its invasive potential, the reason that hemochorial placentas developed, and is this the primary reason why homo sapiens were able to develop a larger, better oxygenated brain that allowed this species to predominate and flourish above all others?[83,84] The answers to these and other questions await the results of prospective international clinical trials.

REFERENCES

1. Li M, Hertz D. Effect of methotrexate therapy upon choriocarcinoma and chorioadenoma. Proc Soc Exp Biol Med 1956;93:361–6.
2. Yarris J, Hunter A. Roy Hertz, MD. (1909-2002): the cure of choriocarcinoma and its impact on the development of chemotherapy for cancer. Gynecol Oncol 2003;89: 193–98.
3. Zubrod C. Historic milestones in curative chemotherapy. Semin Oncol 1979;6(4): 490–505.
4. Willis L. Treatment of pernicious anaemia of pregnancy with folinic acid. Indian J Med Res 1930;17:727–30.
5. Skibisz M, Tong S. Of leaves and butterflies: how methotrexate came to be the savior of women. Obstet Gynecol 2011;118(5):1169–73.
6. Shih I-M, Kurman R. The pathology of intermediate trophoblastic tumors and tumor-like lesions. Int J Gyncol Pathol 2001;20(1):31–47.
7. Oldt R, Kurman R, Shih I-M. Molecular genetic analysis of placental site trophoblastic tumors and epithelial trophoblastic tumors confirms their trophoblastic origin. Am J Pathol 161 2002;1033–37.

8. Messaed C, Wafaa W, Slim R, et al. NLRP7 in the spectrum of reproductive wastage [abstract]. Presented at the XVI World Congress of the I.S.S.T.D. Budapest, Hungary, October 2011.

9. Betel C, Atri M, Osborne R, et al. Sonographic diagnosis of gestational trophoblastic disease and comparison to retained products of conception. J Ultrasound Med 2006;25(8):985–93.

10. Sarmadi S, Izadi-Mood N, Abbasi A, et al. P57KIP2 immunohistochemical expression: a useful diagnostic tool in discrimination between complete hydatidiform mole and its mimics. Arch Gynecol Obstet 2011;283(4):743–8.

11. Castrillon D, Sun D, Weremowicz S, et al. Discrimination of complete hydatidiform mole from its mimics by immunohistochemistry of the paternally imprinted gene product p57KIP2. Am J Surg Pathol 2001;25(10):1225–30.

12. Fang F, Wan X, Xiang Y. The value of p57KIP2 and PHLDA2 immunohistochemistry and flow cytometry in the differential diagnosis of placental hydropic diseases [abstract]. Presented at the XVI World Congress of the I.S.S.T.D. Budapest, Hungary, October 2011.

13. Chaing S, Faziollahi L, Nguyen A, et al. Diagnosis of hydatidiform moles by polymorphic deletion probe fluorescence in situ hybridization. J Mol Diagn 2011; 13(4):406–15.

14. Ronnett B, DeScipio C, Murphy K. Hydatidiform moles: ancillary techniques to refine diagnosis. Int J Gynecol Pathol 2011;30(2):101–16.

15. Cole L. Human chorionic gonadotropin tests. Expert Rev Mol Diagn 2009;(7):721–47.

16. Cole L, Dutoit S, Higgins T. Total hCG tests. Clin Chem Acta 2011;412(23–24): 2216–22.

17. Cole L. Human chorionic gonadotropin and associated molecules. Expert Rev Mol Diagn 2009;9(1):51–73.

18. Cole L, Khanlian S. Hyperglycosylated hCG: a variant with separate biological functions to regular hCG. Mol Cell Endocrinol 2007;2:260–262:228–36.

19. Cole L, Shahabi S, Butler S, et al. Utility of commonly used commercial human chorionic gonadotropin immunoassays in the diagnosis and management of trophoblastic diseases. Clin Chem 2001;47(2):308–15.

20. Cole L, Kardana A. Discordant results in human chorionic gonadotropin assays. Clin Chem 1992;38(2):263–70.

21. Hwang D, Hancock B. Management of persistent, unexplained, low-level human chorionic gonadotropin elevation: a report of 5 cases. J Reprod Med 2004;49(7): 559–62.

22. Cole L, Khanian S. Inappropriate management of women with persistent low hCG results. J Reprod Med 2004;49(6):423–32.

23. White S, Harvey R, Mitchell H, et al. Characterization of transient benign hCG elevations in women following chemotherapy for GTT. J Obstet Gynaecol 2011;31(2): 169–72.

24. Knight A, Bingemann T, Cole L, et al. Frequent false positive beta human chorionic gonadotropin tests in immunoglobulin A deficiency. Clin Exp Immunol 2005;14(2): 333–7.

25. Cole L. Case report: phantom hCG and phantom choriocarcinoma. Gynecol Oncol 1998;71:325–29.

26. Snyder J, Haymond S, Parvin C, et al. Diagnostic considerations in the measurement of human chorionic gonadotropin in aging women. Clin Chem 2005;51(10):1830–5.

27. Papapetrou P, Anagnostopoulos N. A gonadotropin and alpha-subunit suppression test for the assessment of the ectopic production of human chorionic gonadotropin and its subunits after the menopause. J Clin Endocrinol Metab 1985;60(6):1187–95.

28. Boafo-Yirenki A, Everard J, Tidy J, et al. A conservative approach in persistent low-level elevation of serum beta-human chorionic gonadotropin following chemotherapy for gestational trophoblastic neoplasia. J Reprod Med 2009;54(5):288–90.

29. Agarwal R, Harding V, Alifrangis C, et al. Uterine artery pulsatility index (UAPI) is a predictor of methotrexate resistance in low-risk GTN (LR-GTN) independent of the FIGO score: a new standard of care? [abstract]. Presented at the XVI World Congress of the I.S.S.T.D. Budapest, Hungary, October 2011.

30. Price J, Lo C, Abdi S, et al. Is there a role for CT thorax scanning when assessing gestational trophoblastic neoplasia? [abstract]. Presented at the XVII World Congress of the I.S.S.T.D. Budapest, Hungary, October 2011.

31. Tidy J, Gillespie A, Bright N, et al. Gestational trophoblastic disease: a study of mode of evacuation and subsequent need for treatment with chemotherapy. Gynecol Oncol 2000;78:309–12.

32. Hammond C, Borchert L, Tyrey I, et al. Treatment of metastatic disease: good and poor prognosis. Am J Obstet Gynecol 1973;115:451–57.

33. Hassadia A, Kew F, Tidy J, et al. Ectopic gestational trophoblastic disease: have we learned from previous experience [abstract]. Presented at the XVI World Congress of the I.S.S.T.D. Budapest, Hungary, October 2011.

34. McGrath S, Short D, Harvey R, et al. The management and outcome of women with post-hydatidiform mole "low-risk" gestational trophoblastic neoplasia, but hCG levels in excess of 100,000 IU/L. Br J Cancer 2010;(102);810–4.

35. Osborne R, Filiaci V, Schink J, et al. Phase III trial of weekly methotrexate and pulsed dactinomycin for low-risk gestational trophoblastic neoplasia: a gynecologic oncology group study. J Clin Oncol 2011;29(7):825–31.

36. Bagshawe K, Dent E, Newlands E, et al. The role of low-dose methotrexate and folinic acid on gestational trophoblastic tumours. Br J Obstet Gynaecol 1989;96:795–802.

37. Hoestra A, Lurain J, Rademaker A, et al. Gestational trophoblastic neoplasia: treatment outcomes. Obstet Gynecol 2008;112(2 Pt 1):251–8.

38. Gilani M, Yarandi F, Eftekhar Z, et al. Comparison of pulse methotrexate and pulse dactinomycin in the treatment of low-risk gestational trophoblastic neoplasia. Aust N Z J Obstet Gyneacol 2005;45(2):161–4.

39. Gleeson N, Finan M, Fiorica J, et al. Nonmetastatic gestational trophoblastic disease. Weekly methotrexate compared with 8-day methotrexate-folinic acid. Eur J Gynaecol Oncol 1993;14(6):461–5.

40. Kang W, Choi H, Kim S. Weekly methotrexate (50mg/m^2) without dose escalation as a primary regimen for low-risk gestational trophoblastic neoplasia. Gynecol Oncol 2010;117(3):477–80.

41. Mousavi A, Cheraghi F, Yarandi F, et al. Comparison of pulsed dactinomycin versus 5-day methotrexate for the treatment of low-risk gestational trophoblastic disease. Int J Gynaecol Obstet 2012;116(1):39–42.

42. Osborne R. Intermediate risk disease: have we made a mistake? [abstract]. Presented at the XVI World Congress of the I.S.S.T.D. Budapest, Hungary, October 2011.

43. Wong L, Ngan H, Cheng K, et al. Methotrexate infusion for low-risk gestational trophoblastic neoplasia. Am J Obstet Gynecol 2000;183(6):1579–82.

44. Elit L, Covens A, Osborne R, et al. High-dose methotrexate for gestational trophoblastic disease. Gynecol Oncol 1994;54(3):282–7.

45. Hitchins R, Holden L, Newlands E, et al. Single agent etoposide in gestational trophoblastic tumours. Experience at Charing Cross Hospital 1978–1987. Eur J Clin Oncol 1988;24(6):1041–6.

46. Eiriksson L, Wells T, Steed H, et al. Combined methotrexate-dactinomycin: an effective therapy for low-risk gestational trophoblastic neoplasia. Gynecol Oncol 2012;124(3):553–7.
47. Limpongsanurak S. Prophylactic dactinomycin for high-risk hydatidiform mole. J Reprod Med 2001;46(2):110–6.
48. Uberti E, Diestel M, Guimaraes F, et al. Single-dose dactinomycin: efficacy in the prophylaxis of postmolar gestational trophoblastic neoplasia in adolescents with high-risk hydatidiform mole. Gynecol Oncol 2006;102(2):325–32.
49. Goldstein D, Berkowitz R. Prophylactic chemotherapy of complete molar pregnancy. Semin Oncol 1995;22:157–160.
50. Roberts J, Lurain J. Treatment of low-risk metastatic gestational trophoblastic tumors with single-agent chemotherapy. Am J Obstet Gynecol 1996;174(6):1917–23.
51. Osborne R. What is the best regimen for low-risk gestational trophoblastic neoplasia? A review. J Reprod Med 2004;49(8):602–16.
52. Alazzam M, Tidy J, Hancock B, et al. First line chemotherapy in low risk gestational trophoblastic neoplasia. Cochrane Database Syst Rev 2009;21(1):CD007102.
53. Soper J, Mutch D, Schink J, et al. Diagnosis and treatment of gestational trophoblastic disease: ACOG Practice Bulletin No. 53. Gynecol Oncol 2004;93(3):575–85.
54. Goldstein D, Garner E, Feltmate C, et al. The role of repeat uterine evacuation in the management of persistent gestational trophoblastic disease. Gynecol Oncol 2004; 95(3):421–22.
55. Massad L, Abu-Rustum N, Lee S, et al. Poor compliance with post-molar surveillance and treatment protocols by indigent women. Obstet Gynecol 2000;96:940–4.
56. Kerkmeijer L, Wielsma S, Massuager L, et al. Recurrent gestational trophoblastic disease after hCG normalization following hydatidiform mole in The Netherlands. Gynecol Oncol 2007;106(1):142–6.
57. Rotmensch J, Rosenshein N, Block B. Comparison of human chorionic gonadotropin regression in molar pregnancies and post-molar nonmetastatic gestational trophoblastic neoplasia. Gynecol Oncol 1988;29(1):82–6.
58. Shigematsu T, Hirakawa T, Yahata H, et al. Identification of persistent trophoblastic diseases based on a human chorionic gonadotropin regression curve by means of a stepwise piecewise linear regression analysis after the evacuation of uneventful moles. Gynecol Oncol 1998;71(3):376–80.
59. Kerkmeijer L, Thomas C, Harvey R, et al. External validation of serum hCG cutoff levels for prediction of resistance to single-agent chemotherapy in patients with persistent trophoblastic disease. Brit J Cancer 2009;(100):979–84.
60. Dobson L, Lorigan P, Coleman R, et al. Persistent gestational trophoblastic disease: results of MEA (methotrexate, etoposide and dactinomycin) as first-line chemotherapy in high risk disease and EA (etoposide and dactinomycin) as second-line therapy for low risk disease. Brit J Cancer 2000;82(9):1547–52.
61. Coleman R, Tidy J, Hancock B. Single agent dactinomycin as second line low risk treatment for gestational trophoblastic neoplasia: a decade of experience at the Sheffield Centre for Trophoblastic Disease, United Kingdom [abstract] Presented at the XVI World Congress of the I.S.S.T.D. Budapest, Hungary, October 2011.
62. Newlands E, Bower M, Holden C, et al. Management of resistant gestational trophoblastic tumours. J Reprod Med 1998;43(2):111–8.
63. Osborne R, Covens A, Gerulath A, et al. Successful salvage of relapsed high-risk gestational trophoblastic neoplasia patients using a novel paclitaxel-containing doublet. J Reprod Med 2005;54(3):320–7.
64. Bower M, Rustin G, Newlands E. Chemotherapy for gestational trophoblastic tumours hastens menopause by 3 years. Eur J Cancer 1998;34(3):1204–7.

65. Ngan H, Chan F, Au V, et al. Clinical outcome of micrometastasis in the lung in stage 1A persistent gestational trophoblastic disease. Gynecol Oncol 1998;70:192–4.

66. Darby S, Jolley I, Pennington S, et al. Does chest CT matter in the staging of GTN? Gynecol Oncol 2009;112(1):155–60.

67. Athanassiou A, Begent R, Newlands E, et al. Central nervous system metastases of choriocarcinoma: 23 years experience at Charing Cross Hospital. Cancer 1983;52: 1728–35.

68. Newlands E, Holden L, Seckl M, et al. Management of brain metastases in patients with high-risk gestational trophoblastic tumours. J Reprod Med 2002;47(6):465–71.

69. Yang J, Xiang Y, Yang X, et al. Emergency craniotomy in patients with intracranial metastatic gestational trophoblastic tumor. Int J Gynaecol Oncol 2005;89(1):35–8.

70. Neubauer N, Latif N, Kalakota K, et al. Brain metastases in gestational trophoblastic neoplasia (GTN): an update [abstract]. Presented at the XVI World Congress of the I.S.S.T.D. Budapest, Hungary, October 2011.

71. Doyle D, Einhorn L. Delayed effects of whole brain radiotherapy in germ cell tumor patients with central nervous system metastases. Int J Oncol Biol Phys 2008;70(5): 1361–4.

72. Azar J, Schneider B, Einhorn L. Is the blood-brain barrier relevant in metastatic germ cell tumor? Int J Radiat Oncol Biol Phys 2007;69(1):163–6.

73. Crawford R, Newlands E, Rustin G, et al. Gestational trophoblastic disease with liver metastases: the Charing Cross experience. Br J Obstet Gynaecol 1997;104(1): 105–9.

74. Clark R, Nevadunsky N, Ghosh S, et al. The evolving role of hysterectomy in gestational trophoblastic neoplasia at the New England Trophoblastic Disease Center. J Reprod Med 2010;55(5–6):194–8.

75. van Trommel N, Massuager L, Verheijen R, et al. The curative effect of a second curettage in persistent trophoblastic disease: a retrospective cohort study. Gynecol Oncol 2005;99:6–13.

76. Pezeshki M, Hancock B, Silcocks P, et al. The role of repeat uterine evacuation in the management of persistent gestational trophoblastic disease. Gynecol Oncol 2004; 95(3):423–29.

77. Osborne R, Filiaci V, Schink D, et al. The role of second curettage in the primary management of persistent gestational trophoblastic neoplasia; a Gynecologic Oncology Group study.

78. Garner E, Meyerovitz M, Goldstein D, et al. Successful term pregnancy after selective arterial embolization of symptomatic arteriovenous malformation in the setting of gestational trophoblastic tumor. Gynecol Oncol 2003;88:69–72.

79. Cockshott W, Hendrickse J. Persistent arteriovenous fistulae following chemotherapy of malignant trophoblastic disease. Radiology 1967;88:329–33.

80. Stern W, Lopez F, Herzig N. Persistent angiographic abnormalities after cure of malignant trophoblastic disease. Radiology 1968;91:1019–21.

81. Method M, Hirschfield M, Averette H. Angiographic-guided embolization of metastatic invasive mole. Gynecol Oncol 1996;61:442–5.

82. Massuager L. Developments in the management of gestational trophoblastic disease in the Netherlands. Are we on the right track? [abstract]. Presented at the XVI World Congress of the I.S.S.T.D. Budapest, Hungary, October 2011.

83. Cole L. HCG and hyperglycosylated hCG in the establishment of hemochorial placentation. J Reprod Immunol 2009;82(2):112–8.

84. Cole L, Khanlian S, Kohorn E. Evolution of the human brain, chorionic gonadotropins and hemochorial implantation of the placenta: insights into the origin of pregnancy failures, preeclampsia and choriocarcinoma. J Reprod Med 2008;53(8):549–57.

Vulvar and Vaginal Cancer

Jori S. Carter, MD, Levi S. Downs Jr, MD, MS*

KEYWORDS

- Vulvar cancer • Vaginal cancer • Epidemiology • Pathology • Treatment
- Prognosis

KEY POINTS

- The incidence of vulvar dysplasia is increasing, particularly in women aged 20 to 35 years, many of whom have a history of genital dysplasia at other sites.
- Vulvar cancer is primarily a disease of the elderly. Most can be cured with surgery and adjuvant radiotherapy. Sentinel lymph node sampling is becoming the new standard of care for women with early stage vulvar cancer.
- Vaginal cancer a is rare cancer affecting elderly women. Treatment involves a combination of external beam radiotherapy and brachytherapy with surgical resection in a small subset of patients. Despite these treatments, prognosis is poor.

This article describes epidemiology, diagnosis, staging, pathology, management, and prognosis for vulvar and vaginal cancers.

VULVAR CANCER

The vulva consists of the external female genital organs that include the mons pubis, labia minora, labia majora, clitoris, vaginal vestibule containing the Skene and Bartholin glands, and the urethral meatus. Squamous cell carcinomas (SCC) make up 85% to 95% of invasive vulvar carcinomas. The remaining 5% to 15% are adenocarcinoma, basal cell carcinoma, sarcoma, melanoma, and undifferentiated carcinoma.[1]

Epidemiology

In the United States, invasive vulvar cancer will be diagnosed in an estimated 4340 women in 2011, making up 4% of female genital tract cancers and .6% of all cancers in women.[2] Most cases occur in white postmenopausal women, and the incidence has risen steadily by 20% over the last 40 years.[3]

The authors have nothing to disclose.
Division of Gynecologic Oncology, Department of Obstetrics, Gynecology, and Women's Health, University of Minnesota Medical School, 420 Delaware Street Southeast, MMC 395, Minneapolis, MN 55455, USA
* Corresponding author.
E-mail address: downs008@umn.edu

Obstet Gynecol Clin N Am 39 (2012) 213–231
http://dx.doi.org/10.1016/j.ogc.2012.04.002
0889-8545/12/$ – see front matter © 2012 Elsevier Inc. All rights reserved.

The etiologic factor responsible for invasive vulvar cancer is not clear, because it is associated with both chronic vulvar inflammatory lesions and vulvar intraepithelial neoplasia (VIN). SCC is associated with adjacent VIN in up to 85%, and lichen sclerosis in 15% to 40% of cases.[4] Human papillomavirus (HPV) DNA has been isolated in 20% to 60% of invasive vulvar carcinoma, and its role in pathogenesis, or the natural history of infection, may be different from cervical cancer.[5,6] HPV type 16 is the most commonly isolated HPV type in vulvar cancer. HPV 16 or 33 is reported in 71% of warty carcinomas, in 100% of basaloid carcinomas, and in only 4% of invasive differentiated (keratinizing) type vulvar carcinoma.[7] HPV-associated vulvar cancer is more common in women younger than 45 years and more often diagnosed at an earlier stage, compared with that associated with vulvar inflammatory disease, which is seen more commonly in older women and often diagnosed at a later stage.[8] The differentiated (keratinizing) type is usually HPV-negative and frequently associated with p53 mutations.[9] This association supports the theory that there are two different causes for vulvar carcinoma.

Noninvasive Vulvar Disease

Benign vulvar diseases are defined by the International Society for the Study on Vulvar Disease (ISSVD) and have gone through changes of terminology over the years. In 1976, the ISSVD classified benign vulvar disease into categories including vulvar dystrophies (including hyperplastic dystrophy, lichen sclerosis, and mixed dystrophy), vulvar atypia, Paget disease, and squamous cell carcinoma in situ.[10] The classification system was revised in 1989 when the term *vulvar dystrophy* was replaced with *nonneoplastic epithelial disorders of skin and mucosa* (including lichen sclerosis, squamous cell hyperplasia, and other dermatoses), and the terms *atypia* and *in situ lesions* were replaced with *vulvar intraepithelial neoplasia*. VIN was graded 1 to 3 for mild, moderate, or severe/in situ dysplasia, respectively.[11] In 2004, the category of VIN I was removed because of low interobserver reliability, and the differentiation between types of VIN was included,[12] listed as follows:

I. VIN, usual type
   a. VIN, warty type
   b. VIN, basaloid type
   c. VIN, mixed (warty/basaloid) type
II. VIN, differentiated type
III. VIN, unclassified type.

Vulvar intraepithelial neoplasia

The incidence of vulvar dysplasia is drastically increasing with a rate of .56 to 2.86 per 100,000 women,[3] and it is becoming more common in younger women aged 20 to 35 years.[13] Approximately 50% of women with vulvar dysplasia have dysplasia at other sites involving the genital tract, most commonly the cervix. Usual type is associated with HPV infection (particularly HPV16) and cigarette smoking, is often multifocal, and has a pathogenesis similar to cervical dysplasia. Differentiated VIN is generally not associated with HPV infection and is morphologically similar to invasive squamous cell carcinoma in appearance.

Most women with vulvar dysplasia are asymptomatic, and the diagnosis is made with a high index of suspicion. When symptomatic, pruritus is common. Other symptoms include burning, dyspareunia, erythema, edema, and pain. Lesions have a raised surface and are pigmented in 25% of cases.[14] Half of VIN lesions become acetowhite after the application of 5% acetic acid, which should be applied for at least 5 minutes before examination. Thorough examination with the colposcope should follow application of acetic acid, and punch biopsies should be taken of each suspicious lesion.

Goals of treating VIN are to prevent progression to invasive cancer, to relieve symptoms, and to preserve normal anatomy. Treatment options include topical agents, laser ablation, and surgical excision. Topical agents are ideal for younger patients, recurrent disease after surgical excision, or those who are not surgical candidates. Imiquimod, a topical immune-response modifier that is effective through the release of local cytokine production and cell-mediated immunity, is the most commonly used topical agent for the treatment of VIN and results in at least a partial response in approximately 80% of patients after treatment for 16 weeks.[15,16] The agent 5-fluorouracil (5-FU) has response rates up to 75%; however, the local side effects are more common, with inflammation lasting for up to 2 weeks after the completion of a 6- to 10-week course.[17] CO_2 laser ablation is useful in the treatment of multifocal VIN, where a large area of the vulva can be treated with this modality resulting in proper wound healing and good cosmetic outcome. Success rates after a single laser treatment are approximately 75%.[18] Surgical excision is the standard treatment of choice for VIN because it allows for thorough histologic examination to rule out invasive carcinoma.

Lichen sclerosis

Lichen sclerosis is the most common inflammatory, noninfectious disorder of the vulva. It most often occurs in postmenopausal white women and its cause is unknown. Vulvar pruritus is the most common presenting symptom. There may be minimal skin changes on examination, but as inflammation progresses, erythematous papules may become confluent and form scaling. Over time, atrophy and hypopigmented, fine, cigarette-paper–type wrinkling may develop, resulting in resorption of the labia and narrowing of the introitus.[19] Treatment includes vulvar hygiene and topical corticosteroid creams. Lichen sclerosis may be associated with VIN (differentiated type) and vulvar carcinoma in 15% to 40% of cases.[4] Biopsy is warranted for diagnosis to ensure the correct diagnosis and to rule out associated invasive disease.

Lichen planus

Lichen planus is a dermatosis most commonly seen in women over 40.[20] When symptomatic, women present with burning and pruritus. It is often associated with similar lacelike plaques in the oral or vaginal mucosa. Histologic appearance is variable, but diagnosis is confirmed by the presence of a bandlike chronic lymphocytic inflammatory infiltrate and the presence of colloid bodies formed as a result of degenerated keratinocytes.[21] Lichen planus can evolve into erosive vulvar disease, which has been associated with invasive vulvar squamous cell carcinoma.[22]

Paget disease

Extramammary Paget disease of the vulva has a distinct clinical presentation and appears as eczematous, red, weeping lesions on the vulva, most commonly seen in older white women. Cutaneous-type Paget disease may rarely be associated with underlying cutaneous adenocarcinoma.[23] Paget cells are large cells with a prominent nucleus with coarse chromatin, a prominent nucleolus, and foamy-appearing cytoplasm. Wide local excision is required for treatment, which commonly results in positive margins, because epithelial involvement often extends beyond what is visible on examination. Recurrence is common, and many patients undergo repetitive procedures.

Table 1	
FIGO staging criteria for carcinoma of the vulva (2009)	
Stage I	Tumor confined to the vulva
IA	Lesions ≤2 cm in size, confined to the vulva or perineum and with stromal invasion ≤1 mm,[a] no nodal metastasis
IB	Lesions >2 cm in size or with stromal invasion >1.0 mm,[a] confined to the vulva or perineum, with negative nodes
Stage II	Tumor of any size with extension to adjacent perineal structures (1/3 lower urethra, 1/3 lower vagina, anus) with negative nodes
Stage III	Tumor of any size with or without extension to adjacent perineal structures (1/3 lower urethra, 1/3 lower vagina, anus) with positive inguinofemoral lymph nodes
IIIA	(i) with 1 lymph node metastasis (≥5 mm), or (ii) 1–2 lymph node metastasis(es) (<5 mm)
IIIB	(i) with 2 or more lymph node metastases (≥5 mm), or (ii) 3 or more lymph metastases (<5 mm)
IIIC	With positive nodes with extracapsular spread
Stage IV	Tumor invades other regional (2/3 upper urethra, 2/3 upper vagina), or distant structures
IVA	Tumor invades any of the following: (i) upper urethra and or vaginal mucosa, bladder mucosa, rectal mucosa, or fixed to pelvic bone, or (ii) fixed or ulcerated inguinofemoral lymph nodes
IVB	Any distant metastasis including pelvic lymph nodes

[a] The depth of invasion is defined as the measurement of the tumor from the epithelial-stromal junction of the adjacent most superficial dermal papilla to the deepest point of invasion.

From Pecorelli S. Revised FIGO staging for carcinoma of the vulva, cervix, and endometrium. Int J Gynaecol Obstet 2009;105:103–4; with permission.

Diagnosis of Invasive Vulvar Carcinoma

Approximately 50% of vulvar cancer cases present with pruritus and a visible lesion.[24] Women may otherwise have pain, bleeding, or be asymptomatic. Many women have symptoms for up to 6 months, and 30% have had up to three medical consultations and have used topical medications before a tissue diagnosis of cancer is made.[25] Suspicious lesions or symptoms merit a tissue biopsy that includes the underlying stroma. This procedure is most commonly performed in the office setting with local anesthesia and a Keyes punch biopsy.

Staging

In 1988, the Federation International de Gynecology et Obstetrique (FIGO) implemented a surgical staging system that emphasized the status of inguinofemoral lymph node involvement, in which unilateral lymph node metastases defined stage III, and bilateral lymph node metastases defined stage IV disease.[26] In 1995, FIGO made revisions dividing stage I into subdivisions to reflect the low risk of inguinofemoral lymph node metastases in patients with depth of invasion no greater than 1 mm and tumor diameter less than 2 cm.[27] The most recent revisions in 2009 (**Table 1**) implemented three major changes to this system: (1) stages I and II have been combined into stage IB, while keeping the criteria for stage IA the same to account for its negligible risk of lymph node metastasis; (2) stage II includes a lesion of any size that has adjacent spread; (3) the number of involved nodes and the morphology of

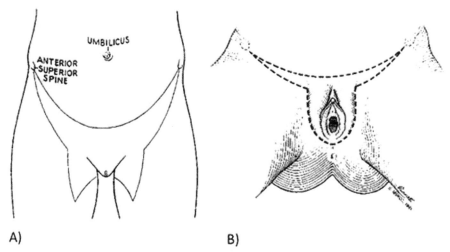

Fig. 1. Traditional en bloc incisional techniques for radical vulvectomy and bilateral inguinofemoral lymphadenectomy. (*A*) Butterfly incision for radical vulvectomy with bilateral inguinofemoral lymphadenectomy which uses convex "wings" over the groins and around the anus to facilitate closure of the defect. (*From* Way S. Malignant disease of the female genital tract. New York: Churchill Livingstone, 1951; with permission.) (*B*) Longhorn incision limits skin resection over the groin to reduce wound breakdown, which uses an arcing superior incision from the lateral margins groins across the mons pubis and the lateral incisions are at the labiocrural folds, and the perianal incision allows resection of the perineal body. (*From* Moore DH, Koh WJ, McGuire WP. Vulva. In: Barakat RR, Markman M, Randall ME, editors. Principles and practice of gynecologic oncology, 5th edition. Baltimore (MD): Lippincott Williams & Williams; 2009; with permission.)

involved nodes are taken into account in stage III, whereas the bilaterally of positive nodes has been discounted.[28]

Pathology

Squamous cell carcinoma

SCC accounts for 85% to 95% of invasive carcinomas of the vulva. Depth of invasion determines the risk of inguinofemoral lymph node metastases, which is approximately 30% overall.[29] Historically, 5-mm depth of invasion defined microinvasion and conferred a 15% to 20% risk of inguinofemoral lymph node involvement. The frequency of lymph node metastasis rises dramatically when depth of invasion is beyond 1 mm.[30,31] The ISSVD therefore defined superficially invasive, stage IA vulvar carcinoma as a single lesion measuring 2 cm or less in diameter and with a depth of invasion of 1 mm or less.[32] Depth of invasion is defined by the Wilkinson method A, which is described as the measurement of the tumor from the epithelial-stromal junction of the most adjacent superficial dermal papilla to the deepest point of invasion **(Fig. 1)**.[31]

In addition to stage and tumor depth of invasion, important pathologic criteria include the presence or absence of vascular space invasion, growth pattern (confluent, compact/pushing, or fingerlike), grade, and histologic type of the tumor.[33] Confluent growth is generally deeply invasive, compact is well-circumscribed and well-differentiated, and fingerlike is poorly differentiated and associated with vascular space involvement. The Gynecologic Oncology Group (GOG) established a well-defined grading system for

SCC of the vulva for grades 1 to 3. Grade 1 tumors are well-differentiated without the presence of any poorly differentiated components. Grade 2 contains both well-differentiated and poorly differentiated components, with the poorly differentiated components not exceeding one half of the tumor. Grade 3 tumors contain both components, with the poorly differentiated component making up greater than one-half of the tumor.[33] The histologic types of vulvar squamous cell carcinoma include the following common types: keratinizing squamous cell, nonkeratinizing squamous cell, basaloid, and warty (condylomatous). The less common types include acantholytic SCC, SCC with giant cells, spindle cell SCC, SCC with sarcomalike stroma, sebaceous carcinoma, verrucous carcinoma, and other rare types.[34]

Verrucous carcinoma

Verrucous carcinoma is a distinct variant of SCC and is associated with HPV type 6. On clinical examination, there are multiple large exophytic, condylomatous lesions. It is usually unresponsive to usual methods of therapy, locally destructive, and rarely lethal. A variant of verrucous carcinoma has been termed *Buschke-Lowenstein* by the World Health Organization. These tumors are well-differentiated and have prominent acanthosis and parakeratosis, with lymphocytic infiltration within the dermal papillae. Treatment is by wide local excision, and it has an excellent prognosis.

Basal cell

Basal cell carcinoma of the vulva makes up only 2% to 4% of vulvar carcinomas, is usually seen in elderly white women, and is often confined to the labia majora. Prognosis is excellent and only wide local excision is necessary. The differential diagnosis includes basaloid SCC, which is locally aggressive and may metastasize; however, it can be differentiated by basaloid SCC's lack of characteristic basal cell growth pattern, the presence of intracellular bridges, and greater nuclear pleomorphism.

Adenocarcinoma

Adenocarcinomas are rare tumors of the vulva. Most cases arise in the Bartholin gland, and 12% of cases are invasive Paget.[23] Bartholin gland carcinoma generally has a poor prognosis because it is deeply infiltrative and difficult to detect in early growth. Approximately 50% are associated with lymph node metastases at the time of diagnosis.[35] Bartholin gland carcinoma is rarely seen in young women, but any enlarged Bartholin cyst/mass detected in a woman over 50 years should be excised and sent for a pathologic diagnosis.

Melanoma

Malignant melanoma of the vulva accounts for 9% of primary malignancies on the vulva. Mean age of diagnosis is 55 years, and it is most common in white women.[36] The tumor may be pigmented, but 25% are amelanotic. Symptoms at presentation include bleeding, pruritus, pain, or dysuria. There are three subtypes: superficial spreading, nodular, and mucosal lentiginous. Mucosal lentiginous is the most common type on the vulva. Malignant melanomas can be histologically diagnosed by the expression of S100 antigen, HMB-45, and Melan-A. The absence of cytokeratin and carcinoembryonic antigen (CEA) will differentiate it from Paget disease. The most important pathologic prognostic factor is the depth of invasion and tumor thickness, as described by Clark level. Local and distant metastases are common, and survival is generally poor.

Sarcoma

Vulvar sarcomas consist of leiomyosarcoma, malignant fibrous histiocytoma, epithelioid sarcoma, and malignant rhabdoid tumor. Leiomyosarcoma is the most common type of primary vulvar sarcoma and is generally larger than 5 cm, localized, and treated by wide local excision. Malignant fibrous histiocytoma is an extremely aggressive tumor associated with early distant metastases. Epithelioid sarcoma occurs in younger women and has slow but progressive growth with a high propensity for local recurrence. Finally, malignant rhabdoid tumors are similar to epithelioid sarcomas, have frequent local recurrence, and have a dismal prognosis associated with distant metastases.

Management of Squamous Cell Carcinoma of the Vulva

Stage IA

Stage IA vulvar carcinoma is considered superficially invasive, has 1 mm or less invasion and less than 2 cm maximum diameter. Because of the negligible risk of lymph node metastases in these patients, they can be managed with wide local excision or radical local excision with 1- to 2-cm negative margins.[24,37] If final pathology result reveals deeper than 1-mm invasion, a second procedure can be scheduled to perform inguinofemoral lymph node dissection (with radical local excision or radical hemivulvectomy if a wide local excision was performed initially).

Stage IB-III

Surgery When greater than 1 mm of invasion is present, superficial and deep inguinofemoral lymph node dissection in combination with radical resection of the vulvar tumor should be performed. Even when groin lymph nodes are not clinically suspicious for metastases, there is a 36% chance that metastasis is present.[38] A randomized study showed that overall survival is improved when lymph node dissection is performed at time of vulvectomy compared with primary radiation of the groins, with a subsequent groin relapse rate of 0% versus 18%, respectively.[39] Therefore, inguinofemoral lymph node dissection is the standard of care when vulvar carcinoma is invasive beyond 1 mm. This dissection was historically performed by en bloc approach with a total radical vulvectomy and bilateral inguinofemoral lymph nodes dissection through butterfly or longhorn incision. The longhorn technique was developed to reduce the amount of skin resection over the groin, but both methods are associated with a 50% rate of wound breakdown (**Fig. 2**).

More conservative procedures using a three-incision approach are associated with reduced morbidity and have been the standard of care for the last several decades.[40] A localized radical excision yields similar rates of local recurrence compared with radical vulvectomy.[41,42] Small focal vulvar cancers can be resected while sparing the rest of the vulva. This procedure is often called *radical wide excision, radical local excision, modified radical vulvectomy,* or *radical hemivulvectomy,* defined as a resection that allows for a 1- to 2-cm margin around the lesion and that is carried to the deep perineal fascia of the urogenital diaphragm. Inguinofemoral lymph node dissection should be performed through separate incisions made over the inguinal ligament. The superficial (8–10 lymph nodes that lie superficial to the cribriform fascia surrounding the saphenous vein) and deep (3–5 lymph nodes medial to the femoral vein beneath the cribriform fascia that continue in the pelvis as the external iliac lymph nodes) lymph nodes should be removed.

Unilateral vulvar tumors, defined as tumors greater than 1 cm from the midline, are at low risk for contralateral lymph node metastases; therefore, it is safe to perform only an ipsilateral inguinofemoral lymph node dissection. Lesions that are in the area of the clitoris and anterior labia minora often have bilateral lymphatic drainage and should have bilateral inguinofemoral node dissection.

Sentinel lymph node mapping and biopsy Over the last decade, sentinel lymph node biopsy has increasingly been used for vulvar cancer as a method to decrease the incidence of wound breakdown and lymphedema associated with inguinofemoral lymph node dissection. The sentinel lymph nodes for vulvar cancer are the superficial inguinofemoral lymph nodes. If these nodes are negative for malignancy, the risk of metastasis to the deep inguinofemoral lymph nodes is insignificant.[43] The first study of sentinel lymph node biopsy for vulvar cancer demonstrated feasibility for detection of the sentinel node using intraoperative isosulfan blue dye.[44] When a technique combining preoperative injection of radioactive tracer (technetium-99 sulfur colloid) and intraoperative blue dye (isosulfan blue or methylene blue) is used, sentinel lymph node biopsy is associated with nearly a 100% negative predictive value.[45]

Sentinel lymph node biopsy is an alternative to complete inguinal lymphadenectomy when tumors have greater than 1-mm invasion, are not greater than 4 cm in size, and groins are clinically negative.[46] The current recommendation is for gynecologic oncologists to establish competency in identifying the sentinel lymph node by following the biopsy with a complete inguinal lymphadenectomy for 10 consecutive cases, with correct identification of the sentinel lymph node and no false-negative rate.[47] An ongoing study by the GOG is evaluating the accuracy of the identification of the sentinel node using a combination of intraoperative blue dye and preoperative radioactive tracer.[48]

Radiation Adjuvant radiation therapy should be given to bilateral groins and lower pelvis for patients who have groin lymph nodes with occult metastases of two or more

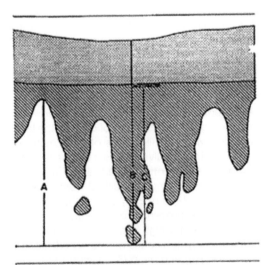

Fig. 2. Methods for measurement for vulvar superficially invasive carcinomas. Method A measures the depth of invasion from the most superficial dermal-epidermal junction of the most superficial adjacent dermal papillae. Method B measures from the surface to the deepest point of invasion. Method C measures from the granular layer to the deepest point of invasion. (*Courtesy of* Edward J Wilkinson MD, Gainesville, FL.)

lymph nodes, macroscopic involvement, or extracapsular spread. The primary tumor bed is generally not given directed radiation therapy because local recurrences are usually cured with local excision,[49] unless the primary tumor pathology shows high-risk prognostic factors such as high tumor grade, presence of lymph vascular space invasion, and positive margins.[50]

It is unusual for vulvar cancer to present initially with clinically palpable inguinal lymph node metastases. Clinical evaluation of the superficial inguinal nodes is inaccurate, with more than 20% of palpably enlarged inguinal lymph nodes resulting in negative histology.[51] Clinically enlarged lymph nodes should have fine-needle biopsy performed to confirm the suspected diagnosis. If the nodes are positive and large, they should be selectively surgically excised (without a full inguinofemoral lymph node dissection) before starting chemoradiation to increase the complete response rate of external beam radiation therapy. Women with extensive, fixed, matted, or ulcerated inguinal lymph node involvement can be treated with concurrent external beam chemoradiation (cisplatin plus 5-FU), with a high probability of having subsequent inguinal dissection, and 32% chance of having no pathologic residual nodal disease.[52]

Stage IVA

Historically, when vulvar disease involves the anus, rectum, rectovaginal septum, proximal urethra, or bladder, primary exenterative procedure resulting in a colostomy and/or urinary diversion was performed. Women who were managed this way had long-term survival rates of up to 70%.[53] The operative morbidity is significant, the frequency of nodal metastases that requires adjuvant therapy is high, and there is a significant impact on quality of life because of loss of sexual and excretive function. Primary chemotherapy cisplatin plus 5-FU with concurrent radiation therapy followed by resection is an alternative to a primary exenterative procedure based on a phase II trial of locally advanced (stage III and IVA) squamous cell carcinoma of the vulva that was not amenable to surgical resection without an exenterative procedure. Of 71 patients in the study who received preoperative chemoradiation, 46.5% had no clinical residual disease, and 31% of these patients had no residual tumor in the pathologic specimen. Only 2.8% had unresectable disease remaining after chemoradiation. After a median follow-up of 50 months, 5 patients underwent pelvic exenteration for recurrent disease, and 55% of patients were alive without evidence of disease.[54]

Based on the success of cervical cancer treatment using cisplatin-containing chemoradiation,[55] and the elimination of treatment breaks, a trial in vulvar cancer using cisplatin concurrent with radiation therapy (180 cGy daily $\times$ 32 fractions = 5760 cGy), resulting in a 20% higher total radiation dose. Preliminary results showed a 64% complete response rate.[56] Pending the final results, clinical practice will likely adapt this regimen of weekly cisplatin with concurrent radiation therapy.

Initial treatment with chemoradiation should be followed with surgical resection in approximately 6 weeks. Residual vulvar cancer is often difficult to distinguish from a healing vulvar tumor site after radiation therapy, so surgical resection with a gross normal tissue margin should be performed to evaluate for pathologic response and to remove visible and residual cancer. Groin dissection should not be performed because the chemoradiation has already treated any subclinical disease that is present, and the likelihood of lymphedema is substantially increased after both inguinal lymph node dissection and radiation to the groin.[57]

Stage IVB

When distant metastatic disease is present at time of vulvar cancer diagnosis, treatment should be individualized and considered palliative. Surgery is not expected to be curative, but may be used judiciously to improve symptoms from pain, or bowel and/or urinary obstructions. Radiation therapy may improve symptoms and shrink tumor size, and chemotherapy may be used as a palliative option. Enrollment in clinical trials, if available, should be encouraged in this cohort of women.

Prognosis and Management of Recurrence

Early stage vulvar cancer has a favorable prognosis. The most important prognostic factor for survival is groin node status (laterality and number). Factors that predict groin metastases include tumor depth of invasion, grade, lymph vascular space invasion, clitoral or perineal location, and clinically suspicious nodes.[51]

Approximately 40% of vulvar carcinomas will recur locally,[58] with a median survival of 52 months.[39] Isolated vulvar recurrences are cured with local excision in 75% of cases.[59] Because most of these patients have had prior surgical excision, primary closure may require the use of rhomboid or myocutaneous (gracilis, gluteus, tensor fascia lata, rectus abdominus) flaps. If recurrent vulvar disease involves the vagina, proximal urethra, or anus, surgical resection can be considered curative with pelvic exenteration in carefully selected individuals with central tumors and no evidence of metastatic disease.[53]

Recurrence in the groin is fatal, with treatment options limited to palliative cytotoxic chemotherapy, and has a median survival of 9 months.[39] This recurrence is more likely to occur if the groin was not adequately evaluated or treated, or if the groins were positive at the time of diagnosis. Untreated groin recurrence predictably results in pain, ulceration, bleeding, and infection. Despite these symptoms, surgical resection is discouraged in the previously radiated patients because wound healing will be hindered and cure is not likely. If groin recurrence occurs in a patient who has not had radiation, surgical resection can be performed by removing bulky disease followed by adjuvant radiation.

VAGINAL CANCER

The vagina is an approximately 7.5-cm dilatable tubular structure that extends from the cervix to the vulva. The majority of invasive vaginal carcinomas are SCC, and the second most common type is melanoma. Adenocarcinoma of the vagina is related to in utero diethylstilbestrol (DES) exposure.

Epidemiology

Primary vaginal cancer accounts for only 1% to 2% of all female genital cancers, and more than 80% are from metastases from other sites (most commonly from the cervix and vulva).[60,61] SCC accounts for 80% to 90% of cases and most commonly arises in the upper portion of the posterior wall of the vagina. The majority of women diagnosed with primary SCC of the vagina are older than 65 years,[62] whereas the majority of women diagnosed with primary adenocarcinoma of the vagina are younger than 20 years of age. The incidence of clear cell adenocarcinoma of the vagina has decreased in recent years because DES is no longer prescribed during pregnancy in the United States. Overall, the 5-year survival rate for primary vaginal carcinoma is approximately 40%, and the most important prognostic factor is stage at diagnosis.[63,64]

The cause of vaginal cancer varies depending on the histology. SCC is associated with a history of invasive or in situ cervical cancer, and prior radiation treatment for a prior anogenital cancer. The association with prior cervical cancer is likely multifactorial, because there is a strong association with HPV 16[62] and prior radiation therapy.[65] Primary vaginal cancer may represent occult residual disease of the cervix; therefore, the definition of a primary vaginal carcinoma is a new vaginal carcinoma developing at least 5 years after cervical cancer. Primary adenocarcinoma of the vagina is most commonly of the clear cell type and has been primarily seen in women who were exposed to DES in utero.[66] The proposed mechanism is that adenocarcinoma arises from vaginal adenosis, which is the sequestration of müllerian glandular epithelium into the vaginal mucosa during embryogenesis.[67]

Noninvasive Vaginal Disease

Vaginal dysplasia is largely asymptomatic. Diagnosis may be made by cytologic abnormalities on a screening Papanicolaou test. If this result occurs in the setting of a surgically absent cervix or a normal cervical colposcopy and biopsy, colposcopy should specifically be performed to evaluate vaginal dysplasia with complete visualization of the vaginal wall, after application of acetic acid and Lugol solution. Abnormal findings should be biopsied.

Various treatment modalities for vaginal intraepithelial neoplasia (VAIN) include surgical excision, topical agents, laser ablation, and radiation therapy. Before treatment with laser or topical therapy, biopsies should be performed to rule out invasive disease. Prospective trials demonstrating the most effective treatment modality of VAIN are sparse in the literature. Surgical resection is the mainstay of the treatment of VAIN because it allows for removal of the diseased tissue while obtaining a histologic diagnosis of the entire lesion. Depending on the extent of disease, surgical excision can be as minimal as a wide local excision, or as extensive as a total vaginectomy, with a recurrence rate of 18%.[68,69]

Topical agents are useful noninvasive treatments for the entire vaginal mucosal surface and multifocal disease and are recommended for low-grade lesions, multifocal disease, and poor surgical candidates. Recommended treatment includes placement of intravaginal suppositories of 5% 5-FU once to twice daily for 5 to 14 days, or once weekly for 10 weeks, resulting in a 7% to 38% recurrence rate after the first course of treatment.[70] The combination of 5-FU with surgical resection has shown improved success compared with 5-FU alone, with success rates of 75% for combination therapy and 29% for 5-FU therapy alone.[17] Data regarding the use of imiquimod for the treatment of VAIN have been more limited in the setting of VAIN, but indicate that it may a promising alternative to 5-FU.[71]

CO_2 laser ablation for the treatment of VAIN is well-tolerated with minimal long-term side effects, but approximately one-third of women will require repeat laser ablation.[72] Intracavitary radiation therapy has been used for the treatment of VAIN,[73] however it is associated with more morbidity than other therapies such as vaginal atrophy, stenosis, and shortening. This option is generally reserved for patients whose disease has failed other therapies, are poor surgical candidates, or have extensive multifocal disease.

Diagnosis of Invasive Vaginal Carcinoma

Most patients with invasive vaginal carcinoma present with painless vaginal discharge and bleeding. When risk factors or symptoms present, a complete examination should be performed that includes speculum examination, digital palpation, colposcopy, cytology, and biopsy of any visible lesions. The speculum should be rotated as it is slowly withdrawn to ensure that the entire vaginal mucosa is visualized. If a lesion is small and located in the lower two-thirds of the vagina, there is a higher chance that

Table 2	
FIGO staging criteria for carcinoma of the vagina (2006)	
Stage 0	Carcinoma in situ, intraepithelial neoplasia
Stage I	Limited to the vaginal wall
Stage II	Involvement of the subvaginal tissue without extension to the pelvic sidewall
Stage III	Extension to the pelvic sidewall
Stage IV	Extension beyond the true pelvis or involvement of the mucosa of the bladder or rectum. Bullous edema as such does not permit a case to be allotted to stage IV
IVA	Spread to adjacent organs and/or direct extension beyond the true pelvis
IVB	Spread to distant organs

From Beller U, Benedet JL, Creasman WT, et al. Carcinoma of the vagina. FIGO 26th annual report on the results of treatment in gynecological cancer. Int J Gynaecol Obstet 2006;95:S29–S42; with permission.

the diagnosis can be missed because of it being obscured by the blades of the speculum. Examination under anesthesia should be performed for difficult office examinations and for thorough clinical staging of histologically proven vaginal cancer. Biopsies of the cervix should be performed to rule out a primary cervical tumor.

Staging

The FIGO staging for vaginal carcinoma is clinically based on bimanual and recto-vaginal examination findings, chest radiograph, cystoscopy, proctoscopy, and intravenous pyelography (**Table 2**). Cystoscopy and/or proctoscopy should be performed when there are findings suggestive of bladder and/or rectal invasion. It can sometimes be difficult to differentiate between disease that is limited to the mucosa (stage I) and disease that invades the subvaginal tissue (stage II).[74] A proposal to subdivide stage II vaginal cancer into stage IIA (tumor infiltrating the subvaginal tissues but not extending into the parametrium) and IIB (tumor infiltrating the parametrium but not extending to the pelvic sidewall) has been considered,[75] but this subclassification has not been widely adopted. Surgical staging is rarely used for vaginal cancer, and evaluation of metastatic disease can be performed by computed tomography, magnetic resonance imaging, or positron emission tomography. If a tumor is present in the vagina that also involves the cervix or vulva, it should be classified respectively as a primary cervical or vulvar cancer.

Pathology

Squamous cell carcinoma
The majority of vaginal cancers are SCCs. Tumors may be graded as well-differentiated, moderately differentiated, or poorly differentiated, but there is no clear correlation between grade and survival.[60] Variants of SCC include keratinizing, nonkeratinizing, basaloid, warty, and verrucous. Verrucous carcinoma is a well-differentiated squamous cell carcinoma that presents grossly with large, cauliflower-like masses. It is a distinct subset of squamous cell carcinoma that commonly recurs locally but rarely metastasizes.

Melanoma
Melanoma is the second most common type of primary vaginal cancer and accounts for approximately 3% of vaginal neoplasms.[76] It usually is diagnosed as a pigmented

lesion in the lower vagina.[77] Melanomas are aggressive tumors. Surgical excision is the primary treatment, but the extent of the surgical resection is debated because patients die of their disease regardless of the extent of surgery.[78]

Adenocarcinoma

Clear cell adenocarcinoma of the vagina is associated with DES exposure in utero. Most cases are located in the upper vagina and exocervix and are diagnosed at early stage.[79] Greater than 95% are associated with vaginal adenosis and exophytic in appearance. Microscopically, clear cell adenocarcinoma is composed of clear and hobnail-shaped cells; clear cells are cuboidal and have glycogen-rich cytoplasm, and the hobnail-shaped cells have large atypical protruding nuclei rimmed by a small amount of cytoplasm.[79] Rarely, clear cell adenocarcinoma of the vagina has been seen in women without DES exposure, and it has been associated with vaginal endometriosis.[80,81] Other than the clear cell variant, primary adenocarcinoma of the vagina is rare, and metastatic sites from other primary carcinomas should be ruled out. Other subtypes reported include mucinous, endometrioid, and mesonephric.[82–84]

Management of Squamous Cell Carcinoma of the Vagina

Surgery

Because vaginal cancer is rare, there is no standard treatment. Radiation therapy is generally the primary and definitive treatment; however, selected stage I to II patients can be treated with surgical resection.[64,74,85] Primary surgical management has been associated with a better prognosis, but this result is likely confounded by selection of the early stage cases that are amenable to surgical resection.[64,86] Appropriate cases for primary surgical management include stage I to II cases in which disease is limited to the upper third of the vagina. These cases may be treated with radical hysterectomy, partial vaginectomy, and pelvic lymphadenectomy.[64,87] Superficial, focal lesions may be removed with wide local excision. Patients requiring exenteration for complete removal of the tumor had worse outcomes than those requiring vulvovaginectomy with or without hysterectomy. Exenteration should be reserved for patients with a centrally recurrent disease after primary treatment with radiation.[88] Several series of small numbers of patients reported disease control rates of 50% after primary surgical approaches, including exenteration for stage III to IV vaginal cancer,[64,74,88] but this technique has not been adapted as the standard therapy, and radiation therapy should continue to be considered the primary therapy in advanced stage patients.

Radiation

A combination of external beam radiation and brachytherapy is beneficial for survival rates in advanced vaginal cancer.[89] Early stages can be treated with brachytherapy alone.[63,89] Larger lesions should be treated with external beam radiotherapy of 5000 cGy to shrink the tumor and treat the pelvic lymph nodes, with subsequent intracavitary treatment to a total tumor doses of 7000 cGY.[63,89] Intracavitary treatment can be delivered by tandem and ovoids if the uterus and cervix are in situ, vaginal cylinder if not present, and interstitial for more deeply invasive tumors.[90] In accord with treatment for cervical cancer, it seems appropriate that chemoradiation regimens including cisplatin and/or 5-FU would be beneficial for vaginal cancer.[91] The rarity of vaginal cancer makes it difficult to conduct randomized trials to prove efficacy for treatment strategies.

Stage IVB

Palliative therapy should be offered for patients with stage IVB vaginal cancer, but curative intent is not realistic. Pain and vaginal bleeding should be managed with palliative radiation therapy to improve quality of life. Intracavitary brachytherapy and split courses of external beam pelvic radiotherapy with a 2-week rest can be administered with reasonable toxicity and with a 42% overall response rate.[92]

The management of metastatic vaginal cancer with chemotherapy is largely anecdotal, and it may be reasonable to extrapolate from data on vulvar cancer to the treatment of vaginal cancer.

Prognosis and Management of Recurrence

The overall 5-year survival rate for all stages of vaginal cancer is approximately 40%. Surveillance Epidemiology and End Results (SEER) data from 1988 to 2001 report the 5-year relative survival rate for patients 20 years of age or older as follows: stage I, 68%; stage II, 54%; stage III, 35%; stage IV, 20%.[93]

Recurrent vaginal cancer has a median time to recurrence of 6 to 12 months, and is associated with a 5-year survival rate of only 12%.[89] Stage I and II disease have a 40% recurrence rate and are local-regional. Recurrence rates vary between 55% and 92% in stage III and IV disease, with 20% to 40% of those recurrences to distant regions.[94] Recurrent vaginal cancer is often difficult to manage. Extent of disease should be carefully evaluated, and the goal of treatment for cure or palliation should be delineated. Generally, the only curable recurrences are those of small volume without metastatic disease. If patients received definitive primary surgery without adjuvant radiotherapy, they may receive external beam radiation and brachytherapy for recurrent disease. For patients who received definitive or adjuvant radiotherapy already, salvage options for central recurrence include radical surgery, usually with exenteration. If small-volume disease recurs after treatment with definitive radiotherapy, options sometimes remain for additional interstitial radiation,[95] conformal three-dimensional external beam radiotherapy, or intraoperative radiation therapy.[96]

SUMMARY

Vulvar cancer is becoming more common as the population ages and is primarily a disease of the elderly. Most vulvar cancers are diagnosed at a localized stage and can be cured with surgery and adjuvant radiotherapy. More conservative therapy has been the mainstay in vulvar cancer treatment, which has lessened short-term and long-term morbidity without sacrificing efficacy. Recent national and international studies continue to prove the value of sentinel lymph node technology, which is moving toward a new standard of care for women with early stage vulvar cancer. Vaginal cancer is a rare cancer that also affects elderly women. Prognosis is poor; however, adequate treatment can be delivered with a combination of external beam radiotherapy and brachytherapy, and with surgical resection for a select group of patients.

REFERENCES

1. Kosary CL. Cancer of the vulva. In: Ries LA, Young JL, Keel GE, et al, editors. SEER survival monographs: cancer survival among adults: U.S. SEER Program, 1988 [NIH Pub. No. 07-6215]. Bethesda (MD): National Cancer Institute; 2007. p. 147–54.
2. American Cancer Society. Vulvar cancer. Available at: http://www.cancer.org/acs/groups/cid/documents/webcontent/003147-pdf.pdf. Accessed August 10, 2011.
3. Judson PL, Habermann EB, Baxter NN, et al. Trends in the incidence of invasive and in situ vulvar carcinoma. Obstet Gynecol 2006;107:1018–22.

4. Zaino, RJ. Carcinoma of the vulva, urethra, and Bartholin's gland. In: Wilkinson EJ, editors. Pathology of the vulva and vagina: contemporary issues in surgical pathology, vol. 9. New York: Churchill Livingstone; 1987. p. 119–53.
5. Rusk D, Sutton GP, Look KY, et al. Analysis of invasive squamous cell carcinoma of the vulva and vulvar intraepithelial neoplasia for the presence of human papillomavirus DNA. Obstet Gynecol 1991;77:918–22.
6. van de Nieuwenhof HP, van Kempen LC, de Hullu JA, et al. The etiologic role of HPV in vulvar squamous cell carcinoma fine tuned. Cancer Epidemiol Biomarkers Prev 2009;18:2061–7.
7. Trimble CL, Hildesheim A, Brinton LA, et al. Heterogeneous etiology of squamous carcinoma of the vulva. Obstet Gynecol 1996;87:59–64.
8. Lanneau GS, Argenta PA, Lanneau MS, et al. Vulvar cancer in young women: demographic features and outcome evaluation. Am J Obstet Gynecol 2009;200: 645e1–5.
9. Flowers LC, Wistuba II, Scurry J, et al. Genetic changes during the multistage pathogenesis of human papillomavirus positive and negative vulvar carcinomas. J Soc Gynecol Investig 1999;6:213–21.
10. Freidrich EG. New nomenclature for vulvar disease: report of the committee on terminology, ISSVD. Obstet Gynecol 1976;47:122–4.
11. Ridley CM, Frankman O, Jones IS, et al. New nomenclature for vulvar disease: International Society for the Study of Vulvar Disease. Hum Pathol 1989;20:495–6.
12. Heler DS. Report of a new ISSVD classification of VIN. J Low Genit Tract Dis 2007;11:46–7.
13. Sturgeon SR, Brinton LA, Devesa SS, et al. In situ and invasive vulvar cancer incidence trends (1973 to 1987). Am J Obstet Gynecol 1992;166:1482–5.
14. Wilkinson EJ. Premalignant and malignant tumors of the vulva. In: Kurman RJ, editor. Blaustein's pathology of the female genital tract. 5th edition. New York: Springer; 2002. p. 99–149.
15. Mathiesen O, Buus SK, Cramers M. Topical imiquimod can reverse intraepithelial neoplasia: a randomised, double-blind study. Gynecol Oncol 2007;107:219–22.
16. van Seters M, van Beurden M, ten Kate FJ, et al. Treatment with vulvar intraepithelial neoplasia with topical imiquimod. N Engl J Med 2008;358:1465–73.
17. Sillman FH, Sedlis A, Boyce JG. A review of lower genital intraepithelial neoplasia and the use of topical 5-fluorouracil. Obstet Gynecol Surv 1985;40:190–220.
18. Penna C, Fallani MG, Fambrini M, et al. CO_2 laser surgery for vulvar intraepithelial neoplasia: excisional, destructive and combined techniques. Reprod Med 2002;47: 913-8.
19. Pincus SH, Stadecker MJ. Vulvar dystrophies and noninfectious inflammatory conditions. In: Wilkinson EJ, editor, Pathology of the vulva and vagina. Contemporary issues in surgical pathology, vol. 9. New York: Churchill Livingstone; 1987. p. 11–23.
20. Lewis FM. Vulval lichen planus. Br J Dermatol 1998;138:569–75.
21. Wilkinson EJ, Xie DL. Benign diseases of the vulva. In: Kurman RJ, editor. Blaustein's pathology of the female genital tract. 5th edition. New York: Springer; 2002. p. 37–98.
22. Kennedy CM, Kaufman RH. Erosive lichen planus of the vulva. Clin Obstet Gynecol 1991;34:605–13.
23. Fanning J, Lambert HC, Hale TM, et al. Paget's disease of the vulva: prevalence of associated vulvar adenocarcinoma, invasive Paget's disease, and recurrence after surgical excision. Am J Obstet Gynecol 1999;180:24–7.
24. Magrina JG, Weaver AL, Gaffey TA, et al. Carcinoma of the vulva stage IA: long term results. Gynecol Oncol 2000;76:24–7.

25. Jones RW, Joura EA. Analyzing prior clinical events at presentation in 102 women with vulvar carcinoma. J Reprod Med 1999;44:766–8.
26. Creasman WT. New gynecologic cancer staging. Obstet Gynecol 1990;75:287–8.
27. Shepherd JH. Cervical and vulva cancer: changes in FIGO definitions of staging. Br J Obstet Gynaecol 1996;103:405–6.
28. Pecorelli S. Revised FIGO staging for carcinoma of the vulva, cervix, and endometrium. Int J Gynaecol Obstet 2009;105:103–4.
29. Podratz KC, Symmonds RE, Taylor WF, et al. Carcinoma of the vulva: analysis of treatment and survival. Obstet Gynecol 1983;61:63–74.
30. Ross MJ, Ehrmann RL. Histologic prognosticators in stage I squamous cell carcinoma of the vulva. Obstet Gynecol 1987;70:774–84.
31. Wilkinson EJ, Rico MJ, Pierson KK. Microinvasive carcinoma of the vulva. Int J Gynecol Pathol 1982;1:29–39.
32. Kneale BL. Microinvasive cancer of the vulva: report of the International Society for the Study of Vulvar Disease Task Force: Proceedings of the 7th World Congress of the ISSVD. J Reprod Med 1983;29:454.
33. Sedlis A, Homesley H, Bundy BN, et al. Positive groin lymph nodes in superficial squamous cell vulvar cancer. A Gynecologic Oncology Group Study. Am J Obstet Gynecol 1987;156:1159–64.
34. Moore DH, Koh WJ, McGuire WP, et al. Vulva. In: Barakat RP, Markman M, Randall ME, editors. Principles and practice of gynecologic oncology. 5th edition. Baltimore (MD): Lippincott Williams & Williams; 2009. p. 555–90.
35. Copeland LJ, Sneige N, Gershenson DM, et al. Bartholin gland carcinoma. Obstet Gynecol 1986;67:794–801.
36. Panizzon RG. Vulvar melanoma. Semin Dermatol 1996;15:67–70.
37. Kelley JL, Burke TW, Tornos C et al. Minimally invasive vulvar carcinoma: an indication for conservative surgical therapy. Gynecol Oncol 1992;44:240–4.
38. Iversen T. The value of groin palpation in epidermoid carcinoma of the vulva. Gynecol Oncol 1981;12:291–5.
39. Stehman FB, Bundy BN, Ball H, et al. Sites of failure and times to failure in carcinoma of the vulva treated conservatively: a Gynecologic Oncology Group study. Am J Obstet Gynecol 1996;174:1128–32.
40. Hacker NF, Leuchter RS, Berek JS, et al. Radical vulvectomy and bilateral inguinal lymphadenectomy through separate groin incisions. Obstet Gynecol 1981;58:574–9.
41. Hacker NF, Berek JS, Lagasse LD, et al. Individualization of treatment for stage I squamous cell vulvar carcinoma. Obstet Gynecol 1984;63:155–62.
42. Siller BS, Alvarez RD, Conner WD, et al. T2/3 vulva cancer: a case-control study of triple incision versus en bloc radical vulvectomy and inguinal lymphadenectomy. Gynecol Oncol 1995;57:335–9.
43. DiSaia PJ, Creasman WT, Rich WM. An alternative approach to early cancer of the vulva. Am J Obstet Gynecol 1979;133:825–32.
44. Levenback C, Burke TW, Gershenson DM, et al. Intraoperative lymphatic mapping for vulvar cancer. Obstet Gynecol 1994;84:163–7.
45. Oonk MH, van de Nieuwenhof HP, de Hullu JA, et al. The role of sentinel node biopsy in gynecological cancer: a review. Curr Opin Oncol 2009;21:425–32.
46. van der Zee AG, Oonk MH, de Hullu JA, et al. Sentinel node dissection is safe in the treatment of early-stage vulvar cancer. J Clin Oncol 2008;28:884–9.
47. Levenback CF, van der Zee AG, Rob L, et al. Sentinel lymph node biopsy in patients with gynecologic cancers: expert panel statement from the International Sentinel Node Society Meeting. Gynecol Oncol 2009;114:151–6.

48. Levenback CF, Tian C, Coleman RL, et al. Sentinel node (SN) biopsy in patients with vulvar cancer: a Gynecologic Oncology Group (GOG) study [abstract 5505]. J Clin Oncol 2009;27(Suppl 15):A5505.
49. Piura B, Masotina A, Murdoch J, et al. Recurrent squamous cell carcinoma of the vulva: a study of 73 cases. Gynecol Oncol 1993;48:189–95.
50. Rutledge FN, Mitchell MF, Munsell MF, et al. Prognostic indicators for invasive carcinoma of the vulva. Gynecol Oncol 1991;42:239–44.
51. Homesley HD, Bundy BN, Sedlis A, et al. Prognostic factors for groin node metastases in squamous cell carcinoma of the vulva (a Gynecologic Oncology Group study). Gynecol Oncol 1993;49: 279–83.
52. Montana GS, Thomas GM, Moore DH, et al. Preoperative chemo-radiation for carcinoma of the vulva with N2/N3 nodes: a Gynecologic Oncology Group study. Int J Radiat Oncol Biol Phys 2000;48:1007–13.
53. Miller B, Morris M, Levenback C, et al. Pelvic exenteration for primary and recurrent vulvar cancer. Gynecol Oncol 1995;58:202–5.
54. Moore DH, Thomas GM, Montana GS, et al. Preoperative chemoradiation for advanced vulvar cancer: a phase II study of the Gynecologic Oncology Group. Int J Radiat Oncol Biol Phys 1998;42:79–85.
55. Rose PG, Bundy BN, Watkins EB, et al. Concurrent cisplatin-based radiotherapy and chemotherapy for locally advanced cervical cancer. N Engl J Med 1999;340: 1144–53.
56. Moore DH, Ali S, Koh WJ, et al. Phase II trial of radiation therapy and weekly cisplatin chemotherapy for the treatment of locally-advanced squamous cell carcinoma of the vulva: a Gynecologic Oncology Group study [abstract]. Gynecol Oncol 2011;120:S1.
57. Gould N, Kamelle S, Tillmanns T, et al. Predictors of complications after inguinal lymphadenectomy. Gynecol Oncol 2001;82:329–32.
58. Maggino T, Landoni F, Sartori E, et al. Patterns of recurrence in patients with squamous cell carcinoma of the vulva: A multicenter CTF Study. Cancer 2000;89: 116–22.
59. Tilmans AS, Sutton GP, Look KY, et al. Recurrent squamous carcinoma of the vulva. Am J Obstet Gynecol 1992;167:1383–9.
60. Herbst AL, Green TH Jr, Ulfelder H. Primary carcinoma of the vagina: an analysis of 68 cases. Am J Obstet Gynecol 1970;106:210–8.
61. Pride GL, Schultz AE, Chuprevich TW, et al. Primary invasive carcinoma of the vagina. Obstet Gynecol 1979;53:218–25.
62. Daling JR, Madeleine MM, Schwartz SM, et al. A population-based study of squamous cell vaginal cancer: HPV and cofactors. Gynecol Oncol 2002;84:263–70.
63. Kirkbride P, Fyles A, Rawlings GA, et al. Carcinoma of the vagina: experience at the Princess Margaret Hospital (1974–1989). Gynecol Oncol 1995;56:435–43.
64. Stock RG, Chen AS, Seski J. A 30-year experience in the management of primary carcinoma of the vagina: analysis of prognostic factors and treatment modalities. Gynecol Oncol 1995;56:45–52.
65. Pride GL, Buchler DA. Carcinoma of vagina 10 or more years following pelvic irradiation therapy. Am J Obstet Gynecol 1977;127:513–7.
66. Herbst AL, Ulfelder H, Poskanzer DC. Adenocarcinoma of the vagina: association of maternal stilbestrol therapy with tumor appearance in young women. N Engl J Med 1971;284:878–81.
67. Robboy SJ, Hill EC, Sandberg EC, et al. Vaginal adenosis in women born prior to the diethylstilbestrol era. Hum Pathol 1986;17:488–92.
68. Cheng D, Ng TY, Ngan HY, et al. Wide local excision (WLE) for vaginal intraepithelial neoplasia (VAIN). Acta Obstet Gynecol Scand 1999;78:648–52.

69. Hoffman MS, DeCesare SL, Roberts WS, et al. Upper vaginectomy for in situ and occult, superficially invasive carcinoma of the vagina. Am J Obstet Gynecol 1992;166: 30–3.

70. Krebs HB. Treatment of vaginal intraepithelial neoplasia with laser and topical 5-fluorouracil. Obstet Gynecol 1989;73:657–60.

71. Buck HW, Guth KJ. Treatment of vaginal intraepithelial neoplasia (primarily low grade) with imiquimod 5% cream. J Low Genit Tract Dis 2003;7:290–3.

72. Diakomanolis E, Rodolakis A, Sakellaropoulos G, et al. Conservative management of vaginal intraepithelial neoplasia (VAIN) by laser CO2. Eur J Gynaecol Oncol 1996;17: 389–92.

73. MacLeod C, Fowler A, Dalrymple C, et al. High-dose-rate brachytherapy in the management of high-grade intraepithelial neoplasia of the vagina. Gynecol Oncol 1997;65:74–7.

74. Ball HG, Berman ML. Management of primary vaginal carcinoma. Gynecol Oncol 1982;14:154–63.

75. Perez CA, Camel HM, Galakatos AE, et al. Definitive irradiation in carcinoma of the vagina: long-term evaluation of results. Int J Radiat Oncol Biol Phys 1998;15: 1283–90.

76. Weinstock MA. Malignant melanoma of the vulva and vagina in the United States: patterns of incidence and population-based estimates of survival. Am J Obstet Gynecol 1994;171:1225–30.

77. Reid GC, Schmidt RW, Roberts JA, et al. Primary melanoma of the vagina: a clinicopathologic analysis. Obstet Gynecol 1989;74:190–9.

78. Miner TJ, Delgado R, Zeisler J, et al. Primary vaginal melanoma: a critical analysis of therapy. Ann Surg Oncol 2004;11:34–9.

79. Herbst AL, Robboy SJ, Scully RE, et al. Clear-cell adenocarcinoma of the vagina and cervix in girls: analysis of 170 registry cases. Am J Obstet Gynecol 1974;119:713–24.

80. Watanabe Y, Ueda H, Nozaki K, et al. Advanced primary clear cell carcinoma of the vagina not associated with diethylstilbestrol. Acta Cytol 2002;46:577–81.

81. Shah C, Pizer E, Veljovich DS, et al. Clear cell adenocarcinoma of the vagina in a patient with vaginal endometriosis. Gynecol Oncol 2006;103:1130–2.

82. Ebrahim S, Daponte A, Smith TH, et al. Primary mucinous adenocarcinoma of the vagina. Gynecol Oncol 2001;80:89–92.

83. Haskel S, Chen SS, Spiegel G. Vaginal endometrioid adenocarcinoma arising in vaginal endometriosis: a case report and literature review. Gynecol Oncol 1989;34: 232–6.

84. Hinchey WW, Silva EG, Guarda LA, et al. Paravaginal wolffian duct (mesonephros) adenocarcinoma: a light and electron microscopic study. Am J Clin Pathol 1983;80: 539–44.

85. Tjalma WA, Monaghan JM, de Barros Lopes A, et al. The role of surgery in invasive squamous carcinoma of the vagina. Gynecol Oncol 2001;81:360–5.

86. Creasman WT, Phillips JL, Menck HR. The National Cancer Data Base report on cancer of the vagina. Cancer 1998;83:1033–40.

87. Davis KP, Stanhope CR, Garton GR, et al. Invasive vaginal carcinoma: analysis of early-stage disease. Gynecol Oncol 1991;42:131–6.

88. Rubin SC, Young J, Mikuta JJ. Squamous carcinoma of the vagina: treatment, complications, and long-term follow-up. Gynecol Oncol 1985;20:346–53.

89. Chyle V, Zagars GK, Wheeler JA, et al. Definitive radiotherapy for carcinoma of the vagina: outcome and prognostic factors. Int J Radiat Oncol Biol Phys 1996;35:891–905.

90. Tewari KS, Cappuccini F, Puthawala AA, et al. Primary invasive carcinoma of the vagina: treatment with interstitial brachytherapy. Cancer 2001;91:758–70.
91. Dalrymple JL, Russell AH, Lee SW, et al. Chemoradiation for primary invasive squamous carcinoma of the vagina. Int J Gynecol Cancer 2004;14:110–7.
92. Spanos WJ Jr, Clery M, Perez CA, et al. Late effect of multiple daily fraction palliation schedule for advanced pelvic malignancies (RTOG 8502). Int J Radiat Oncol Biol Phys 1994;29:961–7.
93. Kosary CL. Cancer of the vagina. In: Ries LA, Young JL, Keel GE, et al, editors. SEER survival monographs: cancer survival among adults: U.S. SEER Program, 1988 [NIH Pub. No. 07-6215]. Bethesda (MD): National Cancer Institute; 2007. p. 155–60.
94. Perez CA, Grigsby PW, Garipagaoglu M, et al. Factors affecting long-term outcome of irradiation in carcinoma of the vagina. Int J Radiat Oncol Biol Phys 1999;44:37–45.
95. Gupta AK, Vicini FA, Frazier AJ, et al. Iridium-192 transperineal interstitial brachytherapy for locally advanced or recurrent gynecological malignancies. Int J Radiat Oncol Biol Phys 1999;43:1055–60.
96. Gemignani ML, Alektiar KM, Leitao M, et al. Radical surgical resection and high-dose intraoperative radiation therapy (HDR-IORT) in patients with recurrent gynecologic cancers. Int J Radiat Oncol Biol Phys 2001;50:687–94.

Cervical Cancer

Jayanthi S. Lea, MD*, Ken Y. Lin, MD, PhD

KEYWORDS

- Cervical cancer • Human papillomavirus • Radical hysterectomy
- Cervical cancer treatment

KEY POINTS

- Squamous cell cervical cancer incidence and mortality have been reduced dramatically as a result of successful screening in many countries.
- Cervical cancer is staged clinically, and stage is the most important indicator of long-term survival.
- Treatment is typically dictated by clinical staging.
- Improvements in radiation techniques and molecular targeted therapy are the current research venues in cervical cancer.

Cervical cancer is the most common gynecologic cancer in women. High-risk human papillomavirus (HPV) is implicated as the major etiologic agent. Most invasive cervical cancers are preceded by a severe cervical dysplasia or carcinoma-in-situ.

Common symptoms associated with cervical cancer are postcoital and irregular vaginal bleeding; watery vaginal discharge; and physical signs associated with venous, lymphatic, neural, or ureteral compression. Diagnosis of cervical cancer usually follows a physical examination and histologic evaluation of cervical biopsies.

Cervical cancer is staged clinically, and stage is the most important indicator of long-term survival. Treatment is typically dictated by clinical staging. In general, early-stage disease is treated effectively with either surgery or chemoradiation. Advanced-stage disease is treated primarily with chemoradiation.

Prevention lies mainly in early detection. For this reason, regular Papanicolaou test (Pap smear) screening is recommended by the American College of Obstetricians and Gynecologists (2003) and the U.S. Preventative Task Force (2003). More recently, HPV vaccines have been developed and marketed for cervical cancer prevention.

The authors have nothing to disclose.
University of Texas Southwestern School of Medicine, 5323 Harry Hines Boulevard, Suite E6.102, Dallas, TX 75390-9032, USA
* Corresponding author.
E-mail address: Jayanthi.Lea@UTSouthwestern.edu

Obstet Gynecol Clin N Am 39 (2012) 233–253
doi:10.1016/j.ogc.2012.02.008
0889-8545/12/$ – see front matter Published by Elsevier Inc.

obgyn.theclinics.com

EPIDEMIOLOGY

Cervical cancer is the third most common cancer and the fourth leading cause of cancer death in women worldwide. In 2008, 529,800 women were diagnosed with cervical cancer and 275,100 died from the disease, accounting for 9% of the total new cancer cases and 8% of total care deaths among women.[1] In the United States, approximately 12,710 women are diagnosed with invasive cervical cancer and 4290 will die from the disease in 2011. The majority of cervical cancer now occurs in developing countries and medically underserved populations due to the lack of Papanicolaou smear screening.[2–5] The incidence and mortality are higher among minorities. The incidence of cervical cancer is 30% higher in African Americans than in whites, and mortality is twice as high.[2–5] The disparity of cervical cancer burden in the developing counties and in medically underserved populations reflects a lack of screening for cervical cancer. Screening for cervical cancer and its premalignant lesions by Pap smear has led to a decrease in the incidence of cervical cancer in the United States.

RISK FACTORS
HPV

HPV can be detected in more than 99% of cervical cancers and is essential for the malignant transformation. More than 40 subtypes of HPV have been identified, of which at least 15 are known to be oncogenic. The most common subtypes, HPV 16 and 18, account for about 70% of cervical cancer in the United States.[6]

HPV infection is common. Most HPV infections are transient. When persistent HPV infection does occur, it has been estimated that it takes an average of 15 years from initial infection to the development of cervical intraepithelial neoplasia (CIN) and ultimately invasive cervical cancer.

Lower Socioeconomic Predictors

Lower educational attainment, older age, obesity, smoking, and neighborhood poverty are independently related to lower rates of cervical cancer screening. Specifically, those living in impoverished neighborhoods have limited access to screening and may benefit from outreach programs to decrease rates of cervical cancer.[7]

Cigarette Smoking

Cigarette smoking, both active and passive, increases the risk of cervical cancer. Among HPV-infected women, current and former smokers have a two- to threefold incidence of high grade squamous intraepitheliel lesion (HSIL) or invasive cancer. Passive smoking is also associated with increased risk, but to a lesser extent.[8] Of cervical cancer types, current smoking has been associated with a significantly increased rate of squamous cell carcinoma, but not of adenocarcinoma. Interestingly, squamous cell and adenocarcinomas of the cervix share most risk factors with this exception of smoking. Although the mechanism underlying the association between smoking and cervical cancer is unclear, smoking may alter HPV infection in those who smoke. For example, "ever smoking" was associated with reduced clearance of high-risk HPV infection.[9,10]

Reproductive Behavior

Parity and combination oral contraceptive (COC) pill use has a significant association with cervical cancer. Pooled data from case-control studies indicate that high parity increases the risk of developing cervical cancer. Specifically, women with seven prior full-term pregnancies have an approximately fourfold increased risk, and those with one or two full-term pregnancies have a twofold increased risk compared with nulliparas.[11]

In addition to parity, long-term COC use may be a cofactor. In women who are positive for cervical HPV DNA and who use COCs, risks of cervical carcinoma increase by up to fourfold compared with women who are HPV positive and never users of COC.[12] In addition, current COC users and women who are within 9 years of use have a significantly higher risk of developing both squamous cell and adenocarcinoma of the cervix.[13]

Sexual Activity

An increased number of sexual partners and early age at first intercourse have been shown to increase cervical cancer risks. Having more than six lifetime sexual partners imposes a significant increase in the relative risk of cervical cancer compared with controls.[13] Similarly, early age at first intercourse, before age 20, confers a significantly increased risk of developing cervical cancer, whereas intercourse after age 21 shows only a trend toward an increased risk. Moreover, abstinence from sexual activity and barrier protection during sexual intercourse has been demonstrated to decrease cervical cancer incidence.[13]

SCREENING AND PREVENTION
Pap Smear

Screening for cytologic abnormality by Pap smear has led to significant reduction in the incidence of cervical cancer in the United States. Pap smear has a sensitivity of 55% to 80% on any given test and does not always detect cervical cancer.[14] In addition, in women with stage I cervical cancer, only 30% to 50% of Pap smears are interpreted as positive for malignancy.[14] Therefore, serial screening as prescribed by the clinical guidelines is important.

HPV Vaccines

The advent of HPV vaccines holds promise of reducing the incidence of cervical cancer. The current HPV vaccines provide protection against HPV types 16 and 18, which account for about 70% of cervical cancers. Vaccines are most effective when administered in sexually naïve individuals. The vaccines are indicated for females 9 to 26 years of age for prevention of cervical and other lower genital tract cancers. However, women who have received HPV vaccines must continue to receive Pap smear screening because present vaccines do not provide protection for other high-risk HPV subtypes that can cause cervical and other lower genital tract cancers. Recent U.S. Food and Drug Administration (FDA) approval has been obtained for vaccination of males in the similar age group for prevention of anal cancers and other HPV-mediated dysplasias; however, downstream effect for preventing subsequent infection in women is unknown.

PATHOPHYSIOLOGY

Squamous cell carcinoma of the cervix typically arises within the squamocolumnar junction from a preexisting dysplastic lesion, which in nearly all cases follows infection with high risk HPV.[15] In general, progression from dysplasia to invasive cancer requires several years, but wide variations exist. The molecular alterations involved with cervical carcinogenesis are complex and not fully understood. Carcinogenesis is suspected to result from the interactive effects between environmental insults, host immunity, and somatic cell genomic variations.[16–19]

Lymphatic Spread

Traditional teaching implies that the pattern of tumor spread typically follows cervical lymphatic drainage. The cervix has a rich network of lymphatics, which follow the course of the uterine vein. These channels drain principally into the paracervical and parametrial lymph nodes. From the parametrial and paracervical nodes, lymph subsequently flows into the obturator lymph nodes and the internal, external, and common iliac lymph nodes. In contrast, lymphatic channels from the posterior cervix course through the rectal pillars and the uterosacral ligaments to the rectal lymph nodes.

More recently, sentinel lymph node data in cervical cancer, pursued with the impetus to understand further the lymphatic trafficking of the cervix, indicate that the external iliac region just distal to the common iliac bifurcation was the most common sentinel lymph node location.[20] Para-aortic lymph nodes have also been identified as the sentinel node in a very small percentage of patients with cervical cancer.[21]

Local Tumor Extension

As primary lesions enlarge and lymphatic involvement progresses, local invasion increases and will eventually become extensive. With extension through the parametria to the pelvic sidewall, ureteral blockage frequently develops. In addition, the bladder and rectum may be invaded by direct tumor extension through the vesico-uterine ligaments.

Distant metastasis results from hematogenous dissemination and the lungs, ovaries, liver, and bone are the most frequently affected organs.

HISTOLOGIC SUBTYPES
Squamous Cell Carcinoma

The two most common histologic subtypes of cervical cancer are squamous cell and adenocarcinoma (**Table 1**). Squamous cell carcinoma of the cervix typically arises at the squamocolumnar junction. Squamous cell carcinoma comprises more than 70% of cervical cancer. Over the last 30 years, there has been a decline in the incidence of squamous cell carcinoma and an increase in the incidence of adenocarcinoma. This trend is likely due to screening for premalignant and malignant diseases of the cervix through Pap smear.[6]

Adenocarcinoma

Adenocarcinoma comprises 25% of cervical cancers and arises from the mucus-secreting glandular cells of the endocervix. Because of this origin within the endocervix, adenocarcinomas are often occult and may be advanced before becoming clinically evident. The traditional Pap smears are not reliable for screening for adenocarcinomas of the cervix. The Gynecologic Oncology Group (GOG) is currently conducting a study to determine if a tumor-associated transmembrane glycoprotein (MN), which has demonstrated powerful discriminatory capacity to identify atypical glandular cells associated with high-grade squamous or glandular cervical cells, can be used as a biomarker to identify cervical adenocarcinoma.

There is controversy regarding whether squamous cell carcinoma or adenocarcinoma is associated with a worse prognosis. When adjusted for stage, some series found similar outcomes between squamous cell carcinoma and adenocarcinoma.[22–25]

Table 1 Histologic subtypes of cervical cancer	
Squamous Cell Carcinoma	
Adenocarcinoma	Endocervical type adenocarcinomas
	Endometrioid adenocarcinomas
	Minimal deviation adenocarcinoma
	Papillary villoglandular adenocarcinoma
	Serous adenocarcinoma
	Clear cell adenocarcinoma
	Mesonephric adenocarcinoma
Mixed cervical carcinomas	Adenosquamous carcinoma
	Glassy cell carcinoma
	Adenoid cystic carcinoma
	Adenoid basal epithelioma
Neuroendocrine tumors of the cervix	Large cell neuroendocrine
	Small cell carcinoma
Other malignant tumors	Sarcomas of the cervix
	Malignant lymphomas
	Metastatic cancers

However, most studies have shown that adenocarcinoma has a worse prognosis and that the difference is more pronounced in the advanced stage.[26–32]

Neuroendocrine/Small Cell Carcinoma

Neuroendocrine tumors account for 2% to 5% of cervical cancers. There are four types of neuroendocrine tumors in the cervix: small cell, large cell, carcinoid, and atypical carcinoid tumors, with the small cell neuroendocrine carcinoma (SCNEC) being the most common variant. SCNEC is considered an extrapulmonary variant of small cell lung cancer and has a worse prognosis than squamous cell carcinoma or adenocarcinoma.[33,34]

Other Less Common Subtypes

Adenosquamous carcinoma exhibits both glandular and squamous differentiation and may be associated with a worse prognosis than squamous cell carcinoma or adenocarcinoma. Other subtypes include adenoid cystic carcinoma, adenoid basal epithelioma, glassy cell carcinoma, sarcoma, and lymphoma.

DIAGNOSIS
Presenting Symptoms

Early stage
Many women with cervical cancer are asymptomatic initially. For those with symptoms, early-stage cervical cancer may present with a watery, blood-tinged vaginal discharge or postcoital bleeding.

Late stage
With the enlargement of cervical mass, the vaginal discharge may become mucoid, purulent, and malodorous as the cervical mass becomes necrotic. With parametrial invasion and extension to the pelvic side wall, the tumor may compress pelvic organs to produce symptoms such as pelvic pain, lower back pain, or lower extremity edema.

With ureteral obstruction, hydronephrosis and renal failure can result. Tumor invasion into the bladder or rectum can result in hematuria, hematochezia, or rectal bleeding.

Diagnosis and Workup

Physical examination

A thorough external genital and vaginal examination should be performed during gynecologic examination to search for concomitant lesions. On speculum examination, the cervix may appear grossly normal if the cancer is microinvasive. Visible cancer may appear as an ulcerated lesion, granular or papillary tissue, exophytic growth, polypoid mass, or barrel-shaped cervix. Large lesions may become necrotic and friable. A watery, purulent, or bloody discharge may be present.

A rectovaginal examination is performed to evaluate the extent of tumor and is the only way to adequately assess parametrial involvement. An enlarged uterus may be palpated, as the result of tumor growth. Obstruction of cervical canal by the tumor can result in hematometra or pyometra and lead to an enlarged uterus. Vaginal extension of the tumor can be appreciated on bimanual and rectovaginal examination as obliteration of the vaginal fornices or a thick, firm, irregular rectovaginal septum. Parametrial extension and involvement of pelvic sidewall and uterosacral ligaments can also be palpated on rectovaginal examination. With the parametrial involvement, the tissue feels firm, irregular, and less mobile.

Most women with cervical cancer have normal general physical examination findings. However, with advanced disease, enlarged inguinal or supraclavicular lymph nodes and lower extremity edema may be found.

Colposcopy and biopsy

Evaluation of the cervix with colposcopy is necessary when a Pap smear reveals abnormal cytology including atypical squamous cells cannot rule out high grade lesion (ASC-H), low grade squamous intraepitheliel lesion (LSIL), HSIL, or atypical glandular cells of undetermined significance (AGUS). During colposcopic evaluation, the entire transformation and all lesions must be visualized for the procedure to be considered adequate. The appearance of the cervix is recorded and a biopsy performed for any suspicious lesion with a Tischler biopsy forceps. Endocervical curettage should also be performed. The biopsies of the lesions should explain the abnormal cytology.

Cervical biopsy and endocervical curetting may reveal invasive cancer, premalignant lesions, or benign tissue. Premalignant lesions such as CIN II and III and carcinoma-in-situ need to be evaluated further with cervical conization to evaluate for the possibility of microinvasive disease. By obtaining the entire lesion on conization, maximum depth of invasion can be evaluated properly. Conization also needs to be performed if colposcopy is inadequate. Either cold knife conization or loop electrosurgical excision is acceptable. However, cold knife conization is preferred because thermal artifact can make interpretation of surgical margins difficult.

Staging

Clinical staging

Cervical cancer is staged by clinical criteria, whereas most other gynecologic malignancy is staged by surgical and pathologic findings. The FIGO system for cervical cancer staging was established by the International Federation of Gynecology and Obstetrics (FIGO), in conjunction with World Health Organization (WHO) and the Union for International Cancer Control (UICC). The FIGO staging system for cervical cancer was modified most recently in 2009 to define prognostic groups more accurately. The FIGO Committee on Gynecologic Oncology decided that clinical staging should be continued, while lymph nodal assessment during staging is not necessary because surgical staging cannot be employed worldwide, especially in low-resource countries. Thus, the aforementioned two changes have been approved in the new staging system as follows. First, the subdivision of the tumor size (with a 4 cm cutoff in maximum diameter) has been applied for previous stage IIA. Second, the previous stage 0 has been deleted from the new clinical staging system because it is a preinvasive lesion.[35]

In addition to physical examination, studies and procedures that are allowed for staging include colposcopy, endocervical curettage, conization, hysteroscopy, cystoscopy, proctoscopy, intravenous pyelogram, and radiography of the lungs and skeleton.[36] Other imaging modalities such as computed tomography (CT) and magnetic resonance imaging (MRI) cannot be used for FIGO staging. The rationale is to provide a basis for resource-rich and resource-poor countries to compare data.

The limitations of clinical staging may led to understaging of some patients.[37] For this reason, additional imaging modality such as CT scans and more recently positron emission tomography (PET)/CT scans are frequently employed in the United States for treatment planning purposes. See **Table 2** for the revised 2009 FIGO staging of cervical cancer.

Radiologic Modalities

CT scan

A CT scan is frequently used to supplement physical examination and studies performed for clinical staging. It can help evaluate the tumor size and identify the extent of disease spread, lymph node involvement, and hydronephrosis.

MRI

The utility of MRI lies in its ability to evaluate in greater accuracy the extent of disease spread in early-stage cervical canoer. MRI has been found to be superior to CT scan and clinical examination for measuring tumor size and determining involvement of uterine corpus or parametrium for evaluation of early-stage cervical cancer.[38,39]

PET

PET scan may provide more accurate assessment of metastatic disease than other imaging modalities. This nuclear medicine scan utilizes radioisotope-tagged substrates such as glucose ($[^{18}F]$-fluoro-2-deoxy-D-glucose [FDG]) and generates images based on the uptake and metabolism of the substrate in the tissues. PET scan with FDG is now increasingly being used as part of initial staging and monitoring of the response to therapy of different types of cancers, including cervical cancer.[40,41] FDG–PET is highly sensitive and specific for the detection of para-aortic lymph nodes in locally advanced disease.[42–44] However, its ability to detect pelvic lymph node metastasis is more limited, especially for early-stage disease.[43,45–47]

Integrated PET/CT is a technique in which both PET and CT are performed sequentially on a hybrid PET/CT scanner. The PET and CT images are then combined using computer software, allowing the physiologic data from the PET imaging to be better localized based on the anatomic information from the CT scan. Integrated PET/CT might be more sensitive than PET alone or MRI for detection of lymph node metastasis.[48]

Table 2
Staging of cervical cancer

FIGO Stage	Definition
I	Cervical carcinoma confined to the cervix.
IA	Invasive carcinoma diagnosed only by microscopy. Stromal invasion with a depth of ≤5 mm and a horizontal spread of ≤7 mm.
IA1	Stromal invasion ≤3 mm in depth and horizontal spread ≤7 mm.
IA2	Stromal invasion >3 mm but ≤5 mm in depth and horizontal spread ≤7 mm.
IB	Clinically visible lesion confined to the cervix or microscopic lesion greater than IA2.
IB1	Clinically visible lesion ≤4 cm in greatest dimension.
IB2	Clinically visible lesion >4 cm in greatest dimension.
II	Cervical carcinoma invades beyond the uterus but not to pelvic wall or the lower third of vagina.
IIA1	Clinically visible lesion ≤4 cm or less with involvement of less than the upper two thirds of the vagina.
IIA2	Clinically visible lesion >4 cm with involvement of less than the upper two thirds of the vagina.
IIB	Tumor with parametrial invasion.
III	Tumor involves lower third of vagina, extends to the pelvic wall, or causes hydronephrosis or nonfunctioning kidney.
IIIA	Tumor involves lower third of vagina, but no extension to pelvic wall.
IIIB	Tumor extends to pelvic wall and/or causes hydronephrosis or nonfunctioning kidney.
IV	Tumor has extended beyond the true pelvis or has involve the mucosa of the bladder or rectum.
IVA	Tumor invades mucosa of bladder or rectum and/or extends beyond true pelvis.
IVB	Distant metastasis (including peritoneal spread; involvement of supraclavicular, mediastinal, or para-aortic lymph nodes; lung; liver; or bone).

TREATMENT
Microinvasive Cervical Cancer

Stage IA
The term microinvasive cervical cancer refers to this group of early-stage, small tumors. Criteria by FIGO staging for stage IA tumor limits stromal invasion to no greater than 5 mm and lateral spread to no wider than 7 mm. Microinvasive cervical cancer carries a minor risk of lymph node involvement and excellent prognosis after appropriate treatment.

Stage IA1
These tumors have stromal invasion no deeper than 3mm and horizontal spread no more than 7 mm and are associated with low risk for lymph node involvement. Squamous cervical cancer with stromal invasion less than 1 mm have a 1% risk of nodal metastasis, and patients with 1 to 3 mm of stromal invasion carry a 1.5% risk or nodal metastases. Of 4098 women studied with stage IA1, fewer than 1% died of the disease.[49] Findings such as this provide the basis for less aggressive management

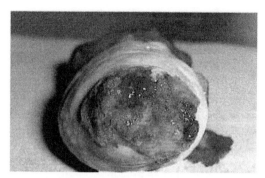

Fig. 1. Stage IB cervical cancer: visible lesion confined to cervix.

of stage IA1 squamous cell carcinoma, if lymphovascular space invasion (LVSI) is absent. Acceptable treatment options include cervical conization or a simple hysterectomy.

The presence of LVSI in stage IA1 cervical cancer increases the risk of lymph node metastasis and cancer recurrence to approximately 5%. Therefore, some gynecologic oncologists manage these cases with modified radical hysterectomy (type II hysterectomy) and pelvic lymphadenectomy.

Stage IA2

Cervical lesions with 3 to 5 mm of stromal invasion have a 7% risk of lymph node metastasis and a greater than 4% risk of cancer recurrence. Therefore, modified radical hysterectomy and pelvic lymphadenectomy are indicated. Alternatively, patients with microinvasive carcinoma (stages IA1 and IA2) and who are poor surgical candidates can be treated with intracavitary brachytherapy alone with excellent results.

Stage IB to IIA1

Cervical stage IB to IIA1 cancer can be treated with either surgery or chemoradiation[50] (**Fig. 1**). In a prospective study of primary therapy, 393 women were randomly assigned to undergo radical hysterectomy and pelvic lymphadenectomy or receive primary radiation therapy. Five-year overall survival and disease-free survival were statistically equivalent (83% and 74%, respectively). Surgical patients, however, had significantly greater severe morbidity rates compared with the radiotherapy group.[50]

Because radiotherapy and surgery are both viable options, the optimum treatment for each woman ideally should assess clinical factors such as menopausal status, age, concurrent medical illness, tumor histology, and cervical diameter. In general, radical hysterectomy for stage IB to IIA tumors is usually selected for young women with low body mass index (BMI) who wish to preserve ovarian function and have concerns about altered sexual functioning following radiotherapy. Surgery is contraindicated in patients with severe cardiac or pulmonary disease or prior thromboembolism. Age and weight are not contraindications to surgery; although in general, older women may have longer hospital stays and heavier women can have longer operative time, greater blood loss, and higher rates of wound complication.

In those electing surgery, oophorectomy may be deferred in younger women. A GOG study evaluated tumor spread to the ovary in those with IB tumors electing radical hysterectomy without adnexectomy. Ovarian metastases were identified in

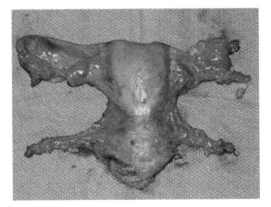

Fig. 2. Radical hysterectomy specimen.

only 0.5% of 770 women with stage IB squamous cell cancers and in 2% of those with adenocarcinomas.[51]

Modified radical hysterectomy (type II)
Modified radical hysterectomy removes the cervix, proximal vagina, and parametrial and paracervical tissue. The ureters are unroofed from the paracervical tunnel until their point of entry into the bladder. They are then retracted laterally to enable removal of the parametrial and paracervical tissue medial to the ureter. This hysterectomy is well suited for tumors with 3- to 5-mm depths of invasion and for smaller stage IB tumors.[52]

Radical hysterectomy (type III)
This hysterectomy requires greater resection of the parametria, and excision extends to the pelvic sidewall (**Fig. 2**). The ureters are completely dissected from their beds and the bladder and rectum are mobilized to permit this more extensive removal of tissue. In addition, at least 2 to 3 cm of proximal vagina is resected. This procedure is performed for larger IB lesions, on patients with relative contraindications to radiation such as diabetes, pelvic inflammatory disease, hypertension, collagen disease, or adnexal masses.

Radical trachelectomy
Some authors have reported management of stage IA2 and IB1 cervical cancer with radical trachelectomy, lymphadenectomy, and placement of cerclage for fertility preservation. These procedures have high cure rates, and successful pregnancies have been reported. Preoperative MRI is recommended for these cases; if the tumor has extended beyond the internal cervical os, then trachelectomy is contraindicated. For selected patients with stage IB1 cervical cancer, fertility-sparing radical trachelectomy appears to have an oncologic outcome similar to that of radical hysterectomy. Lymph vascular space invasion and deep stromal invasion appear to be valuable predictors of outcome.[53,54] The majority of patients can undergo the operation successfully; however, nearly 32% of all selected cases will require hysterectomy or postoperative chemoradiation for oncologic reasons.[55]

Surgical and radiotherapy complication
Complications for early-stage cervical cancer surgery include ureteral stricture, bladder dysfunction, constipation, wound breakdown, lymphocyst, and lymphedema. In addition, adjuvant radiotherapy increases complication risks.

Radiation therapy is also associated with long-term complications. Altered sexual function secondary to shortened vagina, dyspareunia, psychological factors, and vaginal stenosis are often encountered. Late urinary and bowel complications such as fistula formation, enteritis, proctitis, and bowel obstruction may also develop.

Adjuvant treatment after radical hysterectomy

Intermediate risk of recurrence The GOG has defined recurrence risk factors that would identify women who undergo radical surgery for early-stage cervical cancer. Intermediate risk describes those who on average would have a 30% risk of cancer recurrence within 3 years. Factors included in this model are depth of tumor invasion, tumor diameter, and LVSI.

To determine appropriate treatment of these at-risk women, patients with these intermediate-risk factors have been studied. In one study, women were randomly assigned to receive pelvic radiation therapy after radical hysterectomy or radical hysterectomy and observation. A nearly 50% reduced risk of recurrence was found in those who received postoperative adjuvant radiation therapy.[56] However, this adjuvant radiation does not prolong overall survival. In our practice, these intermediate-risk patients are counseled regarding their risk of recurrence and offered the option of adjuvant radiation therapy.

High risk of recurrence A high-risk category of patients who undergo radical surgery for early-stage cervical cancer has also been described. High risk is defined as a 50% to 70% risk of recurrence within 5 years. These women have positive lymph nodes, positive surgical margins, or microscopically positive parametria.[57]

This group is routinely offered adjuvant radiation therapy. Moreover, the GOG recently demonstrated that the addition of concurrent chemotherapy consisting of cisplatin and 5-fluorouracil would be beneficial in significantly prolonging disease-free and overall survival in this group of women with high-risk early-stage cancer.[57]

Stage IIA2 to IVA

Advanced-stage cervical cancers extend past the confines of the cervix and are often found to involve adjacent organs and retroperitoneal lymph nodes (**Fig. 3**). As such, treatment for these tumors must be individualized to maximize patient outcome. The vast majority of advanced-stage tumors have poor prognosis, with 5-year survival rates of less than 50% (**Table 3**). Advanced-stage tumors represent a large proportion

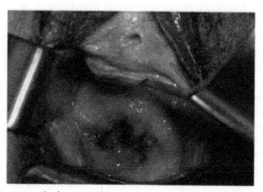

Fig. 3. Advanced-stage cervical cancer: large, ulcerative lesion involving cervix and vagina.

Table 3
Cervical cancer survival rates according to stage

Stage	5-Year Survival (%)
IA	100
IB	88
IIA	68
IIB	44
III	18–39
IVA	18–34

Data from Refs.[79–81]

of invasive cervical cancers treated, depending on the geographic area studied. Untreated, these tumors progress rapidly.

Radiation therapy

This modality forms the cornerstone of advanced-stage cervical cancer management. Both external pelvic radiation and brachytherapy are typically delivered. Of these, external-beam radiation usually precedes intracavitary radiation, which is one form of brachytherapy. External-beam radiation is commonly administered in 25 fractions during 5 weeks. To limit bladder and rectal doses during brachytherapy, bowel and bladder are packed away from the intracavitary source during tandem insertion, using vaginal packing. During staging, if para-aortic nodal metastasis is found, then extended field radiation can be added to treat these affected lymph nodes.

Chemoradiation

Current evidence indicates that concurrent chemotherapy significantly improves overall and disease-free survival of women with advanced cervical cancer. Thus, most patients with stage IIA2-IVA cervical cancer are best treated with chemoradiation. Cisplatin-containing regimens have been associated with the best survival rates.[58,59] For patients without proven para-aortic nodal metastases, a study reported in 1999 demonstrated that pelvic radiation and concurrent chemotherapy was superior to prophylactic extended-field radiation without chemotherapy.[60] Extended-field radiation is used when there is proven common iliac nodal or para-aortic nodal disease, although the dose of concurrent chemotherapy may have to be reduced to manage toxicity. At our institution, cisplatin is given weekly for 5 weeks and is administered concurrently with radiotherapy. Additional doses of chemotherapy, administered after chemoradiation, have also been shown to improve survival outcomes in patients with advanced-stage cervical cancer.[61]

Surgery for advanced stage cervical cancer

Surgical evaluation of retroperitoneal lymph nodes offers accurate detection of pelvic and para-aortic metastasis. In addition, debulking of tumor-laden nodes is also achieved. As a result, lymph node dissection may enhance management of and improve survival rates in patients with advanced-stage cervical cancer. Retrospective studies have suggested a statistically significant survival benefit to extended chemotherapy and/or extended-field radiation therapy if positive pelvic/para-aortic nodes are identified.[62,63]

In addition to its diagnostic power, surgical staging also permits debulking of grossly positive nodes. Evidence supporting a survival benefit from debulking macroscopic para-aortic nodes is contradictory. Although some retrospective studies have shown disease-free survival rates for patients whose macroscopic nodal disease has been resected is similar to that of women with microscopic nodal disease, this benefit does not extend to overall survival rates.[62,64]

Despite these suggested benefits, routine operative staging for advanced-stage cervical cancer has failed to achieve its intended goal of substantially increasing survival. Studies estimate only a 4% to 6% survival benefit.[65,66] These patients often have systemic disease, and failure to control pelvic disease has contributed to the poor overall survival in this group of patients.

Coexistent pelvic mass in advanced-stage cervical cancer

A pelvic mass maybe identified on CT or other imaging. Before radiation, any suspicious adnexal masses should be explored and a histologic diagnosis obtained. Coexistent pyometra or hematometra should be drained and broad-spectrum antibiotics utilized to treat the infection. Active infection may decrease the response to radiation therapy and may exacerbate into a systemic infection when radiation rods are placed for purposes of brachytherapy.

Stage IVB

Patients with stage IVB disease have poor prognosis and are treated for palliative purposes only. Pelvic radiation may be administered for vaginal bleeding or pain. Systemic chemotherapy is offered to palliate symptoms.

SURVEILLANCE

Eighty percent of recurrences are detected within the subsequent 2 years. In addition to pelvic examination, a thorough manual nodal survey should include neck, supraclavicular, infraclavicular, axillary, and inguinal lymph nodes. In addition, a chest radiograph can be obtained yearly. Cervical or vaginal cuff Pap smear should also be collected every 3 months for 2 years and then every 6 months for 3 years. Abnormal Pap smears should prompt further evaluation for recurrent disease. During patient surveillance, identification of an abnormal pelvic mass or abnormal pelvic examination, pain radiating down the posterior thigh, or new-onset lower extremity edema should prompt CT scanning of the abdomen and pelvis.

RECURRENT CERVICAL CANCER DISEASE

Disease recurrence is defined as a new lesion after completion of primary therapy. Cervical cancer that has not completely regressed within 3 months of radiotherapy is considered persistent.

Treatment of persistent or recurrent disease depends on its location and extent. The intent in these cases is usually palliative. However, in certain instances, a woman may qualify for pelvic radiation if she previously had not received this treatment or for a curative-intent surgical procedure. All chemotherapy-based treatments of metastatic disease are administered with a goal of palliation. In these cases, the primary focus is to maximize existing patient quality of life.

Pelvic Exenteration for Secondary Disease

When curative-intent surgery is contemplated, local disease should be biopsy proven. Clinically, a woman may be considered for pelvic exenteration if lower extremity

Table 4
Combination chemotherapy regimens and response rates of cervical cancer

Study	Chemotherapy Agents	Response Rates (%)	PFS	OS
Moore et al[75]	Cisplatin vs cisplatin and taxol (phase III)	19 vs 36	2.8 vs 4.8 mo	No difference
Long et al[76]	Cisplatin vs cisplatin and topotecan (phase III)	13 vs 27	2.9 vs 4.6 mo	6.5 vs 9.4 mo
Morris et al[77]	Cisplatin and vinorelbine (phase II)	30	5.5 mo	
Brewer et al[78]	Cisplatin and gemcitabine (phase II)	22	2.1 mo	

Abbreviations: OS, overall survival; PFS, progression-free survival.

edema, back pain, and hydronephrosis are absent. If present, these suggest disease extension to the pelvic side walls, which would contraindicate surgery. In addition, regional and distant metastasis should be excluded by both physical examination and radiologic imaging.

Pelvic exenteration begins with exploratory laparotomy, biopsies of suspicious lesions and pelvic and para-aortic lymph node evaluation. Exenteration is completed only if there is no disease in frozen section specimens sampled during surgery. A total pelvic exenteration involves enbloc removal of bladder, uterus, rectum, vagina, and at times vulva, depending on the exact site and extent of the recurrent lesion. The reported 5-year survival is approximately 40%, ranging from 18% to 70% in the literature. As part of the total pelvic exenteration, reconstruction can involve diversion of urine utilizing a segment bowel, termed "conduit," a descending colostomy and vaginal reconstruction with placement of flaps or omental pedicle graft.

Alternatively, in highly selected patients radical hysterectomy may be considered an alternative to pelvic exenteration.[67] In these circumstances, women should have small cervical recurrences measuring less than 2 cm and have disease-free pelvic lymph nodes both before and during surgery. With either surgical procedure, intraoperative and postoperative complications can be significant.

Radiotherapy for Recurrent Disease

Patients with central or limited peripheral recurrences who are radiotherapy naive are candidates for curative-intent radiation treatment. In these groups, survival rates of 30% to 70% have been reported.[68–71] Radiotherapy can occasionally be used as salvage treatment after definitive primary radiation in patients with small-volume pelvic disease when there has been a long disease-free interval.

Chemotherapy for Secondary Disease

Antineoplastic drugs are used to palliate both disease and symptoms of advanced, persistent, or recurrent cervical cancer (**Table 4**). Cisplatin is considered the single most active cytotoxic agent in this setting.[72] Overall, response duration to cisplatin is 4 to 6 months, and survival in such women approximates only 7 months.[73] Cisplatin is also combined with paclitaxel or topotecan to offer a survival advantage to this group of patients (see **Table 4**). Ongoing GOG studies aim to determine the best combination cytotoxic chemotherapy for patients with recurrent or persistent cervical cancer.

PALLIATIVE CARE

Palliative chemotherapy is administered only if this treatment does not cause significant decline in patient quality of life. Pain management forms the basis of palliation. Any decision for treatment of cervical cancer in a palliative care setting should be assessed against the benefits of supportive care. We recommend discussion of medical directives if a patient has adequate mental capability. Home hospice is an invaluable part of terminal care for most of these women, who require intense pain management and 100% assistance with daily living activities.

MANAGEMENT DURING PREGNANCY

There is no difference in survival between pregnant and nonpregnant women with cervical cancer when matched by age, stage, and year of diagnosis. As with nonpregnant women, clinical stage at diagnosis is the single most important prognostic factor for cervical cancer during pregnancy. Overall survival is slightly better for cervical cancer in pregnancy because an increased proportion of patients have stage I disease.

Diagnosis

A Pap smear is recommended for all pregnant patients at the initial prenatal visit. In addition, clinically suspicious lesions should be directly biopsied. If Pap test results reveal suspected HSIL or malignancy, then colposcopy is performed and biopsies are obtained. However, endocervical curettage is excluded. If Pap testing indicates malignant cells and colposcopic-directed biopsy fails to confirm malignancy, then diagnostic conization may be necessary. Conization is recommended only during the second trimester and only in patients with inadequate colposcopic findings and extremely strong cytologic evidence of invasive cancer. Conization is deferred in the first trimester, as this surgery is associated with abortion rates of 30% in this part of pregnancy.

Stage I Cancer in Pregnancy

Women with microinvasive squamous cell cervical carcinoma measuring 3 mm or less and containing no LVSI may deliver vaginally and be reevaluated 6 weeks postpartum. Moreover, for those with stage IA or IB disease, studies find no increased maternal risk when treatment is intentionally delayed to optimize fetal maturity regardless of trimester during which cancer was diagnosed. Given the outcomes, a planned treatment delay is generally acceptable for women who are 20 or more weeks gestational age at diagnosis with stage I disease and who desire to continue their pregnancy. However, a patient may be able to delay from earlier gestational ages if she wishes.

Advanced Cervical Cancer in Pregnancy

Women with advanced cervical cancer diagnosed before fetal viability are offered primary chemoradiation. Spontaneous abortion of the fetus tends to follow whole-pelvis radiation therapy. If cancer is diagnosed after fetal viability is reached and a delay until fetal pulmonary maturity is elected, then a classic cesarean delivery is performed. A classic cesarean incision minimizes the risk of cutting through tumor in the lower uterine segment, which can cause serious blood loss. Chemoradiation is administered after uterine involution. For patients with advanced disease and treatment delay, pregnancy may impair prognosis. Women who elect to delay treatment, to provide quantifiable benefit to their fetus, will have to accept an undefined risk of disease progression.

INVASIVE CERVICAL CANCER FOUND AFTER SIMPLE HYSTERECTOMY

Simple hysterectomy for invasive cervical cancer is not curative. The treatment options include either chemoradiation or radical surgery with radical parametrectomy, upper vaginectomy, and pelvic and para-aortic lymphadenectomy. In an exhaustive review of the literature comparing the two options, the weighted average 5-year survival favored radiation therapy over further surgery (68.7% vs 49.2%).[74] Complication rates of either treatment modality after a simple hysterectomy are high. Concurrent cisplatin-based chemoradiation is recommended for gross residual disease, positive imaging, disease in the lymph nodes and/or parametrium, and/or a positive surgical margin.

Survival for patients with no residual cancer after simple hysterectomy is favorable, although the treatment complication rate may be higher than that reported for patients undergoing primary irradiation. Survival for patients with gross disease at the start of posthysterectomy treatment is poor.

SUMMARY

Squamous cell cervical cancer incidence and mortality have been reduced dramatically as a result of successful screening in many countries. The incidence of cervical adenocarcinoma continues to increase. There has been concentrated effort toward improving early detection and screening by utilizing molecular biomarker assays. The FIGO staging system for cervical cancer was revised in 2009. Fertility preservation can be offered to patients with early-stage cervical cancer through radical trachelectomy, although radical hysterectomy remains the surgical standard of care. Concurrent chemotherapy with radiation has been shown to have a survival advantage in patients with advanced-stage disease. Improvements in radiation techniques and molecular targeted therapy are the current research venues in cervical cancer.

REFERENCES

1. Jemal A, Bray F, Center MM, et al. Global cancer statistics. CA Cancer J Clin 2011;61(2):69–90.
2. Barnholtz-Sloan J, Patel N, Rollison D, et al. Incidence trends of invasive cervical cancer in the United States by combined race and ethnicity. Cancer Causes Control 2009;20:1129–38.
3. Wang SS, Carreon JD, Gomez SL, et al. Cervical cancer incidence among 6 Asian ethnic groups in the United States, 1996 through 2004. Cancer 2010;116(4):949–56.
4. Howe HL, Wu X, Ries LA, et al. Annual report to the nation on the status of cancer, 1975–2003, featuring cancer among U.S. Hispanic/Latino populations. Cancer 2006; 107(8):1711–42.
5. Sherman ME, Wang SS, Carreon J, et al. Mortality trends for cervical squamous and adenocarcinoma in the United States: relation to incidence and survival. Cancer 2005;103(6):1258–64.
6. Committee on Practice Bulletins–Gynecology. ACOG practice bulletin. Diagnosis and treatment of cervical carcinomas, number 35, May 2002. Obstet Gynecol 2002;99 (5 Pt 1): 855–67.
7. Datta GD, Colditz GA, Kawachi I, et al. Individual-, neighborhood-, and state-level socioeconomic predictors of cervical carcinoma screening among U.S. black women: a multilevel analysis. Cancer 2006;106(3):664–9.

8. Trimble CL, Genkinger JM, Burke AE, et al. Active and passive cigarette smoking and the risk of cervical neoplasia. Obstet Gynecol 2005;105(1):174–81.

9. Koshiol J, Schroeder J, Jamieson DJ, et al. Smoking and time to clearance of human papillomavirus infection in HIV-seropositive and HIV-seronegative women. Am J Epidemiol 2006;164(2):176–83.

10. Plummer M, Herrero R, Franceschi S, et al. Smoking and cervical cancer: pooled analysis of the IARC multi-centric case-control study. Cancer Causes Control 2003; 14(9):805–14.

11. Muñoz N, Franceschi S, Bosetti C, et al. Role of parity and human papillomavirus in cervical cancer: the IARC multicentric case-control study. Lancet 2002;359(9312):1093–101.

12. Moreno V, Bosch FX, Muñoz N, et al. Effect of oral contraceptives on risk of cervical cancer in women with human papillomavirus infection: the IARC multicentric case-control study. Lancet 2002;359(9312):1085–92.

13. The International Collaboration of Epidemiological Studies of Cervical Cancer. Comparison of risk factors for invasive squamous cell carcinoma and adenocarcinoma of the cervix: collaborative reanalysis of individual data on 8,097 women with squamous cell carcinoma and 1,374 women with adenocarcinoma from 12 epidemiological studies. Int J Cancer 2007;120:885–91.

14. Benoit AG, Krepart GV, Lotocki RJ. Results of prior cytologic screening in patients with a diagnosis of stage I carcinoma of the cervix. Am J Obstet Gynecol 1984;148(5):690–4.

15. Bosch FX, Muñoz N. The viral etiology of cervical cancer. Virus Res 2002;89(2): 183–90.

16. Jones DL, Münger K. Analysis of the p53-mediated G1 growth arrest pathway in cells expressing the human papillomavirus type 16 E7 oncoprotein. J Virol 1997;71(4): 2905–12.

17. Jones EE, Wells SI. Cervical cancer and human papillomaviruses: inactivation of retinoblastoma and other tumor suppressor pathways. Curr Mol Med 2006;6(7):795–808.

18. Helt AM, Funk JO, Galloway DA. Inactivation of both the retinoblastoma tumor suppressor and p21 by the human papillomavirus type 16 E7 oncoprotein is necessary to inhibit cell cycle arrest in human epithelial cells. J Virol 2002;76(20):10559–68.

19. Wontzengen N, Vinokurova S, von Knebel Doeberitz M. Systematic review of genomic integration sites of human papillomavirus genomes in epithelial dysplasia and invasive cancer of the female lower genital tract. Cancer Res 2004;64(11):3878–84.

20. Fader AN, Edwards RP, Cost M, et al. Sentinel lymph node biopsy in early-stage cervical cancer: utility of intraoperative versus postoperative assessment. Gynecol Oncol 2008;111(1):13–7.

21. Cormier B, Diaz JP, Shih K, et al. Establishing a sentinel lymph node mapping algorithm for the treatment of early cervical cancer. Gynecol Oncol 2011;122(2): 275–80.

22. Alfsen GC, Kristensen GB, Skovlund E, et al. Histologic subtype has minor importance for overall survival in patients with adenocarcinoma of the uterine cervix: a population-based study of prognostic factors in 505 patients with nonsquamous cell carcinomas of the cervix. Cancer 2001;92(9):2471–83.

23. Grigsby PW, Perez CA, Kuske RR, et al. Adenocarcinoma of the uterine cervix: lack of evidence for a poor prognosis. Radiother Oncol 1988;12(4):289–96.

24. Kilgore LC, Soong SJ, Gore H, et al. Analysis of prognostic features in adenocarcinoma of the cervix. Gynecol Oncol 1988;31(1):137–53.

25. Lee KB, Lee JM, Park CY, et al. What is the difference between squamous cell carcinoma and adenocarcinoma of the cervix? A matched case-control study. Int J Gynecol Cancer 2006;16(4):1569–73.

26. Davy ML, Dodd TJ, Luke CG, et al. Cervical cancer: effect of glandular cell type on prognosis, treatment, and survival. Obstet Gynecol 2003;101(1):38–45.

27. Eifel PJ, Burke TW, Morris M, et al. Adenocarcinoma as an independent risk factor for disease recurrence in patients with stage IB cervical carcinoma. Gynecol Oncol 1995;59(1):38–44.

28. Eifel PJ, Morris M, Oswald MJ, et al. Adenocarcinoma of the uterine cervix: prognosis and patterns of failure in 367 cases. Cancer 1990;65(11):2507–14.

29. Hopkins MP, Morley GW. A comparison of adenocarcinoma and squamous cell carcinoma of the cervix. Obstet Gynecol 1991;77(6):912–7.

30. Lai CH, Hsueh S, Hong JH, et al. Are adenocarcinomas and adenosquamous carcinomas different from squamous carcinomas in stage IB and II cervical cancer patients undergoing primary radical surgery? Int J Gynecol Cancer 1999;9(1):28–36.

31. Lee YY, Choi CH, Kim TJ, et al. A comparison of pure adenocarcinoma and squamous cell carcinoma of the cervix after radical hysterectomy in stage IB–IIA. Gynecol Oncol 2011;120(3):439–43.

32. Macdonald OK, Chen J, Dodson M, et al. Prognostic significance of histology and positive lymph node involvement following radical hysterectomy in carcinoma of the cervix. Am J Clin Oncol 2009;32(4):411–6.

33. McCusker ME, Coté TR, Clegg LX, et al. Endocrine tumors of the uterine cervix: incidence, demographics, and survival with comparison to squamous cell carcinoma. Gynecol Oncol 2003;88(3):333–9.

34. Chen J, Macdonald OK, Gaffney DK. Incidence, mortality, and prognostic factors of small cell carcinoma of the cervix. Obstet Gynecol 2008;111(6):1394–402.

35. Pecorelli S, Zigliani L, Odicino F. Revised FIGO staging for carcinoma of the cervix. Int J Gynaecol Obstet 2009;105(2):107–8.

36. Benedet JL, Bender H, Jones H 3rd, et al. FIGO staging classifications and clinical practice guidelines in the management of gynecologic cancers. FIGO Committee on Gynecologic Oncology. Int J Gynaecol Obstet 2000;70(2):209–62.

37. Lagasse LD, Creasman WT, Shingleton HM, et al. Results and complications of operative staging in cervical cancer: experience of the Gynecologic Oncology Group. Gynecol Oncol 1980;9(1):90–8.

38. Mitchell DG, Snyder B, Coakley F, et al. Early invasive cervical cancer: tumor delineation by magnetic resonance imaging, computed tomography, and clinical examination, verified by pathologic results, in the ACRIN 6651/GOG 183 Intergroup Study. J Clin Oncol 2006;24(36):5687–94.

39. Sahdev A, Sohaib SA, Wenaden AE, et al. The performance of magnetic resonance imaging in early cervical carcinoma: a long-term experience. Int J Gynecol Cancer 2007;17(3):629–36.

40. Rajendran JG, Greer BE. Expanding role of positron emission tomography in cancer of the uterine cervix. J Natl Compr Canc Netw 2006;4(5):463–9.

41. Wolfson AH. Magnetic resonance imaging and positron-emission tomography imaging in the 21st century as tools for the evaluation and management of patients with invasive cervical carcinoma. Semin Radiat Oncol 2006;16(3):186–91.

42. Lin WC, Hung YC, Yeh LS, et al. Usefulness of (18)F-fluorodeoxyglucose positron emission tomography to detect para-aortic lymph nodal metastasis in advanced cervical cancer with negative computed tomography findings. Gynecol Oncol 2003; 89(1):73–6.

43. Rose PG, Adler LP, Rodriguez M, et al. Positron emission tomography for evaluating para-aortic nodal metastasis in locally advanced cervical cancer before surgical staging: a surgicopathologic study. J Clin Oncol 1999;17(1):41–5.

44. Yen TC, Ng KK, Ma SY, et al. Value of dual-phase 2-fluoro-2-deoxy-d-glucose positron emission tomography in cervical cancer. J Clin Oncol 2003;21(19):3651–8.
45. Amit A, Beck D, Lowenstein L, et al. The role of hybrid PET/CT in the evaluation of patients with cervical cancer. Gynecol Oncol 2006;100(1):65–9.
46. Chou HH, Chang TC, Yen TC, et al. Low value of [^{18}F]-fluoro-2-deoxy-D-glucose positron emission tomography in primary staging of early-stage cervical cancer before radical hysterectomy. J Clin Oncol 2006;24(1):123–8.
47. Wright JD, Dehdashti F, Herzog TJ, et al. Preoperative lymph node staging of early-stage cervical carcinoma by [^{18}F]-fluoro-2–deoxy-D-glucose-positron emission tomography. Cancer 2005;104(11):2484–91.
48. Loft A, Berthelsen AK, Roed H, et al. The diagnostic value of PET/CT scanning in patients with cervical cancer: a prospective study. Gynecol Oncol 2007;106(1): 29–34.
49. Östör AG, Rome RM. Micro-invasive squamous cell carcinoma of the cervix: a clinico-pathologic study of 200 cases with long-term follow-up. Int J Gynecol Cancer 1994;4(4):257–64.
50. Landoni F, Maneo A, Colombo A, et al. Randomised study of radical surgery versus radiotherapy for stage Ib–IIa cervical cancer. Lancet 1997;350(9077):535–40.
51. Sutton GP, Bundy BN, Delgado G, et al. Ovarian metastases in stage IB carcinoma of the cervix: a Gynecologic Oncology Group study. Am J Obstet Gynecol 1992;166 (1 Pt 1):50–3.
52. Landoni F, Maneo A, Cormio G, et al. Class II versus class III radical hysterectomy in stage IB–IIA cervical cancer: a prospective randomized study. Gynecol Oncol 2001; 80(1):3–12.
53. Diaz JP, Sonoda Y, Leitao MM, et al. Oncologic outcome of fertility-sparing radical trachelectomy versus radical hysterectomy for stage IB1 cervical carcinoma. Gynecol Oncol 2008;111(2):255–60.
54. Abu-Rustum NR, Sonoda Y, Black D, et al. Fertility-sparing radical abdominal trachelectomy for cervical carcinoma: technique and review of the literature. Gynecol Oncol 2006;103(3):807–13.
55. Abu-Rustum NR, Neubauer N, Sonoda Y, et al. Surgical and pathologic outcomes of fertility-sparing radical abdominal trachelectomy for FIGO stage IB1 cervical cancer. Gynecol Oncol 2008;111(2):261–4.
56. Sedlis A, Bundy BN, Rotman MZ, et al. A randomized trial of pelvic radiation therapy versus no further therapy in selected patients with stage IB carcinoma of the cervix after radical hysterectomy and pelvic lymphadenectomy: a Gynecologic Oncology Group study. Gynecol Oncol 1999;73(2):177–83.
57. Peters WA 3rd, Liu PY, Barrett RJ 2nd, et al. Concurrent chemotherapy and pelvic radiation therapy compared with pelvic radiation therapy alone as adjuvant therapy after radical surgery in high-risk early-stage cancer of the cervix. J Clin Oncol 2000;18(8):1606–13.
58. Rose PG, Adler LP, Rodriguez M, et al. Positron emission tomography for evaluating para aortic nodal metastasis in locally advanced cervical cancer before surgical staging: a surgicopathologic study. J Clin Oncol 1999;17(1):41–5.
59. Whitney CW, Sause W, Bundy BN, et al. Randomized comparison of fluorouracil plus cisplatin versus hydroxyurea as an adjunct to radiation therapy in stage IIB–IVA carcinoma of the cervix with negative para-aortic lymph nodes: a Gynecologic Oncology Group and Southwest Oncology Group study. J Clin Oncol 1999;17(5): 1339–48.

60. Morris M, Eifel PJ, Lu J, et al. Pelvic radiation with concurrent chemotherapy compared with pelvic and para-aortic radiation for high-risk cervical cancer. N Engl J Med 1999;340(15):1137–43.

61. Dueñas-González A, Zarbá JJ, Patel F, et al. Phase III, open-label, randomized study comparing concurrent gemcitabine plus cisplatin and radiation followed by adjuvant gemcitabine and cisplatin versus concurrent cisplatin and radiation in patients with stage IIB to IVA carcinoma of the cervix. J Clin Oncol 2011;29(13):1678–85.

62. Hacker NF, Wain GV, Nicklin JL. Resection of bulky positive lymph nodes in patients with cervical carcinoma. Int J Gynecol Cancer 1995;5(4):250–6.

63. Holcomb K, Abulafia O, Matthews RP, et al. The impact of pretreatment staging laparotomy on survival in locally advanced cervical carcinoma. Eur J Gynaecol Oncol 1999;20(2):90–3.

64. Cosin JA, Fowler JM, Chen MD, et al. Pretreatment surgical staging of patients with cervical carcinoma: the case for lymph node debulking. Cancer 1998;82(11):2241–8.

65. Kupets R, Thomas GM, Covens A. Is there a role for pelvic lymph node debulking in advanced cervical cancer? Gynecol Oncol 2002;87(2):163–70.

66. Petereit DG, Hartenback EM, Thomas GM. Para-aortic lymph node evaluation in cervical cancer: the impact of staging upon treatment decisions and outcome. Int J Gynecol Cancer 1998;8:353–64.

67. Coleman RL, Keeney ED, Freedman RS, et al. Radical hysterectomy for recurrent carcinoma of the uterine cervix after radiotherapy. Gynecol Oncol 1994;55(1):29–35.

68. Ijaz T, Eifel PJ, Burke T, et al. Radiation therapy of pelvic recurrence after radical hysterectomy for cervical carcinoma. Gynecol Oncol 1998;70(2):241–6.

69. Ito H, Shigematsu N, Kawada T, et al. Radiotherapy for centrally recurrent cervical cancer of the vaginal stump following hysterectomy. Gynecol Oncol 1997;67(2):154–61.

70. Lanciano R. Radiotherapy for the treatment of locally recurrent cervical cancer. J Natl Cancer Inst Monogr 1996;(21):113–5.

71. Potter ME, Alvarez RD, Gay FL, et al. Optimal therapy for pelvic recurrence after radical hysterectomy for early-stage cervical cancer. Gynecol Oncol 1990;37(1):74–7.

72. Thigpen JT, Vance R, Puneky L, et al. Chemotherapy as a palliative treatment in carcinoma of the uterine cervix. Semin Oncol 1995;22(2 Suppl 3):16–24.

73. Vermorken JB. The role of chemotherapy in squamous cell carcinoma of the uterine cervix: a review. Int J Gynecol Cancer 1993;3(3):129–42.

74. Münstedt K, Johnson P, von Georgi R, et al. Consequences of inadvertent, suboptimal primary surgery in carcinoma of the uterine cervix. Gynecol Oncol 2004;94(2):515–20.

75. Moore DH, Blessing JA, McQuellon RP, et al. Phase III study of cisplatin with or without paclitaxel in stage IVB, recurrent, or persistent squamous cell carcinoma of the cervix: a Gynecologic Oncology Group study. J Clin Oncol 2004;22(15):3113.

76. Long HJ 3rd, Bundy BN, Grendys EC Jr, et al. Randomized phase III trial of cisplatin with or without topotecan in carcinoma of the uterine cervix: a Gynecologic Oncology Group study. J Clin Oncol 2005;23(21):4626.

77. Morris M, Blessing JA, Monk BJ, et al. Phase II study of cisplatin and vinorelbine in squamous cell carcinoma of the cervix: a Gynecologic Oncology Group study. J Clin Oncol 2004;22(16):3340.

78. Brewer CA, Blessing JA, Nagourney RA, et al. Cisplatin plus gemcitabine in previously treated squamous cell carcinoma of the cervix: a phase II study of the Gynecologic Oncology Group. Gynecol Oncol 2006;100(2):385.

79. Grigsby PW, Perez CA. Radiotherapy alone for medically inoperable carcinoma of the cervix: stage IA and carcinoma in situ. Int J Radiat Oncol Biol Phys 1991;21(2):375.
80. Komaki R, Brickner TJ, Hanlon AL, et al. Long-term results of treatment of cervical carcinoma in the United States in 1973, 1978, and 1983: Patterns of Care Study (PCS). Int J Radiat Oncol Biol Phys 1995;31(4):973.
81. Webb MJ, Symmonds RE. Site of recurrence of cervical cancer after radical hysterectomy. Am J Obstet Gynecol 1980;138(7 Pt 1):813–7.

Endometrial Cancer

Kimberly K. Leslie, MD[a],*, Kristina W. Thiel, PhD[a],
Michael J. Goodheart, MD[a,b], Koen De Geest, MD[a,b], Yichen Jia[a],
Shujie Yang, PhD[a]

KEYWORDS

- Endometrial cancer • Risk factors • Diagnosis • Treatment • Progesterone
- Estrogen • Chemotherapy

KEY POINTS

- Incidence of endometrial cancer is on the rise, with an estimated 46,470 new diagnoses in 2011 and a lifetime risk of ~3%. Survival for endometrial cancer is significantly worse than 30 years ago.
- Endometrial cancer is most commonly diagnosed at endometrial biopsy in symptomatic patients.
- In 2009, the International Federation of Gynecology and Obstetrics revised the staging system for carcinomas of the endometrium; major changes include grouping stages IA and IB together as IA and the division of Stage IIIC (metastasis to the pelvic and/or paraaortic lymph nodes) into stage IIIC1 (positive pelvic nodes) and IIIC2 (positive paraaortic lymph nodes).
- Studies from LAP2 and other large clinical trials demonstrate no survival benefit for patients that undergo lymphadenectomy.
- Currently, there is no well-established treatment protocol for patients with advanced-stage disease, though chemotherapy is the treatment of choice. The targeted inhibitors of mTOR (temsirolimus, everolimus) and VEGF (bevacizumab) were the first molecular agent to demonstrate activity as single agents in advanced endometrial cancers.
- Emerging novel therapeutic strategies that are being explored in pre-clinical and clinical studies include addition of a molecular inhibitor to increase the efficacy of chemotherapy and use of epigenetic modulators to restore sensitivity to progesterone-based therapy.

Endometrial cancer is the fourth most common cancer in women, with an estimated 46,470 new diagnoses and over 8000 deaths in 2011. Incidence of endometrial

DISCLOSURES
Funding sources: Dr Leslie: National Institutes of Health (NIH) CA99908, the Department of Obstetrics and Gynecology Academic Enrichment Fund, the Gynecologic Oncology Group Core Laboratory for Receptors and Targets funded by NIH CA27469.
Conflict of Interest: The authors declare no competing interests.
[a] Department of Obstetrics and Gynecology, University of Iowa, 200 Hawkins Drive, Iowa City, IA 52242, USA; [b] Division of Gynecologic Oncology, University of Iowa, Iowa City, IA, USA
* Corresponding Author.
E-mail address: kimberly-leslie@uiowa.edu

Obstet Gynecol Clin N Am 39 (2012) 255–268
http://dx.doi.org/10.1016/j.ogc.2012.04.001
0889-8545/12/$ – see front matter © 2012 Elsevier Inc. All rights reserved.

cancer is on the rise, with a lifetime risk of approximately 3%. Most strikingly, 5-year survival is currently significantly worse than 30 years ago (84% survival in 2006 vs 88% survival in 1975), making endometrial cancer only one of two cancers with increased mortality.[1] This rate is stark in comparison with breast and prostate cancer, for which 5-year survival has substantially improved to over 90% for breast and 100% for prostate cancer. For patients with early stage disease, hysterectomy is considered curative. By contrast, advanced stage and high-grade endometrial cancers are lethal. Certain risk factors have been well-characterized, such as menopausal status, obesity, diabetes, hypertension, and unopposed estrogen, although for some of these risk factors, such as obesity, the mechanisms by which these risk factors promote endometrial cancer are not completely understood.[2] In this article the authors describe the current practices for diagnosis and treatment of endometrial cancer and discuss emerging therapeutic strategies that are hoped to improve survival and reverse the alarming rising trend of this disease.

DIAGNOSIS

Unlike breast and prostate cancer, for which screening tests are available to the general population, endometrial cancer is most commonly diagnosed at endometrial biopsy in symptomatic patients; in other words, after a postmenopausal patient reports vaginal bleeding. No generally applicable screening test is available. For patients who receive a pelvic ultrasound for another indication, an enlarged endometrial stripe or other intrauterine anomaly such as a polyp may prompt biopsy in the absence of vaginal bleeding. However, most experts agree that ultrasound is not recommended as a screening tool in asymptomatic patients.

Common noncancerous histologic findings include both simple and complex hyperplasia (both with and without atypia). If left untreated, the incidence of progression to endometrial cancer ranges from 1% to 29% of cases depending on the type of hyperplasia (simple vs complex) and the degree of cytologic atypia.[3] In addition to the risk of cancer progression with a diagnosis of endometrial hyperplasia made in the community setting, a recent study performed within the Gynecologic Oncology Group (GOG) demonstrated that a large percentage of patients (42%) with a biopsy diagnosis of atypical endometrial hyperplasia have a concurrent endometrial cancer at the time of hysterectomy.[4] A similar study performed within an academic medical center examined the incidence of endometrial adenocarcinoma within hysterectomy specimens from patients with a preoperative diagnosis of atypical hyperplasia. This study noted a slightly higher incidence (48%) of endometrial adenocarcinoma in patients with a preoperative diagnosis of endometrial hyperplasia.[5] This result is in contrast to other smaller studies that reported rates of coexistence of endometrial hyperplasia and endometrial cancer as low as 10% of cases.[6] These data suggest at a minimum close observation for women with atypical endometrial hyperplasia with strong consideration given to hysterectomy in women who have completed childbearing or who are not interested in reproduction and progestin therapy in women who wish to maintain fertility.

STAGING

In 2009, the International Federation of Gynecology and Obstetrics (FIGO) revised the staging system for carcinomas of the vulva, cervix, and endometrium.[7,8] The primary changes made for endometrial cancer included the grouping of stages IA and IB together as stage IA, with the loss of prior IC and the division of stage IIIC (metastasis to the pelvic and/or para-aortic lymph nodes) into stage IIIC1 (positive pelvic nodes) and IIIC2 (positive para-aortic lymph nodes). Specifically the old staging system defined stage IA as no invasion into the myometrium, stage IB as less than 50% invasion into the myometrium, and stage IC as equal to or greater than 50% invasion into the myometrium, whereas the new FIGO 2009 system defines stage IA as cancer confined to the uterus with less than 50% myometrial invasion and stage IB as equal to or greater than 50% myometrial invasion, with both IA and IB including any tumor grade. This system was modified after data from the FIGO Annual Report showed no difference in survival between previous stage IA grade 1 or 2 and stage IB grade 1 or 2 tumors.[9] The other significant change involved patients with positive pelvic or para-aortic lymph nodes. Under the old FIGO guidelines, patients with positive pelvic and/or para-aortic lymph nodes were staged as IIIC, and under the new system patients with positive pelvic lymph nodes are separated from those with positive para-aortic with or without positive pelvic lymph nodes, stage IIIC1 and IIIC2, respectively. This change was made because many studies demonstrated worse survival for patients with positive para-aortic lymph nodes when compared with positive pelvic lymph nodes.[10,11]

SURGICAL PROCEDURE FOR ENDOMETRIAL CANCER

Endometrial cancer is initially staged and treated at surgery. Standard treatment for this cancer in the United States consists of removal of the uterus, cervix, both fallopian tubes, and ovaries, as well as selective pelvic and para-aortic lymphadenectomy.

Information regarding the need for lymph node dissection in all cases is difficult to decipher with data supporting both views. It seems that it is reasonable to determine the risk of nodal metastasis in order to assign patients to a low risk group and a high risk group. A recent publication reporting the risk for lymph node metastasis in low versus high risk patients from a secondary analysis of GOG study LAP2 indicates only .8% of patients in the low risk group had nodal involvement.[12] Thus, unnecessary lymphadenectomy may be avoidable in those patients with very low risk for nodal disease. Based on data from GOG study 33, the two factors most important in determining lymph node involvement are depth of tumor invasion and tumor grade.[10] Previous studies examining patients with early stage disease have demonstrated higher recurrence rates in patients with positive lymph nodes as well as decreased survival rates.[14,15] However, two large prospective studies that examined the value of lymph node dissection found no survival difference between groups who did or did not undergo lymphadenectomy. Yet, there were limitations to both of these studies, specifically the inclusion of postoperative therapy and the lack of complete pelvic and para-aortic lymph node dissection.[16,17]

The long-term risks of lymph node dissection are rather uncommon.[18] Relatively recent data from the LAP2 trial have demonstrated the safe use of minimally invasive techniques for lymph node dissection when compared with an open procedure.[19] Although the intraoperative complication rates were similar between these two groups, this study did not specifically examine the complication rates of lymph node dissection. A publication from the Mayo Clinic proposes the identification of a low risk subset of patients in which lymph node dissection can be avoided.[20] No patients in this group had positive lymph nodes, thus demonstrating and confirming the belief that lymph node dissection may be best performed in patients with a high risk for nodal involvement.

For women who are not surgical candidates, primary radiation therapy (RT) may be recommended instead of surgery. As an alternative for younger women wishing to preserve fertility, progestin-containing intrauterine devices have been used with reasonable safety and efficacy,[21,22] although this treatment has predominantly been performed in patients with grade 1 disease. However, one case of grade 2 has been reported to be successfully treated.[21]

RISK STRATIFICATION AND ADJUVANT THERAPY

For those patients who have undergone an appropriate staging and treatment surgery, adjuvant RT (vaginal brachytherapy or external beam), chemotherapy, or hormonal therapy may be recommended depending on risk factors.

Patients are categorized based on risk stratification in the postoperative period.[23] Low risk and low-intermediate risk patients may not require postsurgical therapy; however, molecular risk factors such as p53 mutations and so forth, if known, may impact this decision. Given the potential side effects of adjuvant therapy, it is important to distinguish between patients who would benefit from adjuvant therapy and those who would be better served simply by close clinical follow-up.

Those of high-intermediate risk require postsurgical treatment with RT to reduce local recurrence based on the fact that 75% of recurrences are in the pelvis. Currently there is no well-established treatment protocol for patients with advanced stage disease, although this protocol is the subject of clinical trials. Patients at high risk require adjuvant treatment, which is most often RT for high risk cases confined to the uterus and chemotherapy for cases with extrauterine disease. Large prospective clinical trials have demonstrated that postoperative pelvic RT does decrease local recurrences but has no overall impact on survival.[23,24]

Many clinicians had concerns regarding the side effects of whole pelvic radiation in treating patients with early stage endometrial cancer. Recent evidence from the (PORTEC-2) Post-Operative Radiation Therapy for Endometrial Cancer trial demonstrates that the use of vaginal brachytherapy is no worse than whole pelvic RT, and as a result of this trial, many centers within the United States have shifted to the use of vaginal brachytherapy for their patients in whom adjuvant RT is warranted.[25] Long-term follow-up studies for PORTEC-1 and PORTEC-2 have demonstrated more urinary and bowel dysfunction for patients treated with whole pelvic RT (PORTEC-1) and, as expected, patients who received vaginal brachytherapy exhibited fewer adverse effects than those who received pelvic radiation (PORTEC-2).[26,27]

Obesity is clearly a risk factor for the development of endometrial cancer, but the mechanisms by which obesity promotes endometrial cancer are not well understood.[2] Whereas production of estrone from the adipose tissue with local conversion to estradiol in the endometrium is one hypothesis, recent publications point to a genetic link between obesity and endometrial cancer. For example, an association between single nucleotide polymorphisms in genes related to obesity and endometrial cancer was recently made.[28,29] Much information remains to be understood about the relationship between obesity and endometrial cancer, and support for these efforts are being recognized by the National Cancer Institute (NCI) and other funding agencies, as is reflected by the NCI's recent request for applications directly related to obesity.

CHEMOTHERAPY

Chemotherapy is the treatment of choice for metastatic disease. The choice of the regimen has evolved over the past decade. The most active agents are anthracyclines, platinum compounds, and taxanes. As single agents, these drugs result in a response rate greater than 20%. Single agent chemotherapy is an option for patients who are likely to have unacceptable side effects with multiple agents. However, for the majority of patients, multiple agents are used. Response rates for triple therapy with doxorubicin, cisplatin, and paclitaxel were 57% in GOG 177; however, side effects were prominent.[30] Phase II trials indicate that the double combination of cisplatin and paclitaxel results in a relatively high rate of response, and this regimen seems to be better tolerated.[31–33] A comparison between the triple and double combination regimens with and without doxorubicin is currently under way in GOG 209, and the results are pending.

MOLECULAR THERAPIES FOR ENDOMETRIAL CANCER

We are in an age of renewed hope about cancer treatment with increasing numbers of available agents beyond standard chemotherapeutics.[34–37] A plethora of new molecules that block important signaling and transcriptional/translational pathways in cancer cells are now in use, with many more in development. Although molecular agents have been rapidly deployed to treat other types of malignancies, use in endometrial cancer seems to lag. Endometrial tumors are biologically highly diverse. To realize the benefit these newer drugs may provide, it is our challenge to match individual targeted agents with the tumors most likely to respond. This challenge requires a more complete understanding of uterine carcinogenesis and the molecular events that allow malignant cells to escape normal growth controls. In addition, we must find creative ways to use targeted molecules not only individually, but together and/or with chemotherapy.

Overview of Type I and II Endometrial Cancer

For simplicity, endometrial tumors have been divided into two main subtypes, I and II.[38] Type I endometrial cancer is of endometrioid morphology; it occurs most often in obese postmenopausal women and occasionally in anovulatory premenopausal women. Type I tumors are classically estrogen-related with relatively low grade features and carry a good prognosis. The lesions are commonly well-differentiated, preceded by endometrial hyperplasia, and compose approximately 80% of sporadic tumors. On a molecular level, type I cancers are linked to mutations or down-regulation of the tumor suppressor phospatase and tensin homology (*PTEN*), among other targets, leading to constitutive activation of Akt protein kinase (Akt) and mammalian target of rapamycin (mTOR).[39–43] In comparison, type II tumors comprise a heterogeneous, poorly differentiated group of tumors of high grade endometrioid, serous papillary, or clear cell morphology that primarily occurs in older postmenopausal women. Type II tumors may be estrogen-independent, and they are often accompanied by surrounding endometrial atrophy. Type II cancers have been reported to be associated with abnormalities in *TP53*, *ErbB2*, and *P16*, where high immunostaining indicates mutated nonfunctional proteins.[37,42–47] These tumors are often locally advanced and/or metastatic, and they carry a very poor prognosis.[48] For such lesions, survival is often less than 6 months despite aggressive chemotherapy and radiation.

From this discussion, it is clear that we are beginning to uncover the molecular differences between endometrial cancer subtypes, yet we have not adequately put these findings to use as they pertain to the choice of therapy. In actuality, endometrial tumors often display characteristics of both type I and II cancers in a single lesion. Thus, the challenge for the future will be to find ways to best incorporate targeted molecular therapies for patients with such heterogeneous tumors.

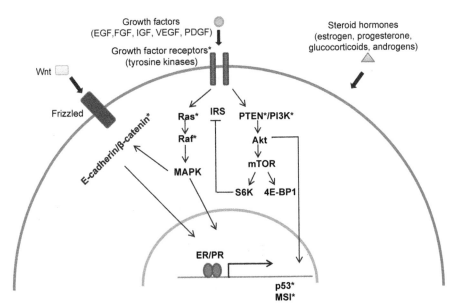

Fig. 1. Critical pathways in endometrial cancer. The major pathways that have been targeted with molecular agents to date. Mutations in key proteins that lead to dysregulation of function are indicated with an asterisk. Activating mutations include those in the tyrosine kinase receptor FGFR2, K-ras, B-raf, PI3K, and β-catenin. Inactivating mutations/deletions have been identified in the tumor suppressors PTEN and p53. Mutations in mismatch repair genes lead to microsatellite instability (MSI).

Central Pathways Controlling Growth in the Endometrium

Endometrial proliferation is controlled by steroid hormones in concert with a complex set of signaling pathways downstream of growth factors and their tyrosine kinase receptors. As shown in **Fig. 1**, cross-talk between steroid hormone and growth factor signaling occurs and is critical for cellular function. The preeminent regulatory signaling pathway consists of two arms: ras/raf/MAPK and PTEN/PI3K/Akt/mTOR (see **Fig. 1**).

Predominance of PI3K/Akt/mTOR signaling in endometrial cancer results from the fact that 30% to 50% of sporadic endometrial carcinomas carry somatically acquired inactivating mutations and/or deletions of PTEN.[49,50] A more recent study reports PTEN inactivation in up to 83% of endometrioid endometrial adenocarcinomas.[41] PTEN is a dual specificity phosphatase that negatively regulates the PI3K/Akt signaling pathway. Mutations that activate PI3K also result in constitutive signaling through this pathway. The protein kinase mTOR is downstream of PTEN and both upstream and downstream of Akt in signaling pathways. It is a member of the phosphatidylinositol kinase-related kinases. Its catalytic activity is regulated by the mitogen activated phosphatidylinositol 3 kinase (PI3K)/Akt pathway. Its principal downstream targets, p70S6 kinase and 4E-binding protein 1 (4E-BP1), control translation. Another of mTOR's targets, eukaryotic initiation factor 4e, induces transformation when overexpressed in experimental models.[51]

Microsatellite instability (MSI), as well as mutations in K-ras, B-raf, FGFR2, PI3K, and beta-catenin, are other genetic alterations common in endometrioid endometrial cancer.[37,43,52,53] Activating K-ras and FGFR mutations result in high levels of activated MAPK, which phosphorylates progrowth transcription factors such as estrogen receptor (ER) and positively regulates beta-catenin activity. ER binds to the promoters of progrowth genes and induces transcription and eventual enhancement of cellular proliferation. The importance of estrogen signaling unopposed by the differentiating effects of progesterone as a risk for endometrial cancer cannot be overstated; this concept has been proved by over 50 years of research indicating that when women receive estrogen-only hormonal replacement therapy there is a resultant significant increase in the rate of endometrial cancer.[54]

For patients with somatic mutations in the germline of the DNA mismatch repair gene, MMR, the disease is called hereditary nonpolyposis colorectal cancer or Lynch syndrome. Mutations in MMR, which occur in endometrioid endometrial cancers, lead to MSI, and patients with Lynch syndrome are diagnosed with endometrial cancer approximately 2 decades younger than patients with sporadic cancer development.[43]

Hormonal Therapy—the First of the Targeted Agents

The uterine endometrium is exquisitely sensitive to hormonal stimulation. Estrogen enhances epithelial proliferation, and progesterone causes epithelial differentiation. In several recent reviews, the application of progestin therapy to endometrial cancer has been described.[55–57] To achieve the antitumor effect, progestins are thought to induce differentiation of tumor cells as well as allow for activation of apoptotic pathways or block active cell division. Not surprisingly, prognosis and response to progestin therapy positively correlates with expression of progesterone receptor (PR). In patients with high PR expression, the overall response rate is 72% compared with 12% in patients with tumors lacking PR.[58] It is important to note, however, that patients who initially responded to progestin therapy frequently relapse. One potential reason for this lack of sustained benefit is because progestins promote downregulation of ER and PR.[59,60] It is thought that a pulse of estrogen can either upregulate both ER and PR (permitting more durable responses to progestin therapy), or recruit neoplastic cells into the cell cycle in a synchronous fashion, enhancing sensitivity to chemotherapy. The Leslie group demonstrated, however, that reexpression of progesterone receptor B (PRB) in PR-negative endometrial cancer cells restores progestin control of cell growth.[61] The addition of an estrogenlike molecule such as tamoxifen and the intermittent use of the progestin have been used by the GOG in study 119 for the purpose of attempting to prevent the progestin-dependent downregulation of PR.[62] The response rate in advanced disease for this study was 33% and segregated with the expression of hormone receptors.[63]

We now understand that one additional mechanism of PR down-regulation is epigenetic via promoter methylation, with one study documenting PRB promoter methylation in 75% of endometrial tumors.[64] Toward developing an alternative treatment strategy, in preclinical studies DNA methyltransferase (DNMT) inhibitors have been explored as a novel approach to restore PR expression.[65,66] One group reported a decrease in proliferation of endometrial cancer cells in response to treatment with a DNMT inhibitor[65]; however, no studies have been reported that examined progestin sensitivity after treatment with an epigenetic modulator in the clinical setting. The authors propose that the combination of progestin therapy with epigenetic modulators that enhance and maintain PR levels is an attractive regimen that offers the opportunity to enhance sensitivity to progestin therapy.[55,56] If hormonal and epigenetic combinations can be created that result in response rates that are the same or better than chemotherapy, but without the substantial side effects, older, frail patients would be particularly benefited.

Given the known relationship between unopposed estrogen stimulation and endometrial cancer risk, it is surprising that compared with progestin treatment, antiestrogen therapy has been disappointing. Tamoxifen alone has limited activity in advanced disease with response rates of 10% in phase II studies.[67] The study of both leuprolide, a gonadotrophin-releasing hormone agonist that results in profound hypoesterogenism,[68] and fulvestrant (GOG 188), the pure antiestrogen,[69] failed to demonstrate sufficient clinical activity to support their widespread use. Likewise, aromatase inhibitors do not demonstrate response rates as high as those obtained with progestins.[70,71] Thus, progestin therapy (at least as a component of the regimen) remains the preferred hormonal treatment for endometrial cancer.

Hormonal Therapy Compared with Chemotherapy

Despite the relatively high response rates with combined chemotherapy, significant side effects are associated with chemotherapy. The negative effects of chemotherapy must be considered given that a majority of the patients with endometrial cancer are elderly and often have comorbidities (ie, obesity, diabetes, and cardiovascular disease). In addition, patients may have had previous RT. Only minor adverse effects have been associated with hormonal therapy (ie, weight gain, edema, and thrombophlebitis), although there is an increased risk of thromboembolism. Thus, for older, frail patients, hormonal therapy is a preferable option, particularly in cases where ER and PR expression are present. However, it is noted that patients without robust ER and PR expression may also respond.[63]

Inhibitors of Growth Factors and Growth Factor Receptor Signaling

Our expanding knowledge of signaling pathways relating cell growth, cell cycle progression, and apoptosis has led to an improved understanding of the molecular events involved in carcinogenesis. Cancer cells require growth factors and their tyrosine kinase receptors to promote angiogenesis, proliferation, invasion, and metastasis. This mechanism sets the stage for expanded therapeutic options, which include blocking the growth factors or receptors with therapeutic inactivating antibodies or with tyrosine kinase inhibitors. For endometrial cancer, agents that block epidermal growth factor receptor (EGFR) (gefitinib, GOG 229C; lapatinib, GOG 229D; erlotinib; cetuximab), human epidermal growth factor receptor 2 (HER-2) (lapatinib, GOG 229D), vascular endothelial growth factor (VEGF) (bevacizumab, GOG 229E; VEGF-trap, GOG 229F), VEGFR (VEGF receptor) (cediranib, GOG 229J), platelet-derived growth factor receptor (PDGFR) (cediranib, GOG 229J), fibroblast growth factor receptor (FGFR) (brivanib, GOG 229I and cediranib, GOG 229J) and mTOR (temsirolimus, National Cancer Institute of Canada; temsirolimus, GOG 248) are under investigation.

In this decade we have reached an important milestone with targeted inhibitors as single agents. The mTOR inhibitors (temsirolimus and everolimus) and bevacizumab were the first molecular therapies other than progestins deemed to have notable clinical benefit in advanced endometrial cancer.[72–74] The response rate for temsirolimus alone in patients with advanced chemonaïve endometrial cancer was 26%.[73] For bevacizumab, the response rate was modest (13.5%) in patients who recurred after chemotherapy and were treated on GOG 229E, yet 40.4% demonstrated progression-free survival beyond 6 months.[72] Trials using tyrosine kinase inhibitors against angiogenic growth factor pathways (VEGFR, PDGFR, FGFR) have yet to be reported, yet it is promising that these trials have achieved the preliminary level of activity required to initiate the second stage of patient accrual in a two-stage phase II design. Thus, it is anticipated that additional drugs with activity will be reported in the coming months. Inhibitors of EGFR and HER-2 have not been impressive thus far as single agents; erlotinib treatment resulted in only one partial response out of 27 cases.[75] Nevertheless, a number of these trials are still ongoing.

Agents on the Horizon

A number of agents are in preclinical testing using models of endometrial cancer. Some have shown remarkable activity alone, whereas others have been combined to achieve true therapeutic synergy. As a biomarker, high expression of the molecular target itself may or may not predict for response. For example, HER-2 amplification in breast cancer predicts for response to trastuzumab therapy, but the level of EGFR expression may not predict response to gefitinib in lung cancer where response has been reported to segregate with EGFR mutations. Similarly, VEGFA levels were not predictive of response to bevacizumab in colorectal cancer[76] but did positively correlate with response to bevacizumab in endometrial cancer as reported from GOG 229E.[72] Regardless of whether the molecular target itself is predictive, the authors hypothesize that other downstream markers will be useful, and the molecular fingerprint of a responsive versus a resistant tumor can be derived. Further research is urgently needed to explore the relationship between marker expression and outcome, the role of surrogate markers, and the best use of accessible tissue.

Clinical benefit may also be achieved using a combinatorial strategy in which one agent improves the efficacy of another. For example, in a recent preclinical study from the Leslie group, combination of the mTOR inhibitor temsirolimus with either a dual PI3K/mTOR inhibitor BEZ235 or a "pure" PI3K inhibitor ZSTK474 resulted in synergistic cell death of endometrial cancer cells.[77] For the BEZ235 and temsirolimus combination in particular, the synergy resulted from blockage of one arm of mTOR signaling, ribosomal 6S kinase, with temsirolimus, whereas BEZ235 inhibited the compensatory Akt activation that occurs in response to temsirolimus as well as a second arm of mTOR signaling, 4E-BP1. This study also identified the molecular fingerprint of cells most likely to respond to temsirolimus treatment alone: loss of PTEN and high basal Akt phosphorylation. However, all cells, regardless of PTEN and Akt phosphorylation status, responded to the BEZ235 and temsirolimus combination treatment.

Another area in which a combination approach may be beneficial is to improve sensitivity to chemotherapy. The first effort by the GOG to combine a molecular inhibitor (either temsirolimus or bevacizumab) with chemotherapy is GOG study 086-P, and the results have not been released. Another more recent GOG trial is studying how sensitivity to chemotherapy (docetaxel and gemcitabine plus granulocyte colony-stimulating factor [G-CSF]) can be restored or increased with a molecular inhibitor, bevacizumab (GOG 250). This strategy is being explored in many other types of solid tumors, and future endometrial cancer trials that pair other molecular inhibitors with chemotherapy are anticipated. These combination strategies will likely be based on results from preclinical experiments analogous to the temsirolimus and BEZ235 study.

Combination of a molecular inhibitor, temsirolimus, with progestin is under study in GOG 248, although the results are not yet available. Given that progestin therapy is so safe for patients as compared with chemotherapy, the authors also propose that strategies to restore PR expression will expand the utility of progestin therapy. One approach is through use of DNMT inhibitors to reverse PR promoter methylation and thereby restore functional PR expression. However, cells may have other mechanisms in place to suppress PR expression, such as histone deacetylation, which also serves as a cellular cue to prevent PR transcription. In other tumors, combination of histone deacetylase (HDAC) inhibitors with DNMT inhibitors has been shown to produce synergistic effects, although the mechanisms are still being teased out.

Other possible inhibitors, including those of heat shock proteins, the proteasome, and poly ADP ribose polymerase (PARP), and controllers of the mitotic machinery, such as polo-like kinase 1, are on the horizon and may be useful in many tumor types, including those of the endometrium. Application of molecular inhibitors in the treatment of solid tumors is still in its infancy as compared with other treatment modalities, and certain obstacles must be overcome to fully realize their potential. First, a better understanding of the types of tumors that are more likely to respond to each inhibitor is necessary. For example, PARP inhibitors may be more effective in type II tumors based on activity in p53-deficient mouse models of breast cancer.[78] Second, studies will need to determine if targeted agents provide benefit in the neoadjuvant setting, such as use of epigenetic modulators to restore PR expression. Finally, with respect to combination strategies, a careful analysis of the timing and sequence of administration must be undertaken.

SUMMARY

Despite the questions and barriers, the incorporation of molecular therapy into treatment regimens in endometrial cancer is an exciting area of investigation with the potential to improve outcomes. Outside of the development of a reliable screening test for endometrial cancer, converting the disease to a chronic state and improving progression-free survival is our best hope to reverse the concerning trend of decreasing 5-year survival for this disease.

CLINICAL UPDATE

The results of GOG 209 (Randomized Phase III Noninferiority Trial of First Line Chemotherapy for Metastatic or Recurrent Endometrial Carcinoma: A Gynecologic Oncology Group Study) were recently reported at the 2012 Society of Gynecologic Oncology Meeting.[79] This study found that addition of a third chemotherapy, doxorubicin, to the combination of cisplatin/carboplatin and paclitaxel, does not improve survival, and, in fact, the two-chemotherapy regimen was better tolerated.

REFERENCES

1. American Cancer Society. Cancer Facts and Figures 2011. Available at: http://www.cancer.org/acs/groups/content/@epidemiologysurveilance/documents/document/acspc-029771.pdf. Accessed November 21, 2011.
2. Schmandt RE, Iglesias DA, Co NN, et al. Understanding obesity and endometrial cancer risk: opportunities for prevention. Am J Obstet Gynecol 2011;205(6):518–25.
3. Kurman RJ, Kaminski PF, Norris HJ. The behavior of endometrial hyperplasia. A long-term study of "untreated" hyperplasia in 170 patients. Cancer 1985;56(2):403–12.
4. Trimble CL, Kauderer J, Zaino R, et al. Concurrent endometrial carcinoma in women with a biopsy diagnosis of atypical endometrial hyperplasia: a Gynecologic Oncology Group study. Cancer 2006;106(4):812–9.
5. Shutter J, Wright TC Jr. Prevalence of underlying adenocarcinoma in women with atypical endometrial hyperplasia. Int J Gynecol Pathol 2005;24(4):313–8.
6. Hahn HS, Chun YK, Kwon YI, et al. Concurrent endometrial carcinoma following hysterectomy for atypical endometrial hyperplasia. Eur J Obstet Gynecol Reprod Biol 2010;150(1):80–3.

7. Pecorelli S. Revised FIGO staging for carcinoma of the vulva, cervix, and endometrium. Int J Gynaecol Obstet 2009;105(2):103–4.
8. Mutch DG. The New FIGO staging system for cancers of the vulva, cervix, endometrium, and sarcomas. Gynecol Oncol 2009;115:325–8.
9. Creasman WT, Odicino F, Maisonneuve P, et al. Carcinoma of the corpus uteri. FIGO 26th Annual Report on the Results of Treatment in Gynecological Cancer. Int J Gynaecol Obstet 2006;95(Suppl 1):S105–43.
10. Gultekin M, Yildiz F, Ozyigit G, et al. Comparison of FIGO 1988 and 2009 staging systems for endometrial carcinoma. Med Oncol 2012. [Epub ahead of print].
11. Page BR, Pappas L, Cooke EW, et al. Does the FIGO 2009 endometrial cancer staging system more accurately correlate with clinical outcome in different histologies?: revised staging, endometrial cancer, histology. Int J Gynecol Cancer 2012. [Epub ahead of print].
12. Milam MR, Java J, Walker JL, et al. Nodal metastasis risk in endometrioid endometrial cancer. Obstet Gynecol 2012;119(2 Pt 1):286–92.
13. Creasman WT, Morrow CP, Bundy BN, et al. Surgical pathologic spread patterns of endometrial cancer. A Gynecologic Oncology Group Study. Cancer 1987;60(8 Suppl):2035–41.
14. Morrow CP, Bundy BN, Kurman RJ, et al. Relationship between surgical-pathological risk factors and outcome in clinical stage I and II carcinoma of the endometrium: a Gynecologic Oncology Group study. Gynecol Oncol 1991;40(1):55–65.
15. Lurain JR, Rice BL, Rademaker AW, et al. Prognostic factors associated with recurrence in clinical stage I adenocarcinoma of the endometrium. Obstet Gynecol 1991;78(1):63–9.
16. Kitchener H, Swart AM, Qian Q, et al. Efficacy of systematic pelvic lymphadenectomy in endometrial cancer (MRC ASTEC trial): a randomised study. Lancet 2009;373(9658):125–36.
17. Benedetti Panici P, Basile S, Maneschi F, et al. Systematic pelvic lymphadenectomy vs. no lymphadenectomy in early-stage endometrial carcinoma: randomized clinical trial. J Natl Cancer Inst 2008;100(23):1707–16.
18. Orr JW Jr, Holloway RW, Orr PF, et al. Surgical staging of uterine cancer: an analysis of perioperative morbidity. Gynecol Oncol 1991;42(3):209–16.
19. Walker JL, Piedmonte MR, Spirtos NM, et al. Laparoscopy compared with laparotomy for comprehensive surgical staging of uterine cancer: Gynecologic Oncology Group Study LAP2. J Clin Oncol 2009;27(32):5331–6.
20. Mariani A, Dowdy SC, Cliby WA, et al. Prospective assessment of lymphatic dissemination in endometrial cancer: a paradigm shift in surgical staging. Gynecol Oncol 2008;109(1):11–8.
21. Brown AJ, Westin SN, Broaddus RR, et al. Progestin intrauterine device in an adolescent with grade 2 endometrial cancer. Obstet Gynecol 2012;119(2 Pt 2):423–6.
22. Leslie KK, Thiel KW, Yang S. Endometrial cancer: potential treatment and prevention with progestin-containing intrauterine devices. Obstet Gynecol 2012;119(2 Pt 2):419–20.
23. Keys HM, Roberts JA, Brunetto VL, et al. A phase III trial of surgery with or without adjunctive external pelvic radiation therapy in intermediate risk endometrial adenocarcinoma: a Gynecologic Oncology Group study. Gynecol Oncol 2004;92(3):744–51.
24. Creutzberg CL, van Putten W, Koper PC, et al. Surgery and postoperative radiotherapy versus surgery alone for patients with stage-1 endometrial carcinoma: multicentre randomised trial. PORTEC Study Group. Post Operative Radiation Therapy in Endometrial Carcinoma. Lancet 2000;355(9213):1404–11.

25. Nout RA, Smit VT, Putter H, et al. Vaginal brachytherapy versus pelvic external beam radiotherapy for patients with endometrial cancer of high-intermediate risk (PORTEC-2): an open-label, non-inferiority, randomised trial. Lancet 2010;375(9717):816–23.

26. Nout RA, van de Poll-Franse LV, Lybeert ML, et al. Long-term outcome and quality of life of patients with endometrial carcinoma treated with or without pelvic radiotherapy in the post operative radiation therapy in endometrial carcinoma 1 (PORTEC-1) trial. J Clin Oncol 2011;29(13):1692–700.

27. Nout RA, Putter H, Jurgenliemk-Schulz IM, et al. Five-year quality of life of endometrial cancer patients treated in the randomised Post Operative Radiation Therapy in Endometrial Cancer (PORTEC-2) trial and comparison with norm data. Eur J Cancer 2011. [Epub ahead of print].

28. Delahanty RJ, Beeghly-Fadiel A, Xiang YB, et al. Association of obesity-related genetic variants with endometrial cancer risk: a report from the Shanghai Endometrial Cancer Genetics Study. Am J Epidemiol 2011;174(10):1115–26.

29. Chen X, Xiang YB, Long JR, et al. Genetic polymorphisms in obesity-related genes and endometrial cancer risk. Cancer 2011. [Epub ahead of print].

30. Fleming GF, Brunetto VL, Cella D, et al. Phase III trial of doxorubicin plus cisplatin with or without paclitaxel plus filgrastim in advanced endometrial carcinoma: a Gynecologic Oncology Group Study. J Clin Oncol 2004;22(11):2159–66.

31. Hoskins PJ, Swenerton KD, Pike JA, et al. Paclitaxel and carboplatin, alone or with irradiation, in advanced or recurrent endometrial cancer: a phase II study. J Clin Oncol 2001;19(20):4048–53.

32. Sorbe B, Andersson H, Boman K, et al. Treatment of primary advanced and recurrent endometrial carcinoma with a combination of carboplatin and paclitaxel-long-term follow-up. Int J Gynecol Cancer 2008;18(4):803–8.

33. Sovak MA, Dupont J, Hensley ML, et al. Paclitaxel and carboplatin in the treatment of advanced or recurrent endometrial cancer: a large retrospective study. Int J Gynecol Cancer 2007;17(1):197–203.

34. Itamochi H. Targeted therapies in epithelial ovarian cancer: Molecular mechanisms of action. World J Biol Chem 2010;1(7):209–20.

35. Temkin SM, Fleming G. Current treatment of metastatic endometrial cancer. Cancer Control 2009;16(1):38–45.

36. Leslie KK, Laidler LL, Albitar L, et al. Tyrosine kinase inhibitors in endometrial cancer. Int J Gynecol Cancer 2005;15:409–11.

37. Zagouri F, Bozas G, Kafantari E, et al. Endometrial cancer: what is new in adjuvant and molecularly targeted therapy? Obstet Gynecol Int 2010;2010:749579.

38. Sherman ME, Sturgeon S, Brinton L, et al. Endometrial cancer chemoprevention: implications of diverse pathways of carcinogenesis. J Cell Biochem Suppl 1995;23: 160–4.

39. Enomoto T, Inoue M, Perantoni AO, et al. K-ras activation in premalignant and malignant epithelial lesions of the human uterus. Cancer Res 1991;51(19):5308–14.

40. Risinger JI, Hayes AK, Berchuck A, et al. PTEN/MMAC1 mutations in endometrial cancers. Cancer Res 1997;57(21):4736–8.

41. Mutter GL, Lin MC, Fitzgerald JT, et al. Altered PTEN expression as a diagnostic marker for the earliest endometrial precancers [see comments]. J Natl Cancer Inst 2000; 92(11):924–30.

42. Ryan AJ, Susil B, Jobling TW, et al. Endometrial cancer. Cell Tissue Res 2005;322(1): 53–61.

43. Okuda T, Sekizawa A, Purwosunu Y, et al. Genetics of endometrial cancers. Obstet Gynecol Int 2010;2010:984013.

44. Moll UM, Chalas E, Auguste M, et al. Uterine papillary serous carcinoma evolves via a p53-driven pathway. Hum Pathol 1996;27(12):1295–300.
45. Zheng W, Cao P, Zheng M, et al. p53 overexpression and bcl-2 persistence in endometrial carcinoma: comparison of papillary serous and endometrioid subtypes. Gynecol Oncol 1996;61(2):167–74.
46. Kounelis S, Kapranos N, Kouri E, et al. Immunohistochemical profile of endometrial adenocarcinoma: a study of 61 cases and review of the literature. Mod Pathol 2000;13(4):379–88.
47. Singh M, Darcy KM, Brady WE, et al. Cadherins, catenins and cell cycle regulators: impact on survival in a Gynecologic Oncology Group phase II endometrial cancer trial. Gynecol Oncol 2011;123(2):320–8.
48. Leslie KK, Stein MP, Kumar NS, et al. Progesterone receptor isoform identification and subcellular localization in endometrial cancer. Gynecol Oncol 2005;96(1):32–41.
49. Ali IU, Gatekeeper for endometrium: the PTEN tumor suppressor gene. J Natl Cancer Inst 2000;92(11):861–3.
50. Tashiro H, Blazes MS, Wu R, et al. Mutations in PTEN are frequent in endometrial carcinoma but rare in other common gynecological malignancies. Cancer Res 1997; 57(18):3935–40.
51. Rosenwald IB, Rhoads DB, Callanan LD, et al. Increased expression of eukaryotic translation initiation factors eIF-4E and eIF-2 alpha in response to growth induction by c-myc. Proc Natl Acad Sci U S A 1993;90(13):6175–8.
52. Byron SA, Gartside M, Powell MA, et al. FGFR2 point mutations in 466 endometrioid endometrial tumors: relationship with MSI, KRAS, PIK3CA, CTNNB1 mutations and clinicopathological features. PLoS One 2012;7(2):e30801.
53. Horst D, Chen J, Morikawa T, et al. Differential WNT activity in colorectal cancer confers limited tumorigenic potential and is regulated by MAPK signaling. Cancer Res 2012;72(6):1547–56.
54. Furness S, Roberts H, Marjoribanks J, et al. Hormone therapy in postmenopausal women and risk of endometrial hyperplasia. Cochrane Database Syst Rev 2009;2: CD000402.
55. Yang S, Thiel KW, De Geest K, et al. Endometrial cancer: reviving progesterone therapy in the molecular age. Discov Med 2011;12(64):205–12.
56. Yang S, Thiel KW, Leslie KK. Progesterone: the ultimate endometrial tumor suppressor. Trends Endocrinol Metab 2011;22(4):145–52.
57. Kim JJ, Chapman-Davis E. Role of progesterone in endometrial cancer. Semin Reprod Med 2010;28(1):81–90.
58. Ehrlich CE, Young PC, Stehman FB, et al. Steroid receptors and clinical outcome in patients with adenocarcinoma of the endometrium. Am J Obstet Gynecol 1988; 158(4):796–807.
59. Satyaswaroop PG, Clarke CL, Zaino RJ, et al. Apparent resistance in human endometrial carcinoma during combination treatment with tamoxifen and progestin may result from desensitization following downregulation of tumor progesterone receptor. Cancer Lett 1992;62(2):107–14.
60. Mortel R, Zaino RJ, Satyaswaroop PG. Designing a schedule of progestin administration in the control of endometrial carcinoma growth in the nude mouse model. Am J Obstet Gynecol 1990;162(4):928–34 [discussion: 934–6].
61. Dai D, Kumar NS, Wolf DM, et al. Molecular tools to reestablish progestin control of endometrial cancer cell proliferation. Am J Obstet Gynecol 2001;184(5):790–7.
62. Whitney CW, Brunetto VL, Zaino RJ, et al. Phase II study of medroxyprogesterone acetate plus tamoxifen in advanced endometrial carcinoma: a Gynecologic Oncology Group study. Gynecol Oncol 2004;92(1):4–9.

63. Singh M, Zaino RJ, Filiaci VJ, et al. Relationship of estrogen and progesterone receptors to clinical outcome in metastatic endometrial carcinoma: a Gynecologic Oncology Group Study. Gynecol Oncol 2007;106(2):325–33.

64. Sasaki M, Dharia A, Oh BR, et al. Progesterone receptor B gene inactivation and CpG hypermethylation in human uterine endometrial cancer. Cancer Res 2001;61(1):97–102.

65. Ren Y, Liu X, Ma D, et al. Down-regulation of the progesterone receptor by the methylation of progesterone receptor gene in endometrial cancer cells. Cancer Genet Cytogenet 2007;175(2):107–16.

66. Xiong Y, Dowdy SC, Gonzalez Bosquet J, et al. Epigenetic-mediated upregulation of progesterone receptor B gene in endometrial cancer cell lines. Gynecol Oncol 2005;99(1):135–41.

67. Thigpen T, Brady MF, Homesley HD, et al. Tamoxifen in the treatment of advanced or recurrent endometrial carcinoma: a Gynecologic Oncology Group study. J Clin Oncol 2001;19(2):364–7.

68. Covens A, Thomas G, Shaw P, et al. A phase II study of leuprolide in advanced/recurrent endometrial cancer. Gynecol Oncol 1997;64(1):126–9.

69. Covens AL, Filiaci V, Gersell D, et al. Phase II study of fulvestrant in recurrent/metastatic endometrial carcinoma: a Gynecologic Oncology Group study. Gynecol Oncol 2011;120(2):185–8.

70. Rose PG, Brunetto VL, VanLe L, et al. A phase II trial of anastrozole in advanced recurrent or persistent endometrial carcinoma: a Gynecologic Oncology Group study. Gynecol Oncol 2000;78(2):212–6.

71. Ma BB, Oza A, Eisenhauer E, et al. The activity of letrozole in patients with advanced or recurrent endometrial cancer and correlation with biological markers–a study of the National Cancer Institute of Canada Clinical Trials Group. Int J Gynecol Cancer 2004;14(4):650–8.

72. Aghajanian C, Sill MW, Darcy KM, et al. Phase II trial of bevacizumab in recurrent or persistent endometrial cancer: a Gynecologic Oncology Group study. J Clin Oncol 2011;29(16):2259–65.

73. Oza AM, Elit L, Tsao MS, et al. Phase II study of temsirolimus in women with recurrent or metastatic endometrial cancer: a trial of the NCIC Clinical Trials Group. J Clin Oncol 2011;29(24):3278–85.

74. Oza AM, Elit L, Biagi J, et al. Molecular correlates associated with a phase II study of temsirolimus (Temsirolimus) in patients with metastatic or recurrent endometrial cancer–NCIC IND 160. Proc Am Soc Clin Oncol 2006;24(18s):121s [abstr: 3003].

75. Oza AM, Eisenhauer EA, Elit L, et al. Phase II study of erlotinib in recurrent or metastatic endometrial cancer: NCIC IND-148. J Clin Oncol 2008;26(26):4319–25.

76. Jubb AM, Hurwitz HI, Bai W, et al. Impact of vascular endothelial growth factor-A expression, thrombospondin-2 expression, and microvessel density on the treatment effect of bevacizumab in metastatic colorectal cancer. J Clin Oncol 2006;24(2):217–27.

77. Yang S, Xiao X, Meng X, et al. A mechanism for synergy with combined mTOR and PI3 kinase inhibitors PLoS One 2011;6(10):e26343.

78. Hay T, Matthews JR, Pietzka L, et al. Poly(ADP-ribose) polymerase-1 inhibitor treatment regresses autochthonous Brca2/p53-mutant mammary tumors in vivo and delays tumor relapse in combination with carboplatin. Cancer Res 2009;69(9):3850–5.

79. Miller DS. Randomized Phase III Noninferiority Trial of First Line Chemotherapy for Metastatic or Recurrent Endometrial Carcinoma: A Gynecologic Oncology Group Study, in Society of Gynecologic Oncology Meeting. Austin, TX; 2012.

Epithelial Ovarian Cancer

Ahmed N. AL-Niaimi, MD[a,]*, Mostafa Ahmed, BS[b],
Chase B. Petersen, MD[c]

KEYWORDS

- Ovarian cancer • Chemotherapy • Staging • Surgery • Pathology

KEY POINTS

- Ovarian cancer is the second most common cancer of the female genital tract, yet is the deadliest of all.
- Most ovarian cancers are diagnosed in later stages, this is caused by both the absence of screening method and atypical presenting symptoms.
- Treatment includes optimal surgical debunking, followed by chemotherapy.
- The 5 years survival varied between 20–39%.

Epithelial ovarian cancer is the deadliest gynecologic malignancy, constituting the fourth most common cause of death in women and the fifth most common among United States women, after cancers of the lung, breast, colon, and uterus.[1] More than 21,550 cases of ovarian cancer are diagnosed annually in the United States, with approximately 14,500 dying from this disease.[1] A woman's overall lifetime risk for epithelial ovarian cancer is 1.7 % unless increased because of familial risk.

PATHOLOGY AND STAGING

Nearly 80% of epithelial cancers are of serous histologic type. Less frequently encountered histologic types include mucinous (10%), endometrioid (10%), and either clear cell, Brenner, or undifferentiated carcinomas (fewer than 1%).

Regardless of the histology, the behaviors of ovarian cancer cells are categorized into three distinct clinical types; borderline tumors, low-grade tumors, and invasive cancer.

Borderline tumors, which account for 15% of epithelial ovarian tumors, occur more frequently in premenopausal women and overall have a favorable prognosis.[2–4]

[a] Division of Gynecologic Oncology, Department of Obstetrics and Gynecology, University of Wisconsin School of Medicine and Public Health, H4/636 Clinical Science Center, 600 Highland Avenue, Madison, WI 53792–6188, USA; [b] University of Wisconsin School of Medicine and Public Health, Madison, WI, USA; [c] Department of Obstetrics and Gynecology, University of Wisconsin School of Medicine and Public Health, Madison, WI, USA
* Corresponding author.
E-mail address: alniaimi@wisc.edu

Obstet Gynecol Clin N Am 39 (2012) 269–283
http://dx.doi.org/10.1016/j.ogc.2012.03.003
0889-8545/12/$ – see front matter © 2012 Elsevier Inc. All rights reserved.

obgyn.theclinics.com

Borderline tumors, however, can have metastatic implants categorized as invasive and noninvasive implants. Invasive implants are more likely to proliferate in the peritoneal cavity, leading to intestinal obstruction and death.[3,4]

Low-grade ovarian epithelial cancers are usually either serous or mucinous cancers that are generally unresponsive to chemotherapy. Low-grade mucinous tumors may have corresponding pseudomyxoma peritonei, or "jelly belly," which is characterized by copious production of gelatinous mucin, which alone can cause functional bowel obstruction. Low-grade serous carcinomas frequently arise from a borderline precursor and are molecularly distinct from high-grade serous tumors. These tumors contain B-raf and K-ras mutations as compared with p53 mutations seen in high-grade serous cancers.[5,6] Compared with high-grade serous carcinomas (grades 2 and 3), low-grade serous carcinomas have a significantly longer progression-free survival (PFS; 45 vs 19.8 months).[7]

CAUSES

Risk factors for ovarian cancer have been widely studied. Ovarian cancer incidence varies with geographic location. Low parity, infertility, early menarche, and late menopause are associated with elevated ovarian cancer risk.[8,9] One possible mechanism for raising the risk level is repeated cycles of disruption and repair of the ovarian surface epithelium leading to a high rate of p53 overexpression.[10,11] Other risk factors are obesity in adolescence, fertility-enhancing medications,[12] and hormone replacement therapy.[13] Genetic predisposition is seen in approximately 10% to 15% of patients with ovarian cancer, the majority of those women possessing a BRCA1 or BRCA2 gene mutation.[14] For those with BRCA mutation, the use of oral contraceptives or prophylactic removal of the ovaries and fallopian tubes is essential to minimize the cancer risk.

SCREENING

To date there is no effective method of screening for ovarian cancer. In premenopausal women, transvaginal ultrasonography and CA125 have a high rate of false-positives Routine annual pelvic examinations have provided poor results. Recent data from the Prostate, Lung, Colorectal and Ovarian Cancer Screening randomized controlled trial in postmenopausal women confirmed that routine screening in the general population did not reduce ovarian cancer mortality. In fact, in 3285 women with false-positive tests, 1080 underwent surgical management of whom 163 (15%) experienced at least one major complication.[15]

CA125 increases the early diagnosis of epithelial ovarian cancer.[16–24] Sensitivity of CA125 is 50% for stage I disease and 60% for stage II.[24] Specificity improves when CA125 is used in conjunction with transvaginal ultrasonography.[16]

Family history of ovarian cancer increases a woman's risk of the disease over the general population. Of the two BRCA gene mutations, BRCA1 predisposes a woman to a lifetime risk between 28% and 44%, and BRCA2 carries a 27% lifetime risk. When combined there is an 82% lifetime risk of breast cancer.[14,25–27]

Lynch II syndrome and hereditary nonpolyposis colorectal cancer syndrome (HNPCC syndrome) are autosomal dominant genetic causes of ovarian cancer.[28] HNPCC syndrome involves familial colon cancer (known as Lynch I syndrome) and increased rates of ovarian, endometrial, and breast cancers.[28]

Management of Women at High Risk for Ovarian Cancer

The American Society of Clinical Oncologists strongly recommends that women at high risk for ovarian cancer undergo careful evaluation by geneticists. BRCA1 and

BRCA2 testing is clearly beneficial; however, it must be conducted in conjunction with genetic counseling.[29] For those who test positive for a BRCA mutation, the National Institutes of Health Consensus Conference on Ovarian Cancer recommends screening with transvaginal ultrasonography or CA125 levels starting at the age of 35 or 10 years earlier than the youngest age that a family member was diagnosed with ovarian or breast cancer. Beyond screening, prophylactic bilateral salpingo-oophorectomy reduces ovarian cancer risk by 92% and breast cancer risk between 50% and 80%.[30]

CLINICAL PRESENTATION

With early diagnosis of ovarian cancer, cure is possible. Prompt detection and treatment are essential to decreasing disease morbidity and mortality. Unfortunately, the signs and symptoms of ovarian cancer are vague and initially subtle, which often can delay diagnosis.

Symptoms

Most symptoms of ovarian cancer are nonspecific; however, nearly all women will have at least one symptom that is pelvic, abdominal, or menstrual in nature.[31–33] One recent study[34] developed an ovarian cancer symptom index that illustrates many of the common symptoms of ovarian cancer including pelvic or abdominal pain, urinary frequency or urgency, increased abdominal size or bloating, and difficulty eating or feeling full. The overall sensitivity for early disease with this index was 56.7% and 79.5% for advanced stage cancer. Other symptoms can include fatigue, weight changes, indigestion, nausea, anorexia, constipation, back pain, and pain with intercourse.[34] These symptoms are typically insidious in onset and occur daily. It is uncommon for ovarian cancer to present with acute symptoms such as torsion.

Signs

Several signs are typical of ovarian cancer. A mass found on examination that is solid, fixed, or irregular could be malignant. Masses can sometimes be palpated on abdominal examination due to omental caking or peritoneal disease. Another hallmark of ovarian cancer is the presence of ascites, which can occur with pleural effusions and dyspnea. The combination of more than one of these findings raises the possibility for pelvic neoplasm and bears further workup. As with any malignancy, there is increased risk of thromboembolic disease, which may present as deep venous thrombosis, pulmonary embolus, or cerebrovascular accident.

Diagnosis

Combining history, physical examination, laboratory findings, and radiologic findings supports the diagnosis of ovarian cancer. Definitive diagnosis is made via tissue or cytologic diagnosis. A thorough abdominal and pelvic examination, especially a rectovaginal examination, is key to suspecting a diagnosis of ovarian cancer. A delayed diagnosis often results because patients complain about abdominal symptoms, so pelvic examinations are not performed.

A bimanual and rectovaginal examination that reveals an adnexal mass that is fixed, solid, and irregular may indicate cancer; however, tubo-ovarian abscesses and endometriomas can present similarly. A rectovaginal exam can help detect rectal masses and can be enhanced by performing a guaiac test for occult blood. The ovaries are also often better evaluated on rectovaginal examination, because they can lie posterior to the uterus.

The abdominal examination may reveal peritoneal masses, omental caking in the mid to left upper abdomen, or grossly enlarged adnexal masses on palpation. Evaluating for a fluid wave can aid in identifying ascites. Groin and supraclavicular lymph nodes should also be evaluated.

Serum markers and radiology

Routine screening of low-risk women by serum markers and imaging have not been shown to be cost-effective because of a high false-positive rate. However, ultrasound and serum level of CA125 are essential to the evaluation of symptomatic patients.

Transvaginal ultrasound provides better resolution than an abdominal one for evaluation of adnexal masses.[35–38] Complex adnexal features favor malignancy and include irregular borders; solid components (especially those with color Doppler flow); multiple, thick septations (>2–3 mm); and masses that are complex and bilateral or large (>8–10 cm in diameter).[39–41] Simple cysts are more commonly benign. Morphologic features that may indicate malignant neoplasia include large, mostly solid, relatively fixed, or irregularly shaped.

Any significant intraperitoneal ascites, especially in postmenopausal women, is typically abnormal. Additionally, enlarged lymph nodes, peritoneal masses, or carcinomatosis noted on ultrasound suggests malignancy. In patients with a definite pelvic mass, abdominopelvic computed tomography (CT) or magnetic resonance imaging (MRI) provides little addition to characterizing the mass.[42,43] (CT or CT/positron emission tomography [PET] scan, however, is helpful to evaluate distant disease, adenopathy, intraparenchymal metastases, or extraperitoneal disease, all of which may alter the possibility of optimal cytoreductive surgery, favoring a neoadjuvant chemotherapy approach.)

Serology

CA 125 greater than the institutional normal when an adnexal mass is present should be interpreted with caution. When evaluating an adnexal mass, this value must be taken in context to avoid false-positive results, because it is widely distributed in adult tissues. CA125 can be elevated for numerous reasons:

- Physiologically in menstruation, ovulation, and pregnancy
- Other gynecologic causes, including pelvic inflammatory disease, endometriosis, and fibroids
- Any disease causing inflammation of the pleura, pericardium, or peritoneum
- Malignancies, including breast, endometrial, pancreatic, colon, and lung cancers
- Other diseases including hepatitis, cirrhosis, ascites, and tuberculosis.

More than 80% of patients with epithelial ovarian cancer have elevated CA125 levels. When thoughtfully applied, this test can detect 50% of patients with stage I disease and over 90% of those with disease in stages II to IV.[36] CA125 specificity can be further improved when combined with transvaginal ultrasound or when these levels are followed over time.[23] Jacobs and colleagues[16] developed a Risk of Malignancy Index, which combines menopausal status, transvaginal ultrasound findings, and CA125 level to determine high or low risk of malignancy[44] (**Table 1**).

Surgical staging of ovarian cancer is a methodologic process that includes removing or sampling all the tissues that might harbor the tumor. Accordingly the surgery should include:

1. Peritoneal washing with normal saline for cytology analysis.
2. Hysterectomy with bilateral salpingo-oophorectomy.

Table 1		
Ovarian cancer surgical staging and debulking		
Stage I		Cancer limited to the ovaries.
	IA	Cancer is present in one ovary.
	IB	Cancer is present in both ovaries.
	IC	Cancer is present in one or both ovaries and one or more of the following is true: cancer is found on the outside surface of one or both ovaries, the outer covering of the tumor has ruptured, or cancer cells are found in the fluid or tissue linings of the abdomen.
Stage II		Cancer is present in one or both ovaries, and has spread to other parts of the pelvic region.
	IIA	Cancer has spread to the uterus and/or fallopian tubes.
	IIB	Cancer has spread to other organs in the pelvic region such as the bladder, rectum, or sigmoid colon.
	IIC	Cancer has spread to the uterus, fallopian tubes, bladder, sigmoid colon, or rectum. Additionally, cancer may be present in tissue and fluid samples of the lining of the abdominal cavity.
Stage III		Cancer is found in one or both ovaries and has spread to the abdomen.
	IIIA	Cancer is found in one or both ovaries and has microscopically spread to other parts of the abdominal peritoneum.
	IIIB	Cancer has spread to the peritoneum in an amount less than 2 centimeters.
	IIIC	Cancer has spread to the peritoneum more than 2 centimeters and/or has spread to the lymph nodes.
Stage IV		Stage IV ovarian cancer is the most advanced stage of the disease. In this stage, cancer is found in one or both ovaries and has spread to parts of the body beyond the abdomen, or in the liver parenchyma.

Ovarian cancer is staged according to International Federation of Gynecology and Obstetrics (FIGO) staging.

3. Bilateral pelvic and para-aortic lymphadenectomy.
4. Omentectomy.
5. Peritoneal biopsies from the pelvis, paracolic gutters, and diaphragm. This step should be done if the tumor is limited to one of two ovaries or to the pelvis.

A careful initial surgical staging is very important. A national study[45] has shown that up to 28% of patients initially thought to have stage I disease were "upstaged" when reexplored for proper staging, as well as 43% of those thought to have stage II disease.

Surgical debulking of ovarian cancer, on the other hand, means a surgical approach that includes the removal of all ovarian cancer, regardless where the cancer has spread. This approach may include bowel resection, splenectomy, and removal of the peritoneum, or even segmental liver resection.

What is considered an optimal debulking has also evolved with time. In 1969 a study showed that debulking an ovarian tumor to no palpable status showed a dramatic effect on survival. It was not until 1975 that Griffiths,[46] in a secondary analysis of a study for adjuvant chemotherapy, showed a median overall survival increase of 27 months when the debulking surgery was done to a no-residual status. Further studies in the 1980s and 1990s set the mark to 2 cm for an optimal debulking. Combined studies from the Gynecologic Oncology Group (GOG)[40,41] showed that debulking to a microscopic status produced a dramatic effect on both the median progression-free and overall survival. It has since been decided that debulking to a microscopic status is optimal for ovarian cancer.

ADJUVANT TREATMENT

Mainline treatment after optimal ovarian cancer surgery is chemotherapy. Other modalities of treatment for early ovarian cancer, including radiotherapy, have been used to supplement chemotherapy; however, this treatment is not the standard of care in the United States.

Early Ovarian Cancer

Early ovarian cancer is defined as stages I and II. The stages are further classified by pathology to early low-risk ovarian cancer (stage IA, grade 1 or 2) and early high-risk ovarian cancer (stage IA, grade 3 or stage IB–II with any grade).

Patients with early low-risk ovarian cancer (stage IA, grade 1 or 2) need no further treatment after surgery. A study published by Young and colleagues[47] has shown that compared with no treatment there is no survival benefit when patients are treated with melphalan after surgery. Similarly, Trope and colleagues[48] have shown that treating with carboplatin offers no survival benefit compared with observation.

Patients with early high-risk ovarian cancer (stage IA, grade 3, or stage IB–II with any grade) need three cycles of chemotherapy after surgery. A study published by Trimbos and colleagues[49] showed that treating patients with chemotherapy improves overall survival to 82% compared with 72% for patients who did not get any chemotherapy. A GOG study 157[50] showed that six cycles of carboplatin and paclitaxel did not add survival when compared with three cycles. A recent GOG study 175[51] also showed that maintenance chemotherapy after the three cycles is not necessary.

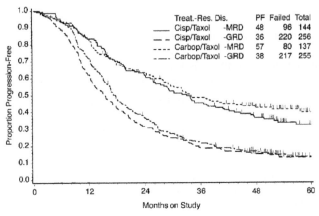

Fig. 1. Superior PFS of the combination carboplatin/paclitaxel. (*From* Katsumata N, Yasuda M, Takahashi F, et al. Dose-dense paclitaxel once a week in combination with carboplatin every 3 weeks for advanced ovarian cancer: a phase 3, open-label, randomised controlled trial. Lancet 2009, 374(9698), 1331–1338; with permission.)

Advanced Ovarian Cancer

Many trials have been published that showed combination chemotherapy after ovarian cancer surgery is needed to achieve a better survival compared with single agent chemotherapy.[52] A series of studies[53–58] has compared combinations of chemotherapy; the latest[58] has concluded that six cycles of combination chemotherapy with carboplatin and paclitaxel are superior (**Fig. 1**), and that is now the standard of care in the United States. The main side effects of this combination include hair loss, bone marrow suppression, and neuropathy. The modalities of administering this combination of chemotherapy are evolving.

Two modalities are the most commonly used now in the United States. The first is intravenous chemotherapy and the second is a combination of intravenous and intraperitoneal chemotherapy.

The "conventional" intravenous chemotherapy modality involves giving the carboplatin in a dose of 5 AUC and the paclitaxel in a dose of 175 mg/m2 every 3 weeks.[58] A recently published modified version of the latter, called "dose-dense" chemotherapy,[59] combines carboplatin (5 AUC) given every 3 weeks with weekly paclitaxel (80 mg/m2). Results of this study showed the dose-dense chemotherapy outcome was progression-free survival of 28 months versus 17 months ($P = 0.0015$) for the conventional course (**Fig. 2**). The dose-dense chemotherapy, however, caused more anemia as a side effect compared with the conventional approach.

Intraperitoneal chemotherapy is the second modality of treatment. The results of many trials[60–63] have been published, but most recently, the GOG-172 trial[62] showed

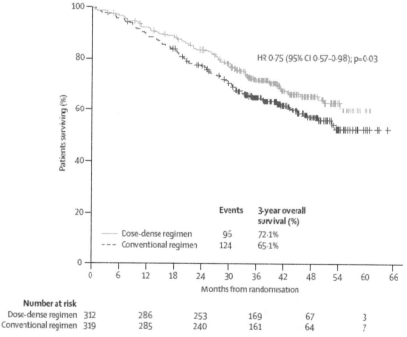

Fig. 2. Superior PFS of the dose-dense chemotherapy. CI, confidence interval; HR, hazard ratio. (*From* Katsumata N, Yasuda M, Takahashi F, et al. Dose-dense paclitaxel once a week in combination with carboplatin every 3 weeks for advanced ovarian cancer: a phase 3, open-label, randomised controlled trial. Lancet 2009, 374(9698), 1331–1338; with permission.)

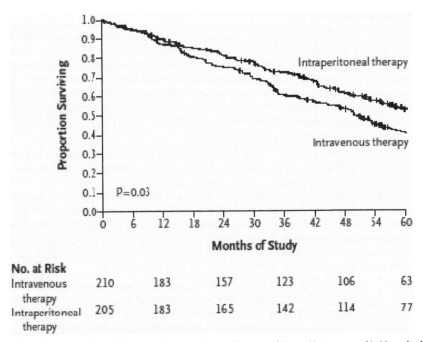

No. at Risk

Intravenous therapy	210	183	157	123	106	63
Intraperitoneal therapy	205	183	165	142	114	77

Fig. 3. The superiority of intraperitoneal chemotherapy. (*From* Katsumata N, Yasuda M, Takahashi F, et al. Dose-dense paclitaxel once a week in combination with carboplatin every 3 weeks for advanced ovarian cancer: a phase 3, open-label, randomised controlled trial. Lancet 2009, 374(9698), 1331–1338; with permission.)

the superiority of giving intraperitoneal/intravenous chemotherapy compared with intravenous conventional chemotherapy. The former modality offered an overall survival of 65 months versus 49 months ($P = 0.03$) for the conventional approach (**Fig. 3**). However, the intraperitoneal/intravenous chemotherapy regimen has more toxicity and side effects, and therefore a high rate of chemotherapy incompletion with lower quality of life. Those factors should be weighed against the increased survival benefit. There is an ongoing GOG randomized clinical trial comparing outcomes of the three modalities.

Bone marrow suppression is the most frequent side effect that causes both significant morbidity and mortality. Carboplatin or paclitaxel doses can be lowered to ameliorate those side effects, or the therapy can be delayed for a week or two to allow proper recovery of the bone marrow. Neuropathy is a more permanent side effect; if it is detected early in the treatment, the paclitaxel can be changed to docetaxel[56] or liposomal doxorubicin[63] without compromising the survival outcome to reduce the incidence of neuropathy.

A randomized European study[64] has shown that neoadjuvant chemotherapy can lower the operative morbidities compared with the conventional adjuvant chemotherapy (upfront surgery followed by the same chemotherapy). This study also has shown the modalities have a similar survival outcome, but unfortunately the survival outcome is much lower than what has been shown in United States randomized trials. Neoadjuvant therapy can be an option to improve surgical outcomes for patients with a high level of preoperative morbidity, understanding that it might lower patients' overall survival.

NEW MOLECULAR TARGETED THERAPY

A new molecular targeted treatment for ovarian cancer includes many medications, the most important of which is a vascular endothelial growth factor inhibitor, also called bevacizumab. Two studies have been published looking at the effect of bevacizumab as an additive treatment to traditional chemotherapy for ovarian cancer. The first study, GOG 218,[65] used bevacizumab with chemotherapy in the adjuvant setting and as maintenance afterward. This study showed a net gain of 4 months of progression-free survival with use of bevacizumab during and up to 10 months after carboplatin and paclitaxel chemotherapy, with no effect on overall survival in early survival analysis. The other international study is ICON-7,[66] which similarly showed a gain of 2 months of progression-free survival without affecting overall survival.

Although the effect of bevacizumab is only on progression-free survival, it is still being studied in current GOG studies. Further studies are needed to delineate the true effect of bevacizumab on long-term survival. Adding bevacizumab to conventional chemotherapy in both trials, however, added more side effects. The most important ones are bowel perforation and additional bone marrow suppression.

POSTTREATMENT SURVEILLANCE

After completion of the adjuvant chemotherapy, a systematic follow-up is needed. **Table 2**[67] outlines the necessary follow-up. Clinical examination is done accordingly, with a CT scan of the abdomen and pelvis to be performed only if a clinical suspicion is raised.

Serum levels of CA125 increase early in cancer recurrence. Although results of a recent randomized blinded trial United Kingdom study of early versus delayed chemotherapy indicate that diagnosing and treating recurrent disease earlier based on the knowledge of high CA125 serum levels does not increase the patient's overall survival, rather patients who initiated chemotherapy when CA125 levels reached twice the upper limit of normal had more chemotherapy and a worse quality of life compared with women who initiated treatment at the time of symptoms.[68,68] In the United States, CA125 serum level is still routinely used in patient follow-up because It might trigger a CT scan that detects cancer recurrence that can be surgically removed, which was not considered in the Rustin study.[69] In the event of an isolated high level of serum CA125 with the absence of radiologic evidence of cancer recurrence, reinitiating chemotherapy should be decided on an individual patient basis.

RECURRENCE

The overall recurrence rate of ovarian cancer is 62%; however, recurrence varies from 10% for stage I to 85% for stage IV with suboptimal debulking. The mean time of recurrence also varies from 12 months for a suboptimal debulked Stage III ovarian cancer to 24 months when optimal debulking is achieved. More important, the timing of recurrence largely determines how the patient is to be treated, and hence recurrence is classified as follows:

1. Platinum-refractory recurrence: the tumor continues to progress during the adjuvant chemotherapy.
2. Platinum-resistant recurrence: the tumor recurs less than 6 months after completing chemotherapy.
3. Platinum-sensitive recurrence: the tumor recurs more than 6 months after completing chemotherapy.

Table 2
Surveillance for ovarian cancer after completion of therapy

Variable	Months			Years		
	0–12	12–24	24–36	3–5	>5	
Review of symptoms and physical examination	Every 3 mo	Every 3 mo	Every 4–6 mo	Every 6 mo	Yearly	
Papanicolaou test/cytologic evidence	Not indicated	Not indicated	Not indicated	Not indicated	Not indicated	
Cancer antigen 125	Optional	Optional	Optional	Optional	Optional	
Radiographic imaging (chest radiograph, PET/CT/MRI)	Insufficient data to support routine use	Insufficient data to support routine use	Insufficient data to support routine use	Insufficient data to support routine use	Insufficient data to support routine use	
Recurrence suspected	CT/or PET scan	CT and/or PET scan	CT and/or PET scan	CT and/or PET scan	CT and/or PET scan	
	Cancer antigen 125	Cancer antigen 125	Cancer antigen 125	Cancer antigen 125	Cancer antigen 125	

Both platinum-refractory and platinum-resistant recurrence are to be treated with second line chemotherapy, because further surgical resection is of no benefit. Chemotherapy options include paclitaxel, topotecan, liposomal doxorubicin (PLD), or gemcitabine. The patient should know that the best case response to chemotherapy is 12% after PLD, and that the longest median survival is 10 months as reported after topotecan.[70,71]

For platinum-sensitive recurrence, surgical intervention can be considered if the recurrence is limited to a few accessible lesions and if at least 12 months have lapsed since the completion of the chemotherapy. The longer the progression-free survival and the fewer the lesions, the more successful the surgical debulking will be. The GOG is performing the first randomized trial in an attempt to answer the question of the true impact of secondary cytoreduction at the time of first recurrence in platinum-sensitive patients. With or without surgery, second line chemotherapy is also considered the mainstay of treatment for platinum-sensitive recurrence. Because the recurrence is considered platinum-sensitive, carboplatin-based chemotherapy can be initiated. Carboplatin and paclitaxel can be considered,[72] or carboplatin and PLD, because the CALYPSO study has shown that combination offers a superior overall survival when compared with carboplatin and paclitaxel.

REFERENCES

1. Jemal A, Siegel R, Ward E, et al. Cancer statistics, 2009. CA Cancer J Clin 2009; 59(4):225–49.
2. Barnhill DR, Kurman RJ, Brady MF, et al. Preliminary analysis of the behavior of stage I ovarian serous tumors of low malignant potential: a Gynecologic Oncology Group study. J Clin Oncol 1995;13(11):2752–6.
3. Seidman JD, Kurman RJ. Subclassification of serous borderline tumors of the ovary into benign and malignant types. A clinicopathologic study of 65 advanced stage cases. Am J Surg Pathol 1996;20(11):1331–45.
4. Bell DA, Weinstock MA, Scully RE. Peritoneal implants of ovarian serous borderline tumors. Histologic features and prognosis. Cancer 1988;62(10):2212–22.
5. McCluggage WG. Morphological subtypes of ovarian carcinoma: a review with emphasis on new developments and pathogenesis. Pathology 2011;43(5):420–32.
6. Jones S, Wang TL, Kurman RJ, et al. Low-grade serous carcinomas of the ovary contain very few point mutations. J Pathol 2012;226(3):413–20.
7. Bodurka DC, Deavers MT, Tian C, et al. Reclassification of serous ovarian carcinoma by a 2-tier system: A Gynecologic Oncology Group Study. Cancer 2011 Nov 9 [epub ahead of print].
8. Negri E, Franceschi S, Tzonou A, et al. Pooled analysis of 3 European case-control studies: I. Reproductive factors and risk of epithelial ovarian cancer. Int J Cancer 1991;49(1):50–6.
9. Franceschi S, La Vecchia C, Booth M, et al. Pooled analysis of 3 European case-control studies of ovarian cancer: II. Age at menarche and at menopause. Int J Cancer 1991;49(1):57–60.
10. Purdie DM, Bain CJ, Siskind V, et al. Ovulation and risk of epithelial ovarian cancer. Int J Cancer 2003;104(2):228–32.
11. Schildkraut JM, Bastos E, Berchuck A. Relationship between lifetime ovulatory cycles and overexpression of mutant p53 in epithelial ovarian cancer. J Natl Cancer Inst 1997;89(13):932–8.
12. Ness RB, Cramer DW, Goodman MT, et al. Infertility, fertility drugs, and ovarian cancer: a pooled analysis of case-control studies. Am J Epidemiol 2002;155(3):217–24.

13. Lacey JV Jr, Mink PJ, Lubin JH, et al. Menopausal hormone replacement therapy and risk of ovarian cancer. JAMA 2002;288(3):334–41.

14. Whittemore AS, Gong G, Itnyre J. Prevalence and contribution of BRCA1 mutations in breast cancer and ovarian cancer: results from three U.S. population-based case-control studies of ovarian cancer. Am J Hum Genet 1997;60(3):496–504.

15. Buys SS, Partridge E, Black A, et al. Effect of screening on ovarian cancer mortality: the Prostate, Lung, Colorectal and Ovarian (PLCO) Cancer Screening Randomized Controlled Trial. JAMA 2011;305(22):2295–303.

16. Jacobs I, Oram D, Fairbanks J, et al. A risk of malignancy index incorporating CA 125, ultrasound and menopausal status for the accurate preoperative diagnosis of ovarian cancer. Br J Obstet Gynaecol 1990;97(10):922–9.

17. Jacobs I, Davies AP, Bridges J, et al. Prevalence screening for ovarian cancer in postmenopausal women by CA 125 measurement and ultrasonography. BMJ 1993; 306(6884):1030–4.

18. Rustin GJ, van der Burg ME, Berek JS. Advanced ovarian cancer. Tumour markers. Ann Oncol 1993;4 Suppl 4:71–7.

19. Jacobs IJ, Skates S, Davies AP, et al. Risk of diagnosis of ovarian cancer after raised serum CA 125 concentration: a prospective cohort study. BMJ 1996;313(7069): 1355–8.

20. Einhorn N, Sjovall K, Knapp RC, et al. Prospective evaluation of serum CA 125 levels for early detection of ovarian cancer. Obstet Gynecol 1992;80(1):14–8.

21. Jacobs IJ, Oram DH, Bast RC Jr. Strategies for improving the specificity of screening for ovarian cancer with tumor-associated antigens CA 125, CA 15-3, and TAG 72.3. Obstet Gynecol 1992;80(3 Pt 1):396–9.

22. Berek JS, Bast RC Jr. Ovarian cancer screening. The use of serial complementary tumor markers to improve sensitivity and specificity for early detection. Cancer 1995;76(10 Suppl):2092–6.

23. Skates SJ, Xu FJ, Yu YH, et al. Toward an optimal algorithm for ovarian cancer screening with longitudinal tumor markers. Cancer 1995;76(10 Suppl):2004–10.

24. Boyd J. Specific keynote: hereditary ovarian cancer: what we know. Gynecol Oncol 2003;88(1 Pt 2):S8–10 [discussion: S11–3].

25. Frank TS, Manley SA, Olopade OI, et al. Sequence analysis of BRCA1 and BRCA2: correlation of mutations with family history and ovarian cancer risk. J Clin Oncol 1998;16(7):2417–25.

26. Lerman C, Narod S, Schulman K, et al. BRCA1 testing in families with hereditary breast-ovarian cancer. A prospective study of patient decision making and outcomes. JAMA 1996;275(24):1885–92.

27. King MC, Marks JH, Mandell JB. Breast and ovarian cancer risks due to inherited mutations in BRCA1 and BRCA2. Science 2003;302(5645):643–6.

28. Lynch HT, Cavalieri RJ, Lynch JF, et al. Gynecologic cancer clues to Lynch syndrome II diagnosis: a family report. Gynecol Oncol 1992;44(2):198–203.

29. Burke W, Daly M, Garber J, et al. Recommendations for follow-up care of individuals with an inherited predisposition to cancer. II. BRCA1 and BRCA2. Cancer Genetics Studies Consortium. JAMA 1997;277(12):997–1003.

30. Averette HE, Nguyen HN. The role of prophylactic oophorectomy in cancer prevention. Gynecol Oncol 1994;55(3 Pt 2):S38–41.

31. Goff BA, Mandel L, Muntz HG, et al. Ovarian carcinoma diagnosis. Cancer 2000; 89(10):2068–75.

32. Olson SH, Mignone L, Nakraseive C, et al. Symptoms of ovarian cancer. Obstet Gynecol 2001;98(2):212–7.

33. Vine MF, Calingaert B, Berchuck A, et al. Characterization of prediagnostic symptoms among primary epithelial ovarian cancer cases and controls. Gynecol Oncol 2003; 90(1):75–82.

34. Goff BA, Mandel LS, Drescher CW, et al. Development of an ovarian cancer symptom index: possibilities for earlier detection. Cancer 2007;109(2):221–7.

35. Campbell S, Royston P, Bhan V, et al. Novel screening strategies for early ovarian cancer by transabdominal ultrasonography. Br J Obstet Gynaecol 1990;97(4): 304–11.

36. van Nagell JR Jr, Higgins RV, Donaldson ES, et al. Transvaginal sonography as a screening method for ovarian cancer. A report of the first 1000 cases screened. Cancer 1990;65(3):573–7.

37. van Nagell JR Jr, Gallion HH, Pavlik EJ, et al. Ovarian cancer screening. Cancer 1995;76(10 Suppl):2086–91.

38. van Nagell JR Jr, DePriest PD, Reedy MB, et al. The efficacy of transvaginal sonographic screening in asymptomatic women at risk for ovarian cancer. Gynecol Oncol 2000;77(3):350–6.

39. Ueland FR, DePriest PD, Pavlik EJ, et al. Preoperative differentiation of malignant from benign ovarian tumors: the efficacy of morphology indexing and Doppler flow sonography. Gynecol Oncol 2003;91(1):46–50.

40. Cohen LS, Escobar PF, Scharm C, et al. Three-dimensional power Doppler ultrasound improves the diagnostic accuracy for ovarian cancer prediction. Gynecol Oncol 2001;82(1):40–8.

41. Kurjak A, Kupesic S, Sparac V, et al. The detection of stage I ovarian cancer by three-dimensional sonography and power Doppler. Gynecol Oncol 2003;90(2):258–64.

42. Bristow RE, Duska LR, Lambrou NC, et al. A model for predicting surgical outcome in patients with advanced ovarian carcinoma using computed tomography. Cancer 2000;89(7):1532–40.

43. Togashi K. Ovarian cancer: the clinical role of US, CT, and MRI. Eur Radiol 2003;13 Suppl 4:L87–104.

44. Chia YN, Marsden DE, Robertson G, et al. Triage of ovarian masses. Aust N Z J Obstet Gynaecol 2008;48(3):322–8.

45. Young RC, Decker DG, Wharton JT, et al. Staging laparotomy in early ovarian cancer. JAMA 1983;250(22):3072–6.

46. Griffiths CT. Surgical resection of tumor bulk in the primary treatment of ovarian carcinoma. Natl Cancer Inst Monogr 1975;42:101–4.

47. Young RC, Walton LA, Ellenberg SS, et al. Adjuvant therapy in stage I and stage II epithelial ovarian cancer. Results of two prospective randomized trials. New Engl J Med 1990;322(15):1021–7.

48. Trope C, Kaern J, Hogberg T, et al. Randomized study on adjuvant chemotherapy in stage I high-risk ovarian cancer with evaluation of DNA-ploidy as prognostic instrument. Ann Oncol 2000;11(3):281–8.

49. Trimbos JB, Parmar M, Vergote I, et al. International Collaborative Ovarian Neoplasm trial 1 and Adjuvant ChemoTherapy In Ovarian Neoplasm trial: two parallel randomized phase III trials of adjuvant chemotherapy in patients with early-stage ovarian carcinoma. J Natl Cancer Inst 2003;95(2):105–12.

50. Bell J, Brady MF, Young RC, et al. Randomized phase III trial of three versus six cycles of adjuvant carboplatin and paclitaxel in early stage epithelial ovarian carcinoma: a Gynecologic Oncology Group study. Gynecol Oncol 2006;102(3):432–9.

51. Mannel RS, Brady MF, Kohn EC, et al. A randomized phase III trial of IV carboplatin and paclitaxel x 3 courses followed by observation versus weekly maintenance

low-dose paclitaxel in patients with early-stage ovarian carcinoma: a Gynecologic Oncology Group Study. Gynecol Oncol 2011;122(1):89–94.

52. McGuire WP, Hoskins WJ, Brady MF, et al. Cyclophosphamide and cisplatin compared with paclitaxel and cisplatin in patients with stage III and stage IV ovarian cancer. New Engl J Med 1996;334(1):1–6.

53. Piccart MJ, Bertelsen K, Stuart G, et al. Long-term follow-up confirms a survival advantage of the paclitaxel-cisplatin regimen over the cyclophosphamide-cisplatin combination in advanced ovarian cancer. Int J Gynecol Cancer 2003;13 Suppl 2:144–8.

54. Muggia FM, Braly PS, Brady MF, et al. Phase III randomized study of cisplatin versus paclitaxel versus cisplatin and paclitaxel in patients with suboptimal stage III or IV ovarian cancer: a gynecologic oncology group study. J Clin Oncol 2000;18(1):106–15.

55. Ozols RF, Markman M, Thigpen JT. ICON3 and chemotherapy for ovarian cancer. Lancet 2002;360(9350):2086–7 [author reply: 2088].

56. Vasey PA, Paul J, Birt A, et al. Docetaxel and cisplatin in combination as first-line chemotherapy for advanced epithelial ovarian cancer. Scottish Gynaecological Cancer Trials Group. J Clin Oncol 1999;17(7):2069–80.

57. Pilotti S, Oggionni M, Bohm S, et al. ICON3 and chemotherapy for ovarian cancer. Lancet 2002;360(9350):2087–8 [author reply: 2088].

58. Bookman MA, Brady MF, McGuire WP, et al. Evaluation of new platinum-based treatment regimens in advanced-stage ovarian cancer: a Phase III Trial of the Gynecologic Cancer Intergroup. J Clin Oncol 2009;27(9):1419–25.

59. Katsumata N, Yasuda M, Takahashi F, et al. Dose-dense paclitaxel once a week in combination with carboplatin every 3 weeks for advanced ovarian cancer: a phase 3, open-label, randomised controlled trial. Lancet 2009;374(9698):1331–8.

60. Alberts DS, Liu PY, Hannigan EV, et al. Intraperitoneal cisplatin plus intravenous cyclophosphamide versus intravenous cisplatin plus intravenous cyclophosphamide for stage III ovarian cancer. New Engl J Med 1996;335(26):1950–5.

61. Markman M, Bundy BN, Alberts DS, et al. Phase III trial of standard-dose intravenous cisplatin plus paclitaxel versus moderately high-dose carboplatin followed by intravenous paclitaxel and intraperitoneal cisplatin in small-volume stage III ovarian carcinoma: an intergroup study of the Gynecologic Oncology Group, Southwestern Oncology Group, and Eastern Cooperative Oncology Group. J Clin Oncol 2001;19(4):1001–7.

62. Armstrong DK, Brady MF. Intraperitoneal therapy for ovarian cancer: a treatment ready for prime time. J Clin Oncol 2006;24(28):4531–3.

63. Pignata S, Scambia G, Ferrandina G, et al. Carboplatin plus paclitaxel versus carboplatin plus pegylated liposomal doxorubicin as first-line treatment for patients with ovarian cancer: the MITO-2 randomized phase III trial. J Clin Oncol 2011;29(27):3628–35.

64. Vergote I, Trope CG, Amant F, et al. Neoadjuvant chemotherapy or primary surgery in stage IIIC or IV ovarian cancer. New Engl J Med 2010;363(10):943–53.

65. Burger RA, Brady MF, Bookman MA, et al. Incorporation of bevacizumab in the primary treatment of ovarian cancer. New Engl J Med 2011;365(26):2473–83.

66. Perren TJ, Swart AM, Pfisterer J, et al. A phase 3 trial of bevacizumab in ovarian cancer. New Engl J Med 2011;365(26):2484–96.

67. Salani R, Backes FJ, Fung MF, et al. Posttreatment surveillance and diagnosis of recurrence in women with gynecologic malignancies: Society of Gynecologic Oncologists recommendations. Am J Obstet Gynecol 2011;204(6):466–78.

68. Rustin GJ. Follow-up with CA125 after primary therapy of advanced ovarian cancer has major implications for treatment outcome and trial performances and should not be routinely performed. Ann Oncol 2011;22 Suppl 8:viii45–8.
69. Rustin G, van der Burg M, Griffin C, et al. Early versus delayed treatment of relapsed ovarian cancer. Lancet 2011;377(9763):380–1.
70. Bookman MA, Malmstrom H, Bolis G, et al. Topotecan for the treatment of advanced epithelial ovarian cancer: an open-label phase II study in patients treated after prior chemotherapy that contained cisplatin or carboplatin and paclitaxel. J Clin Oncol 1998;16(10):3345–52.
71. Gordon AN, Fleagle JT, Guthrie D, et al. Recurrent epithelial ovarian carcinoma: a randomized phase III study of pegylated liposomal doxorubicin versus topotecan. J Clin Oncol 2001;19(14):3312–22.
72. Kurtz JE, Kaminsky MC, Floquet A, et al. Ovarian cancer in elderly patients: carboplatin and pegylated liposomal doxorubicin versus carboplatin and paclitaxel in late relapse: a Gynecologic Cancer Intergroup (GCIG) CALYPSO sub-study. Ann Oncol 2011;22(11):2417–23.

What is Integrative Oncology and Can It Help My Patients?

Mario Javier Pineda, MD, PhD, Diljeet K. Singh, MD, DrPH*

KEYWORDS

- Integrative Oncology • Complementary and alternative medicine
- Gynecologic oncology • Quality of life

KEY POINTS

- Complementary and alternative medicine practices are widely used by gynecologic oncology patients.
- Integrative medicine describes the combination of conventional medicine with complementary medical practices for which there is evidence for safety and efficacy.
- While still a nascent field, integrative oncology techniques can be incorporated into comprehensive gynecologic cancer care to improve the quality and quantity of cancer patients' lives.
- Multiple studies have demonstrated cancer patient quality of life is predictive of survival.

Integrative oncology is both a science and a philosophy that focuses on the well-being of cancer patients and proposes multiple approaches to accompany conventional therapies to facilitate health. In addition, integrative oncologists strive to support the innate healing abilities of the individual, utilizing techniques for self-empowerment, individual responsibility, and lifestyle changes that could potentially reduce both cancer recurrence and second primary tumors.[1]

The words *complementary* or *alternative* medicine can evoke a visceral response in the gynecologic oncologist who has had patients who have wasted time, money, and perhaps their chance at curative therapy on a "natural" approach, which came with false promises of cure and no side effects. As long as there is disease, there will be supposed "miracle cures"; however, these charlatan practices have no place in true integrative oncology.

The authors have nothing to disclose.
Division of Gynecologic Oncology, Northwestern University Feinberg School of Medicine, 250 East Superior Street, Suite 5-2168, Chicago, IL 60611, USA
* Corresponding author.
E-mail address: diljeet.singh@bannerhealth.com

Obstet Gynecol Clin N Am 39 (2012) 285–312
http://dx.doi.org/10.1016/j.ogc.2012.03.001
0889-8545/12/$ – see front matter © 2012 Elsevier Inc. All rights reserved.

obgyn.theclinics.com

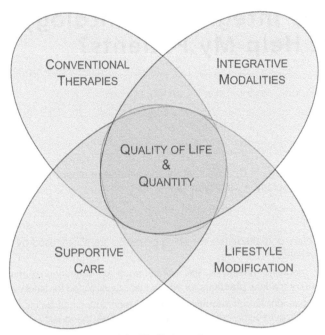

Fig. 1. An integrative oncology model of holistic patient care.

The National Institutes of Health National Center on Complementary and Alternative Medicine defines complementary medicine as "a group of diverse medical and healthcare systems practices, and products that are not generally considered part of conventional medicine," but that are practiced with conventional care. "Alternative" therapies are typically promoted as a substitute for mainstream care, and by definition have not been scientifically proven, often have no scientific foundation, and have sometimes even been disproved.[2] The concept of integrative medicine has evolved to describe the combination of conventional medicine with complementary medical practices for which there is evidence of safety and efficacy. Consistent with current usage, the authors use the acronym CAM (complementary and alternative medicine) as synonymous with integrative medicine.

The Consortium of Academic Health Centers for Integrative Medicine defines integrative medicine as "the practice of medicine that reaffirms the importance of the relationship between practitioner and patient, focuses on the whole person, is informed by evidence, and makes use of all appropriate therapeutic approaches, healthcare professionals, and disciplines to achieve optimal health and healing".[3] Integrative oncology focuses on the complex health of people with cancer and proposes an array of approaches to accompany the conventional therapies.[4] As physicians trained in the comprehensive care of our patients, gynecologic oncologists are ideally suited to appreciating the "whole patient" philosophy of integrative oncology and to its adopting tools and techniques to improve our patients' outcomes (**Fig. 1**).

Whereas categorization of many integrative modalities is fluid and some practices fall into multiple categories, the authors have grouped them into six commonly used domains (**Table 1**): (1) diet and lifestyle modifications such as the Mediterranean or antiinflammatory diet, and exercise programs; (2) natural products and supplements

Table 1
Herbs and supplements

Supplement	Common Reasons for Use	Possible Interaction
Chondroitin[a]	Osteoarthritis, joint pain	May increase effects of warfarin, excess manganese in some brands
Coenzyme Q10[a]	Antioxidant, various	Likely safe in low doses
Dong quai	Menopausal symptoms, menstrual cramps	Anticoagulant, may enhance warfarin activity
Echinacea[a]	Prevention and treatment of URI	Likely safe in short-term use, immunostimulatory contraindicated with immunosuppressants
Ephedra (ma huang)	Various, including common cold	Enhanced sympathomimetic effect, potentially interacts with inhaled general anesthetics to cause dysarrhythmias
Evening primrose	Mastalgia, skin disorders	Likely safe, possible anticoagulant activity
Feverfew	Migraines	Antiplatelet activity, may inhibit hepatic metabolism
Fish oil/DHA/omega-3[a]	Decrease triglycerides, prevention of heart disease	Likely safe in low doses, higher doses may increase risk of bleeding
Flaxseed oil[a]	Various	Likely safe in low doses, antiplatelet activity
Garlic supplements[a]	Hypercholesterolemia, prevention of atherosclerosis	Increased effects antiplatelet drugs, warfarin, antihypertensives, and lipid-lowering drugs
Ginger pills	Antiemetic	Antiplatelet activity; increased effects of anticoagulants and antihypertensives
Ginkgo biloba[a]	Memory loss	Antiplatelet activity
Ginseng[a]	Various, DM	Increased INR with warfarin, increased effects of platelet inhibitors
Glucosamine[a]	Arthritis/joint pain	May increase effects of warfarin
Goldenseal	Antiinflammatory, antimicrobial	May inhibit hepatic metabolism, increased effect of antihypertensives and digoxin, decrease effect of anticoagulants
Green tea[a]	Various, including mental alertness, cancer prevention	High doses (tea or extract) result in high doses of caffeine and may increase risk of bleeding

(continued on next page)

	Common Reasons for	
Supplement	**Use**	**Possible Interaction**
Kava kava	Anxiolytic, sleep disorders	May decrease effectiveness of dopaminergic drugs, may inhibit hepatic metabolism, enhances effects of sedatives and hypnotics, may cause liver failure
Licorice	Gastric ulcers	Potassium loss with thiazide diuretics, inhibits hepatic metabolism, decreased effectiveness of antihypertensives and warfarin
Melatonin	Sleep disorders	Likely safe for short-term use, drugs that alter hepatic metabolism may alter melatonin effects
St. John's wort	Antidepressant	Multiple drug-herb interactions due to induction of hepatic metabolism
Valerian	Sleep disorders	Likely safe in short-term use, enhances effects of sedatives and hypnotics
Vitamin E	Antioxidant, various, prevention of atherosclerosis	Safe in low dose, higher doses may increase risk of bleeding

Table 1
(continued)

Abbreviations: DM, diabetes mellitus; INR, international normalized ratio (prothrombin time); URI, upper respiratory infection.

[a] The 10 most commonly used supplements in the National Health Interview Survey 2007. Data from cited sources.[5,6–11]

(discussed later and in **Table 2**); (3) mind-body interventions including yoga, music therapy, and guided imagery; (4) manipulative and body-based interventions such as chiropractic and massage therapy; (5) energy-based interventions including Reiki and therapeutic touch; and (6) alternative medical systems including naturopathic, homeopathic, Ayurvedic, and traditional Chinese medicine, which includes acupuncture. Further examples of each domain are provided in **Table 1**.

The flaws of our current health care system are beyond the scope of this article, but patients' widespread use of alternative and complimentary approaches and their willingness to pay out of pocket for these modalities outside their provider's knowledge speaks to gaps in our current paradigm.[12] Integrative oncology and the model it offers has the potential to address these gaps. The authors hope with this article to describe integrative medicine as it applies to gynecologic oncology. Specifically, they describe the substantial benefits integrative approaches can have on improving quality of life (QoL), which correlates with survival. The authors provide a brief overview of integrative medicine focusing on those areas pertinent to gynecologic oncology and introduce the issues that make research in this area

Table 2	
Integrative medicine domains	
Domain	**Examples**
Diet and lifestyle	Mediterranean diet, antiinflammatory diet, aerobic exercise, resistance training
Natural products and supplements	Herbs, botanicals, vitamins, minerals, antioxidants
Mind-body interventions	Yoga, mindfulness/meditation-based stress reduction, music therapy, hypnosis, meditation, prayer, guided imagery, Qigong/tai chi chuan
Manipulative and body-based interventions	Chiropractic, massage
Alternative medical systems	Traditional Chinese medicine and acupuncture, Ayurveda, Kampo, homeopathy, naturopathic medicine
Energy-based interventions	Reiki, therapeutic touch

difficult. In addition, through the use of examples in lifestyle medicine and symptom management, they seek to provide support for the use of integrative approaches in the gynecologic oncology patient and offer practitioners tools they can incorporate into their practice to improve the quality and perhaps the quantity of their patients' lives.

WHY DOES QUALITY OF LIFE MATTER AND HOW CAN I IMPROVE IT?

A recent metaanalysis using 30 randomized controlled trials from the European Organization for Research and Treatment of Cancer, which included survival data for over 10,000 patients with 11 different cancer sites found that QoL is predictive of survival.[13]

Both clinicians and patients have long understood that maximizing quality of life is as or more important than simply prolonging life; however, in the past we lacked both a comprehensive view of this multidimensional concept and the ability to measure it in an understandable and reproducible fashion. Whereas it now seems self-evident that QoL is an essential outcome in the cancer patient, decades of work have contributed to our ability to measure QoL and to elucidate its relationship to survival.[14,15] In general, quality of life is a patient's own reported status in multiple domains including functional, physical, psychological/emotional, social/sexual, and financial; QoL is affected by disease status and treatment. Integrative approaches are ideal to impact on many of the domains of QoL because they provide tools to address both cancer and treatment-related symptoms.

In gynecologic oncology patients, researchers describe QoL assessments as imperative in assessing cancer burden, treatment, and prognosis.[16] Domains found to be most affected by chemotherapy are physical and functional well-being (PWB, FWB), and these domains are amenable to intervention with integrative techniques.[17,18] The Gynecologic Oncology Group (GOG) phase III trial comparing cisplatin and paclitaxel chemotherapy with or without interval cytoreduction (GOG 152) was the first multicenter ovarian cancer study to examine the prognostic value of QoL and showed that lower midtreatment QoL was predictive of worse overall survival (OS).[17] More recent data from GOG 172, a randomized trial of 400 women with optimally debulked epithelial ovarian cancer receiving primary intravenous or intra-peritoneal chemotherapy found baseline PWB was associated with OS.[16] Further data analysis revealed that lack of energy and being bothered by side effects of treatment were important contributors in women whose overall QoL score was in the lowest quartile.[16,19,20] Additional work in advanced cervical cancer patients demon-strated that the PWB subscale of the Functional Assessment of Cancer Therapy for patients with cervical cancer (FACT-Cx), was significantly associated with OS after accounting for other known prognosticators including performance status, race, prior radiosensitizer use, time to recurrence, and age.[21] These studies suggest there may be indicators within QoL that identify women at risk for reduced OS who could be targeted with specific approaches to improve outcomes.[16]

Temel and colleagues[22] conducted a landmark study that begins to explore our ability to intervene on QoL indicators to improve survival. In patients with metastatic non–small cell lung cancer, early integration of palliative care with a focus on symptom management with standard oncologic care prolonged survival by approx-imately 2 months compared with standard care alone; simultaneously patients reported clinically meaningful improvements in QoL and mood.[22] Thus, QoL is an outcome that is potentially amenable to intervention with integrative modalities focused on symptom management.

WHO IS USING INTEGRATIVE MODALITIES, WHAT ARE THEY USING, AND ARE THEY SAFE?

The extensive use of integrative modalities represents a challenge and an opportunity to our field; we must balance the desire to provide our patients access to all potentially beneficial modalities while not forgoing safety.

Who Is Using CAM and Do Their Providers Know??

Over 60% of gynecologic oncology patients may be using integrative modalities, and many do not discuss their use with their providers.[23]

Both the data and the demographics of gynecologic oncology patients support the high likelihood that our patients are using CAM approaches and that the majority are not revealing this use to their providers. Surveys and clinical studies suggest CAM users are more likely to be female, middle-aged, college-educated and relatively wealthy.[5,24] In addition, significantly more patients with cancer, specifically female cancer patients, use CAM services and practices compared with noncancer patient populations.[5,25] In a study of patients within the first 6 months of diagnosis of ovarian cancer, von Gruenigen and colleagues[26] found that patients who used CAM modal-ities used them expressly to increase QoL. Furthermore, a study that examined CAM use by gynecologic oncology patients revealed that 66% of gynecologic oncology patients used CAM modalities and on average spent more annually on CAM compared with gynecologic patients ($711 vs $622, respectively).[23]

Using data extrapolated from a telephone survey, Eisenberg and colleagues[12] found that estimated expenditures for alternative medicine professional services increased 45.2% between 1990 and 1997. Total 1997 out-of-pocket expenditures relating to alternative therapies were conservatively estimated at $27.0 billion, and the number of CAM provider visits was estimated to be 629 million; these values both exceeded the out-of-pocket expenses for all US physician services for the same year and the number of primary care provider visits.[12] The vast majority (>95%) of CAM use is in conjunction with conventional medicine, with studies showing that more than

18% of prescription drug users are concurrently taking herbal remedies and/or vitamins.[12,27]

Recent work demonstrated that whereas the proportion of respondents who disclosed herb or supplement use to their physician rose from 33.4% in 2002 to 45.4% in 2007, the majority of users still do not report use to their provider.[5] Studies show that most patients are interested in discussing their CAM use with their physician but are concerned that their physician will not understand, approve of, or have interest in these modalities.[28] Furthermore, although increasing numbers of physicians express open attitudes toward CAM therapies, they may be hesitant to discuss them with patients because of their lack of knowledge and a desire not to appear uninformed.[29]

CAM therapies are increasingly being provided by hospitals and conventional practices, taught in medical and allied health professions schools, and covered by insurance.[2,30,31] In 2010, an American Hospital Association report revealed that 42% of responding hospitals offered one or more CAM services, up from 6% in 1998.[30] A study examining the use of CAM among patients with various cancer diagnoses at a comprehensive cancer center showed that the most common CAM therapies were nutritional supplements (91%), dietary changes (27%), exercise (23%), acupuncture (20%), Asian movement therapies such as yoga, tai chi or hi kung (16%), massage (10%), energy therapies (7%), prayer and spirituality practices (6%).[32]

Are These Approaches Safe?? Herbs, Antioxidants/Vitamins and Soy

Several concerns regarding the usage of herbs, antioxidants, and soy are relevant to providers of women with a gynecologic malignancy.

Are these approaches safe: herbs?

Quality of herbal preparations has not been well-governed, and contamination of preparations has been reported. However, reported cases of complications with herb use are quite rare, and with trained guidance, safe, effective products can be identified.

Given their substantial pharmacologic activity, herbs may interact with over-the-counter and prescription drugs. See **Table 1**, which highlights commonly used herbs and supplements, their indication, and possible interactions. Also highlighted are the 10 herbs and supplements identified by the 2007 National Health Interview Survey as the most commonly used by respondents in the 30 days prior to being surveyed.[5] Pharmacodynamic herb-drug interactions include potentiating the sedative effect of anesthetics by kava and valerian, and these may be held perioperatively.[33–35] St John's wort induces cytochrome P450, leading to increased metabolism of many drugs including warfarin, irinotecan, cyclosporine, oral contraceptives, digitalis, midazolam, lidocaine, and calcium channel blockers.[35–37] Echinacea, goldenseal, and licorice may inhibit cytochrome P450, thus increasing circulating concentrations of these same medications.[34] These herbs that induce and inhibit drug metabolism should be used with caution during chemotherapy, as should other drugs known to alter metabolism.

In addition, herbs may have hematologic and cardiovascular effects that practitioners should be aware of. Antiplatelet effects, prolongation of coagulation parameters, and/or interaction with warfarin can theoretically occur with chondroitin, evening primrose, gingko biloba, garlic, ginseng, ginger, green tea concentrated pills, fish and flax seed oils, vitamin E, dong quai, and feverfew (see **Table 1**).[34] Consideration should be given to holding these herbs before surgery; however, it is unlikely that their potential bleeding effects warrant prohibiting their use during chemotherapy.[38] Cardiovascular effects of ephedra include tachycardia, hypertension, and palpitations, and pharmacologic doses of garlic may cause hypotension. Hypoglycemia has been reported with ginseng. All patients should be queried regarding their use of herbs and other supplements.

Are these approaches safe: antioxidants/vitamins?

Whole food approaches to vitamins are recommended for cancer prevention and prognosis. We can't put apples in capsules, but we can encourage our patients to eat 5 to 7 servings of fruits and vegetables a day.

Since the initial epidemiologic studies suggesting decreased rates of cancer with increasing intake of fruits and vegetables were published, we have failed in our efforts to create a pill that would replicate these benefits. Observational evidence demonstrated an inverse relationship between dietary intake of various antioxidants (β-carotene, vitamin C, selenium, and vitamin E) and both cancer and cardiovascular disease incidence.[39,40] Prompted by these dietary intake studies, as well as many in vitro and animal studies demonstrating benefits of antioxidants in malignant processes, numerous clinical trials were undertaken and have failed to demonstrate any prevention benefit to antioxidant supplementation in populations at high risk for specific-site cancers. Clinical trials and metaanalyses have found inconsistent results regarding adverse mortality risks of high-dose antioxidant supplementation.[41–44]

Two large prospective trials have demonstrated risks of high-dose synthetic β-carotene supplementation in participants who smoked. The Alpha-Tocopherol and Beta-Carotene Cancer Prevention Study examined dl-α-tocopheryl acetate and synthetic β-carotene in more than 29,000 male smokers, and at 6 years of follow-up, the study showed an increase in cumulative lung cancer incidence and higher mortality in the β-carotene arm compared with placebo control arm.[45,46] The Beta-Carotene and Retinol Efficacy Trial examined β-carotene and retinyl palmitate in more than 18,000 men and women at high risk for developing lung cancer due to tobacco use or asbestos exposure history. Within 4 years of follow-up, the study showed an increased risk of lung cancer and an increased risk of any-cause mortality in the combination β-carotene and retinol supplementation arm.[47]

The differences in vitamin and micronutrient doses, formulations, and combinations between whole food sources and supplements are possible causes for the discrepancies between the observational studies and the clinical trials.[43] Intake of antioxidants through diets rich in fruits and vegetables is safe and encouraged. For cancer prevention, high-dose supplementation may not be safe and is discouraged in current smokers. Further research is necessary to determine which populations would benefit from supplementation and if different dosages and combinations of vitamins and micronutrients will prove to be beneficial in populations at risk for cancer.

Substantial controversy exists regarding the safety of supplemental antioxidant administration in patients with cancer during chemotherapy and radiation.[48–51] Some practitioners contend that antioxidant supplements are useful in conjunction with chemotherapy because they enhance the efficacy of the chemotherapy and alleviate toxic side effects, allowing patients to tolerate chemotherapy for the full course of treatment and possibly at higher doses.[52] Others have raised the concern that antioxidants may decrease the efficacy of chemotherapy by interfering with its mechanism of action, which includes the formation of free radicals which result in tumor cell damage.[53] Antioxidants function, in part, through a reduction in the effects of free radicals. This concern that antioxidants will decrease the effects of these treatments, however, has not been borne out in most populations undergoing chemotherapy. In the majority of studies, patients receiving antioxidants during chemotherapy do not experience differences in treatment response but are more likely to experience a reduced side effect profile and to tolerate a greater number of chemotherapy cycles.[54]

The data are less conclusive for patients undergoing radiation therapy. In a study examining 540 patients with stage I or II head and neck cancer, Meyer and colleagues[55] demonstrated that antioxidant supplementation using synthetic β-carotene and vitamin E (dl-α-tocopherol) or vitamin E alone during radiation therapy was associated with significant increased incidence of recurrence of initial cancer, all-cause mortality, and mortality from initial cancer in those patients who smoked during supplementation. Nonsmokers had no increased risk of those outcomes with antioxidant supplementation.[55] Clearly, patients undergoing radiation therapy should not combine smoking and antioxidant supplementation; in the nonsmoker, the use of multivitamins to replace nutrients that they are not able to consume in their diet as whole foods is reasonable.

Are these approaches safe: soy?

Whole food approaches to soy (tofu, tempeh, edamame, soy milk) are beneficial for those at risk for cancer and are safe in cancer patients.

Substantial data support preventive benefits of phytoestrogens in the development of hormonally mediated cancers. Phytoestrogens are naturally occurring plant substances with a chemical structure similar to 17-β estradiol. They consist mainly of isoflavones (found in high concentrations in soy beans and other legumes) and lignans (found in a variety of fruits, vegetables, and cereal products). Although tofu is the main source of soy in Asian diets, in Western diets, it is from soy additives to nonsoy foods that likely do not provide the same benefits as whole soy products. Isoflavones (genistein and daidzein) are weak estrogens compared with estradiol. The high soy intake and low rates of breast cancer in Asian populations led to the hypothesis that soy consumption might decrease breast cancer risk by displacing estradiol and functioning as a relative antiestrogen. In a pooled metaanalysis of 18 studies, high soy intake was associated with a modest but significant reduction in breast cancer incidence.[56] A second metaanalysis that separately considered studies conducted in Asian and Western countries concluded that higher intake of isoflavones among Asian populations was associated with a 29% reduction in breast cancer risk with evidence of a dose-response relationship and consistent effects seen across all studies.[57] In contrast, among Western populations there was no association with soy intake, but the highest level was only about .8 mg per day and may not have been high enough to see any effect. An additional metaanalysis found that compared with the lowest soy intake group, the highest soy intake group had a 39% decrease in the risk of all endocrine-related cancers, a 30% decrease in the risk of endometrial cancer, and a 48% decrease for ovarian cancer.[58] A case-control study of 500 women with endometrial cancer found that when comparing highest to lowest intake groups, isoflavone intake was associated with a 41% decrease in risk.[59] In postmenopausal women protection from isoflavones was even stronger, and a 43% reduction in endometrial cancer risk was also seen for lignan intake.

In patients already diagnosed with cancer, safety and potential benefits for soy have been described in breast cancer patients but not gynecologic cancer patients. Researchers have proposed that epigenetic changes explain the results of two recent human studies showing that a moderate consumption of genistein improved prognosis in

Asian breast cancer survivors and showed no increase in breast cancer recurrence in Western women.[56] Thus, evidence confirms that whole soy products and phytoestrogens from whole food sources are at least safe and potentially beneficial in women with hormonally mediated cancers.

Why Is the Research Limited???

1. *Nascent field with recent establishment of centralized source of guidance and funding.*
2. *Compounds are difficult to characterize and study.*
3. *Differing philosophic perspectives on health and disease.*

Data from well-conducted trials on the risks and benefits of complementary modalities are limited for several reasons. First, a consistent source of guidance and funding for research and training in integrative medicine was only recently established in 1992 with relatively limited funding until this decade.[30,31,60,61] Second, researchers have identified lack of quality and substantial variability of dietary supplements as a significant challenge to conducting research.[60] The Food and Drug Administration (FDA) regulates dietary supplements as foods, not drugs, and so does not analyze the content of dietary supplements. This status precludes patenting, limiting pharmaceutical company investment in research; in addition, whereas synthetic, single-entity drugs are relatively easy to characterize, the complexities of herbal preparations and our incomplete knowledge regarding the active components hinder research efforts.[62]

Last, traditional evidence-based medical research focuses on one variable and its impact on one outcome. By definition integrative approaches imply a whole system with multiple component parts that work together toward the maximum benefit of the patient.[63] Thus, the best suited research programs would evaluate a whole systems approach to patients and might include psychological interventions, physical exercises, nutritional variations, and combinations of botanicals.[64] For example, in a series of work with prostate cancer patients, Ornish and colleagues[65–67] used a mixed interventions approach described as comprehensive lifestyle changes including nutritional changes, physical activity, and meditation and found decreases in prostate-specific antigen and cell and serum level changes, which inhibit cancer progression.[65–67]

Clearly a great deal of additional work must be conducted to justify the time and money we are investing in integrative approaches. However, as practitioners engaged in patient-centered care, we must prioritize the needs of our patients and can take a "best available data" approach. As gynecologic oncologists, we often treat patients with highly toxic therapies that have less than a 25% chance of activity. We talk to our patients about their goals of care, about the risks and benefits of an intervention, and together we make best possible choices with potentially limited data. This same approach can be applied to integrative modalities.

WHAT INTEGRATIVE APPROACHES ARE THERE EVIDENCE FOR? LIFESTYLE MODIFICATION: DIET, EXERCISE, AND STRESS MANAGEMENT

The American Cancer Society (ACS) nutrition and activity goals of care: prevent nutrient deficiencies, minimize nutrition-related side effects, preserve lean body mass, initiate/maintain physical activity individualized for each patient to maximize QoL.[68]

Women diagnosed with or at risk for gynecologic malignancies frequently ask questions regarding the impact of lifestyle modification on their cancer-related outcomes. We have all been asked: "Are there foods I should or should not eat?"

"Should I take vitamins or other supplements?" "Is there anything I can do to help my chances?" With existing data, we can make specific recommendations empowering our patients to participate in their health care and potentially improving their outcomes. Strong evidence supports the benefits of good nutrition, increased physical activity, stress management, and social support on both cancer prevention and cancer prognosis. Highly curable endometrial cancer patients represent an ideal opportunity to encourage preventive behaviors given their high risk for metabolic syndrome–associated comorbidities and the motivation for change that a recent cancer diagnosis may provide.

A holistic approach to patient care should include lifestyle modification as part of routine care. Even without trials specifically examining gynecologic malignancies, guiding patients to maintain a healthy diet, perform regular physical exercise, and reduce stress is safe, reasonable, and recommended.[69–71] Cancer patients and survivors at risk for nutritional inadequacies should be referred to specialists for guidance on nutritional supplementation to promote optimum nutritional status, manage tumor-related and treatment-related symptoms, meet increased nutritional needs, and correct any nutritional deficits.[2]

Is There a Cancer-Preventive Diet?

Data exist to support global dietary recommendations to prevent and potentially to improve cancer outcomes and QoL.

Studies of diet, nutrition, and cancer risk are often limited by retrospective collection of data, difficulty in correlating specific nutrients in food diaries, and the inherent restrictions of epidemiologic studies. In addition, advocates of integrative health approaches have objected to the reductionism of studying specific nutrients (vitamin A and β-carotene) instead of whole foods (yellow and orange fruits and vegetables) where the interactions of food components may be important. Studying regional dietary patterns in populations with decreased cancer risks is one way to take a more holistic and practical approach.

What is the Mediterranean diet?
The Mediterranean diet is characterized by consumption of omega-3–containing fats (in the form of olive oil, fish, and nuts), protein predominantly from plant and fish sources, high consumption of fruits and vegetables, low consumption of meat (in particular, red meat), low to moderate dairy consumption, and regular, but moderate, consumption of alcohol (predominantly red wine).[72–74] Mechanistically, researchers have proposed that the health benefits of this diet are based on bioactive compounds and their interactions, specifically (1) monounsaturated to saturated fatty acid ratio, (2) dietary fiber, (3) antioxidant capacity of the whole diet, (4) phytosterol intake.[75] A recent metaanalysis showed that increased adherence to the Mediterranean diet was associated with a significant reduction of overall mortality, cardiovascular incidence and mortality, cancer incidence and mortality, and neurodegenerative diseases.[76] Most recently, data showed that increased adherence with a Mediterranean diet was associated with a significant decrease in cancer incidence and mortality in a cohort that included more than 450,000 individuals with greater than 30,000 incident cancers.[73,77,78]

La Vecchia[79] examined the relationship between the gynecologic cancers and specific components of the Mediterranean diet and found a significant decreased risk for endometrial and ovarian cancer with improved vegetable intake. The risk for ovarian cancer was statistically decreased for women with an increase of 1 g/wk of omega-3 fatty acids. Highest consumption level of whole grain foods was associated with decreased risk of endometrial and ovarian cancer.[79] In addition, an increase in risk of endometrial and ovarian cancer was associated with higher red meat intake.[72]

Do individual dietary components matter?

Additional work has evaluated specific dietary components and gynecologic malignancies. In a review of the literature on variation in meat and fish intake by Kolahdooz and colleagues,[80] they found that low consumption of processed meat and higher consumption of poultry and fish may reduce the risk of ovarian cancer. A case-control study of diet and ovarian cancer in western New York found that compared with women in the lowest quintile of intake, reduced risks were observed for women in the highest quintile of intake of dietary fiber (57% decrease), carotenoids (67% decrease), stigmasterol (58% decrease), total lignans (57% decrease), vegetables (53% decrease), and poultry (55% decrease).[81] A systematic review of the role of diet on the risk of human papillomavirus persistence and cervical neoplasia that included 23 observational studies and 10 randomized clinical trials showed possible protective effects of fruits, vegetables, vitamins C and E, β-carotene, lycopene, lutein/zeaxanthin, and cryptoxanthin.[82]

An association between decreased vitamin D levels and increased rates of cancer has been described.[83] Researchers have postulated that the known north-south gradient in age-adjusted mortality rates of ovarian cancer in the United States are attributable to lower solar irradiance and thus lower serum vitamin D levels.[84] In support of this hypothesis, laboratory findings have suggested that low levels of vitamin D metabolites could contribute to the development of ovarian cancer. A review of the literature found that approximately half of the ecologic and case-control studies reported reductions in incidence or mortality of ovarian cancer with increasing geographic latitude, solar radiation levels, or dietary/supplement consumption of vitamin D, whereas the other half reported null associations with ovarian cancer risk.[85] A case-control serum study of over 7000 subjects from the National Health and Nutrition Examination Surveys found that ovarian cancer cases were three times more likely to have low serum vitamin D.[86] These investigators concluded that deficiency in vitamin D provides a causative link between the long-known ecologic findings regarding latitude.

Can botanicals change outcomes?

Although the data are highly promising, we cannot yet make strong recommendations for individual botanicals.

Several botanicals are being investigated as agents to inhibit cancer development; they include green tea, curcumin, astragalus, and resveratrol. A systematic review of publications on green tea concludes potential cancer preventive benefits and recommended further studies.[87] A case-control study of epithelial ovarian cancer in China showed that habitual green tea intake was protective against cancer development, and the benefit was dose-dependent and duration-dependent.[88] A recent prospective cohort study in over 60,000 Swedish women followed for over 15 years provided evidence that green tea intake reduced the risk for the development of epithelial ovarian cancer in a dose-dependent manner.[89]

Curcumin, a component of turmeric or curry powder, has been shown to down-regulate several pathways of cancer initiation and promotion.[90] Oral curcumin is well-tolerated and has biological activity in some patients with pancreatic cancer.[91] The dried root of Astragalus membranaceus (huang-qi), a traditional Chinese herbal medicine, demonstrated improvements in survival, tumor response, and performance status in a metaanalysis of randomized trials of almost 3000 lung cancer patients on platinum-based chemotherapy.[92] Resveratrol is a polyphenol found in numerous plant species including grapes that has been shown to possess chemopreventive properties against several cancers through apoptosis induction.[93] Additional studies of these agents in gynecologic cancer are warranted.

Researchers analyzed the association between intake of five common dietary flavonoids and the incidence of epithelial ovarian cancer among over 60,000 women in the Nurses' Health Study.[94] Whereas no clear association was found between total intake of the five flavonoids and ovarian cancer, there was a significant 40% decrease in ovarian cancer incidence for the highest versus lowest quintile of kaempferol intake and a significant 34% decrease in incidence for the highest versus lowest quintile of luteolin intake. An inverse association with consumption of non-herbal tea and broccoli, the primary contributors to kaempferol intake in our population, further supported this association.

Does Diet Matter Once Someone Has Cancer?

The relationship between diet and prognosis in gynecologic cancer patients is not well-studied, but the general oncology literature suggests value to improving nutrition even after a cancer diagnosis to support health and healing during treatment. In a longitudinal study of over 300 women with ovarian cancer, longer survival was associated with increased total fruits and vegetables and vegetables separately, with subgroup analyses showing yellow and cruciferous vegetables to be the significant components.[95] In a population-based cohort of over 600 women with epithelial ovarian cancer followed for up to 5 years, death was reduced in women who reported higher intake of vegetables and cruciferous vegetables.[96] Inverse associations were seen between protein, red and white meat, and survival. Although additional studies are required to elucidate its impact on gynecologic cancer prognosis, a recommendation to adhere to the Mediterranean diet is reasonable and achievable for most patients.

In regard to individual dietary components and cancer prognosis, research has been done on vitamin D, green tea, and selenium. Studies in Norway and England found that individuals diagnosed with any cancer in summer or fall, when serum 25-hydroxyvitamin D levels are highest, had a milder clinical course and longer survival than those diagnosed in winter or spring.[97] However, no vitamin D studies focused on gynecologic cancer survival after diagnosis are available. A small cohort study following over 200 women with epithelial ovarian cancer demonstrated that habitual green tea consumption caused a significant dose-dependent increase in survival rate.[98] Researchers evaluated the impact of randomized selenium supplementation in over 30 patients with ovarian cancer undergoing chemotherapy. After 3 months of selenium, increases in white blood cells and a significant decrease of hair loss, abdominal pain, weakness, and loss of appetite were noted among selenium-supplemented patients.[99] Thus, promising data demonstrate the need for additional research to evaluate the potential for dietary modification and supplementation to improve survival and side effects in women with gynecologic malignancies.

What About Physical Activity and Weight?

The ACS recommends that patients with cancer maintain normal weight, increase physical activity, and eat a diet low in fat and refined carbohydrates and high in vegetables and fruits, as a potential aid to some aspects of prognosis, acknowledging lack of definitive data.[100]

Weight, diet, and exercise are interrelated and modifiable risk factors for many diseases including cancer. Examining over 1 million men and women in the Cancer Prevention Study, a prospective observational mortality study, Calle and colleagues[101] demonstrated that mortality rates from all cancers increase with increasing body mass index (BMI) compared with normal BMI. In the subset of women with uterine corpus cancer, this result was most striking, with a relative risk of as high as 6.25 for patients in the highest BMI category compared with patients with a normal BMI.[101] Using 380 early stage endometrial cancer patients enrolled in GOG, von Gruenigen and colleagues[102] found an increase in mortality with increasing BMI that reached statistical significance in patients with BMI at or above 40 kg/m^2.

Independent of BMI, exercise has a role in prevention of endometrial cancer. A recent metaanalysis of five cohort studies with 3463 total cases demonstrated that even after adjusting for BMI, women with the most recreational physical activity had a significantly decreased risk of endometrial cancer compared with women with the least.[103] An independent analysis of 26 studies that examined physical activity and endometrial cancer found a 20% reduction in endometrial cancer risk when comparing those with the highest level of exercise with lowest.[104]

The Women's Healthy Eating and Living Study was a prospective study of women with early stage breast cancer that showed that a combination of eating five or more fruits and vegetables per day and accumulating greater than 540 metabolic tasks-minutes per week (equivalent to walking 30 minutes per day, 6 days per week) were associated with a significant survival advantage.[105] A study of physical activity in ovarian cancer patients demonstrated an inverse association between activity and fatigue, peripheral neuropathy, mood disturbance, and sleep disturbance and a direct association between activity and happiness and sleep quality.[69]

How Does Stress Factor Into Cancer?

Stress-induced immunosuppression or dysregulation may contribute to the development and progression of malignancy.[106]

Clinical and preclinical studies suggest that key psychological factors or stressors influence cancer biology. The most commonly studied psychological factors are stress, depression, and social support or isolation. In ovarian cancer patients, depressed and anxious mood is associated with a greater impairment of the cellular immune response and an increase in tumor progression.[107,108] Stressors disrupt homeostasis, triggering a stress response that result in physiologic and behavioral changes that are mediated by the autonomic nervous system (ANS) and the hypothalamic-pituitary-adrenal axis, which in turn influence tumor behavior.[109–113] In an orthotopic mouse model of ovarian carcinoma, Thaker and colleagues[112] found that chronic stress activated the β-adrenergic pathway, leading to increased tumor growth and angiogenesis. In line with these findings, clinical studies have demonstrated an inverse relationship between social support and plasma concentration of angiogenic vascular-endothelial growth factor and interleukin-6, an inflammatory cytokine that has been linked to ovarian cancer prognosis.[109,114] The catecholamine stress hormone norepinephrine may influence tumor progression by modulating the expression of factors implicated in angiogenesis and metastasis.[115,116] Finally, glucocorticoids and other inflammatory cytokines have also been implicated as stress response mediators that may play a role in tumor biology.[111]

Whereas clinical outcome data exist for the role of stress in tumor initiation, progression, and OS, the most compelling data link psychological stress to cancer progression with evidence of shorter recurrence intervals, increased risk of metastatic disease, and more rapid disease progression in patients undergoing chronic psychological stressors.[113] These data led to studies of psychological interventions in breast cancer patients, which thus far have not shown a survival advantage but consistently show improvements in psychosocial parameters and QoL and demonstrate the feasibility of implementing psychosocial interventions without adverse outcomes for participants.[117,118] Social isolation is associated with an increased risk of death from cancer; thus, support groups and social connection can benefit cancer patients.[119] Oncology care providers are encouraged to conduct routine surveillance for psychological stressors, to refer patients for psychological evaluation and treatment, to recommend patient-specific stress reduction strategies, and to support activities that address social isolation.

Can we manage stress with mind-body interventions?

Integrative strategies to address stress in cancer patients include relaxation training, meditation, graded exercise, yoga, tai chi, and other mind–body interventions that induce the relaxation response.[120]

The use of mind-body interventions in oncology patients is based on the premise that interactions between the mind, behavior, and the body can be manipulated to affect physiological functioning and promote health (examples are given; see **Table 2**, CAM Domains).[121–123] Mind-body interventions are thought to influence health via modification of the stress and relaxation response pathways and neuroendocrine homeostasis. Specifically, the reflexive sympathetic ANS response to stress can be suppressed using techniques to induce parasympathetic ANS tone resulting in a health state that promotes healing.[110,121,124] Many conditions have been documented to respond to mind-body interventions including high blood pressure, headache, and sleep and mood disturbance.[122]

The increasingly commonplace practice of yoga, a mind-body intervention that combines meditation, breathing, and exercise, contributed to an increase in mind-body intervention trials to improve mental and physical health in various patient groups, including cancer patients.[125,126] A mindfulness meditation–based stress reduction (MBSR) program implemented in a Canadian academic hospital used a combination of yoga, guided imagery, home practice, group education, and skill building in a heterogeneous population of 90 cancer patients who were randomized to either an 8-week program or a wait-list control group. Researchers found an improvement in total mood disturbance and total stress in the meditation group compared with the wait-list control group with benefits that were maintained at 6-month follow-up.[127,128] Additionally, a recent metaanalysis of 19 MBSR trials that included 5 randomized controlled trials incorporating more than 400 patients demonstrated moderate improvement in both mood and stress level.[129] In a multicenter study of 410 predominantly breast cancer patients using a program of breathing exercises, 18 gentle yoga postures, and meditation, significant improvements were seen in sleep quality, fatigue, and QoL.[130] Whereas data are limited for gynecologic oncology populations, the substantial potential for benefit of mind-body approaches with little risk of harm supports the use of these techniques.

WHAT INTEGRATIVE APPROACHES ARE THERE EVIDENCE FOR? SYMPTOM MANAGEMENT

Common symptoms and areas for potential intervention that affect QoL in gynecologic oncology patients include sleep, fatigue, nausea/vomiting, depression, anxiety, pain, lymphedema, ascites, and sexual health.[131,132] Given the whole patient approach of integrative modalities, many interventions address multiple cancer-related symptoms. In the largest prospective observational study of massage therapy, researchers in a major cancer center treated 1290 cancer patients with Swedish massage, reflexology/foot massage, or light touch massage and found clinically relevant improvement in multiple areas including pain (improved by 48%), fatigue (43%), stress/anxiety (60%), nausea (51%), and depression (36%).[133] A summary of integrative interventions that can be applied to specific symptoms of gynecologic oncology patients can be found in **Table 3**, CAM Symptom Toolkit.[147]

Insomnia is a common problem in patients with cancer; in a survey of ovarian cancer patients, investigators found the majority of responders reported poor sleep quality, and almost half used a sleep aid at least once in the prior month.[149] Conventional therapies for sleep disturbances include benzodiazepine receptor agonists and behavioral therapies and in the short term, both have comparable efficacy. However, only behavioral therapies demonstrate persistent benefits on sleep quality when intervention is completed.[150] Short-term use of melatonin has been shown to improve sleep outcomes with effect sizes comparable to prescription medications but with fewer side effects.[10,147,148]

Cancer-related fatigue (CRF) has been defined as "a distressing persistent, subjective sense of physical, emotional, and/or cognitive tiredness or exhaustion related to cancer or cancer treatment that is not proportional to recent activity and interferes with usual functioning."[151] CRF is qualitatively different from the fatigue experienced by healthy individuals in its severity, effect on QoL, and inability to be relieved by rest. The most recent National Comprehensive Cancer Network recommendations for CRF incorporate CAM modalities (massage therapy, imagery, fitness, and nutrition) as part of the nonpharmacologic treatments alongside psychosocial interventions, cognitive behavior therapies, and physical and occupational therapy referrals.[151] The two treatment modalities with the best evidence of efficacy for CRF are physical activity and psychosocial interventions.[152] A systematic review and metaanalysis of the role of physical activity on CRF showed a consistent, qualitative improvement in fatigue.[134] Additionally, in a study of 47 cancer patients, investigators demonstrated a decrease in fatigue in an acupuncture-treated group when compared with sham therapy.[135] These trials report small effect sizes, highlighting the need for further work to develop more effective interventions.

Integrative modalities can serve as adjuvants to or substitutes for pharmacologic approaches to nausea and vomiting (N&V).[153] Two recent Cochrane reviews support the efficacy of acupuncture to wrist point P6 to treat postoperative N&V and acupuncture point stimulation for the treatment of chemotherapy-induced N&V.[137,138] In the only trial examining gynecologic oncology patients, You and colleagues[140] performed a randomized trial of 142 women aged 45 to 63 receiving platinum-based chemotherapy for ovarian cancer comparing acupuncture with wrist acupoint PC6 and vitamin B_6 with vitamin B_6 alone or PC6 acupuncture alone. The combination arm had significantly fewest episodes of emesis and the greatest number of emesis-free days; this result was followed in efficacy by acupuncture alone that was superior to B_6 alone.

Table 3				
Symptom tool kit for integrative medicine				
Symptom	**Subjects (n)**	**Intervention**	**Key Outcome(s)**	**Refs**
Cancer Risk				
	Adult women with uterus in situ (3463)	Metaanalysis of recreational physical activity	↓ of risk of EMCA, persistent when controlled for BMI.	103
Fatigue				
	Men and women with various cancers	Systematic review and metaanalysis of physical activity interventions	↓ fatigue during and after treatment.	134
	Men and women with various cancers finished chemotherapy at least 1 month prior, moderate to severe fatigue (47)	RCT acupuncture vs acupressure vs sham acupressure	↓ fatigue in both acupuncture and acupressure groups vs sham. Acupuncture better than acupressure.	135
	Various cancers in three large teaching universities (US and Australia) (162)	RCT medical Qigong	↑ in QoL, ↓ fatigue, ↓ mood disturbance.	136
Nausea and Vomiting				
	CINV in various cancers; chemotherapy of moderate to high risk of emesis (214)	Systematic review of electroacupuncture and manual acupuncture	↓ in acute vomiting, no change in nausea severity.	137
	Postoperative nausea vomiting	Systematic review of stimulation of acupuncture point PC6	↓ in PONV, need for rescue antiemetics.	138
	Females undergoing breast surgery; postoperative nausea vomiting (77)	RCT of P6 electro-acupoint stimulation vs ondansetron vs placebo	↓ in PONV, effect persisted to 24-h follow-up.	139
	CINV ovarian cancer stage II or III (142)	RCT acupuncture to PC6, Vitamin B_6, both	↓ in emesis episodes per day, ↑ in emesis-free days.	140
	Cisplatin chemotherapy (alone or in combination) gynecologic oncology patients (48)	Randomized double blind crossover study of standard of care antiemetics PLUS ginger (250 mg capsules) vs metoclopramide (10 mg)	Equivalent to metoclopramide in delayed nausea.	141

(continued on next page)

Table 3 *(continued)*				
Symptom	**Subjects (n)**	**Intervention**	**Key Outcome(s)**	**Refs**
Oral Mucositis				
	Adults with breast cancer treated with anthracycline-based chemotherapy (326)	RCT of Saforis (proprietary glutamine formulation) with a double crossover design	↓ WHO grade 3 and 4 oral mucositis without evidence of study drug side effects.	142
Pain				
	Primary breast cancer (86)	RCT 5 wk (2x/wk, 30 min per session) Swedish massage	↓ in body pain, persisted 6 wk out.	143
	Advanced cancer with moderate-severe pain, multisite (380)	RCT massage 2 wk (6 sessions 30 min/ session) vs simple touch	↓ in body pain.	145
	Ovary and breast cancer patients undergoing palliative therapy (40)	Single site cohort undergoing 8-wk well-described acupuncture course	↓ in pain, anxiety, fatigue, depression.	145
	Various cancer patients with chronic pain > 1 mo (90)	RCT auricular acupuncture 2 treatments 1 mo apart	↓ in pain, persisted 8 wk.	146
Sleep Disturbance				
	55–80 y old insomnia patients (354)	1 wk, single blind, placebo run-in period followed by a 3-wk double blind treatment period with PR-melatonin or placebo, 1 tablet per day at 2 h before bedtime	↓ sleep latency, ↑ quality of life (comparable effect size to prescription medication).	147
	Patients admitted with medical diagnosis with insomnia other than acute insomnia (32)	RCT comparing short-term melatonin use to placebo	↑ sleep quality, ↓ sleep latency.	148
	Nonmetastatic cancer patients, predominantly breast cancer with 2–24 mo of sleep disturbance, multisite (410)	RCT of 4 wk yoga intervention (2x/wk; 75 min/ session) vs standard of care monitoring	↑ sleep quality, ↓ fatigue, ↑ QoL.	130

Abbreviations: CINV, chemotherapy-induced nausea and vomiting; EMCA, endometrial cancer; PONV, postoperative nausea and vomiting; PR, prolonged release; RCT, randomized controlled trial, WHO, World Health Organization.

Table 4
Integrative medicine internet resources

Organization	Brief Description	Address
American Dietetic Association	Provides patient and provider nutritional resources including a "Find a Nutrition Professional" with expertise in oncology nutrition.	www.eatright.org
Arizona Center for Integrative Medicine	Designed for physicians, nurse practitioners, and physician assistants, the Fellowship in Integrative Medicine at the Arizona Center for Integrative Medicine is a 1000-h, 2-y distance learning program.	http://integrativemedicine.arizona.edu/education/ fellowship/
Consortium of Academic Health Centers for Integrative Medicine	Provides an overview of the principles and practice of integrative health care within academic institutions. Provides a contact information by state/province of the 51 (at time of publication) member academic member institutions.	www.imconsortium.org
Medline Plus	Provides database for prescription and OTC drugs as well as an extensive database on vitamins, supplements, botanical/herbs.	www.nlm.nih.gov/medlineplus/druginformation.html
Memorial Sloan Kettering About Herbs Site	Provides objective information for health care professionals, including clinical summary for each agent, details about constituents, adverse effects, interactions, and potential benefits or problems.	www.mskcc.org/cancer-care/integrative-medicine/about-herbs-botanicals-other-products
The Natural Standard	Subscription-based service that provides peer-reviewed database access for CAM therapies including herbs and nutraceuticals.	www.naturalstandard.com

(continued on next page)

Table 4 (continued)		
Organization	**Brief Description**	**Address**
NIH National Center for Complementary and Alternative Medicine	Includes CAM overview of funding opportunities, a short pharmacopeia of herbs and nutraceuticals.	www.nccam.nih.gov
NIH Office of Dietary Supplements	Provides overview of individual vitamins, minerals, and other dietary supplements. Fact sheets available in Spanish. information for consumers and health care providers	http://ods.od.nih.gov
Society for Integrative Oncology	Dedicated to the studying and facilitating of cancer treatment and recovery process through the use of integrated complementary therapeutic options.	www.integrativeonc.org

Abbreviations: NIH, National Institutes of Health, OTC, over-the-counter.

The physiology of pain in a cancer patient is complex and can result from inflammatory, neuropathic, ischemic, and compression mechanisms.[154] Multiple treatment modalities need to be used and should be tailored to the type of pain being experienced. The World Health Organization analgesic ladder forms the foundation of most treatment guidelines and includes nonsteroidal antiinflammatory drugs, opioids, adjuvant analgesics (antidepressants, anticonvulsants, muscle relaxants, topical anesthetics, and steroids), psychosocial interventions, and complementary integrative medicine therapies.[155] In a multisite randomized clinical trial that included 380 adults with advanced cancer experiencing moderate-severe pain, patients were randomized to six 30-minute massage therapies compared with simple touch, with massage therapy patients showing significant improvement in pain and mood.[144] In a pilot study examining the effect of acupuncture on QoL in patients with advanced breast and ovarian cancer, researchers found statistically significant benefits for pain, mood disturbances, and fatigue.[145] Other representative trials supporting CAM modalities in the treatment of pain are summarized (see **Table 3**, Symptom Toolkit).

Although data are limited on the prevalence of mood disturbances in gynecologic patients, one study revealed that 42% of patients presented with clinically significant anxiety or depression.[131,156] Initial triage should evaluate for problems requiring immediate psychiatric referral including suicidal ideation.[157] Nonpharmacologic treatments may include psychosocial interventions (individual or group psychotherapy) and integrative oncology approaches. Both massage and mind-body interventions have successfully been used as adjuvant therapy for mood.[127,144,158]

SUMMARY

Integrative oncology lends itself to the comprehensive practice of gynecologic oncology with multiple tools and interventions that can impact on QoL and survival.

However, there remains a paucity of well-designed, well-powered randomized control trials on various CAM modalities for gynecologic cancer patients. The reasons for the lack of level 1 evidence include the nascent state of integrative medicine as a science, the limitations on CAM funding, the relative lack of integration of CAM practitioners into the oncology community, and absence of strict regulation of herbs and supplements by the US FDA.[159] The use of CAM as adjunctive therapies will likely continue given the patient-driven trends to date, and given the evidence for at least safety and potentially efficacy, our patients deserve our willingness to use all possible approaches to improving their outcomes. Continued evolution of our ability to specifically measure and describe QoL will further our ability to hone in on domains most important to patients and their survival and allow practitioners to make patient-specific recommendations. Multimodal programs that include physical activity, stress management, and diet have the potential to address demonstrated deficits in PWB and FWB in ovarian cancer patients (see **Fig. 1**, which suggests a model of collaborative gynecologic oncology care). Integrative oncology represents a holistic approach to patient care whose goal is maximization of patient quantity and quality of life. Patients can achieve this optimal outcome through the synergy of conventional care, integrative modalities, lifestyle modifications, and supportive care. Refer to **Table 4** for a listing of integrated medicine Internet resources.

REFERENCES

1. Sagar SM, Lawenda BD. The role of integrative oncology in a tertiary prevention survivorship program. Prev Med 2009;49(2-3):93–8.
2. Deng GE, et al. Evidence-based clinical practice guidelines for integrative oncology: complementary therapies and botanicals. J Soc Integr Oncol 2009;7(3):85–120.
3. Kligler B, et al. Core competencies in integrative medicine for medical school curricula: a proposal. Acad Med 2004;79(6):521–31.
4. Sagar SM. The integrative oncology supplement–a paradigm for both patient care and communication. Curr Oncol 2008;15(4):166–7.
5. Wu CH, Wang CC, Kennedy J. Changes in herb and dietary supplement use in the US adult population: a comparison of the 2002 and 2007 National Health Interview Surveys. Clinical Ther 2011;33(11):1749–58.
6. Kumar NB, Allen K, Bell H. Perioperative herbal supplement use in cancer patients: potential implications and recommendations for presurgical screening. Cancer Control 2005;12(3):149–57.
7. Izzo AA. Ernst E. Interactions between herbal medicines and prescribed drugs: an updated systematic review. Drugs 2009;69(13):1777–98.
8. Kaye AD, Kucera I, Sabar R. Perioperative anesthesia clinical considerations of alternative medicines. Anesthesiol Clin North America 2004;22(1):125–39.
9. Cohen PA, Ernst E. Safety of herbal supplements: a guide for cardiologists. Cardiovasc Ther 2010;28(4):246–53.
10. Lee CO. Complementary and alternative medicines patients are talking about: melatonin. Clin J Oncol Nurs 2006;10(1):105–7.
11. Fugh-Berman A. Herb-drug interactions. Lancet 2000;355(9198):134–8.
12. Eisenberg DM, et al. Trends in alternative medicine use in the United States, 1990–1997: results of a follow-up national survey. JAMA 1998;280(18):1569–75.
13. Quinten C, et al. Baseline quality of life as a prognostic indicator of survival: a meta-analysis of individual patient data from EORTC clinical trials. Lancet Oncol 2009;10(9):865–71.

14. Garcia SF, et al. Standardizing patient-reported outcomes assessment in cancer clinical trials: a patient-reported outcomes measurement information system initiative. J Clin Oncol 2007;25(32):5106–12.

15. Grzankowski KS, Carney M. Quality of life in ovarian cancer. Cancer Control 2011;18(1):52–8.

16. von Gruenigen VE, et al. The association between quality of life domains and overall survival in ovarian cancer patients during adjuvant chemotherapy: a Gynecologic Oncology Group Study. Gynecol Oncol 2012;124(3):379–82.

17. Wenzel L, et al. Quality-of-life comparisons in a randomized trial of interval secondary cytoreduction in advanced ovarian carcinoma: a Gynecologic Oncology Group study. J Clin Oncol 2005;23(24):5605–12.

18. Wenzel LB, et al. Health-related quality of life during and after intraperitoneal versus intravenous chemotherapy for optimally debulked ovarian cancer: a Gynecologic Oncology Group Study. J Clin Oncol 2007;25(4):437–43.

19. von Gruenigen VE, et al. Assessment of factors that contribute to decreased quality of life in Gynecologic Oncology Group ovarian cancer trials. Cancer 2009;115(20): 4857–64.

20. von Gruenigen VE, et al. A comparison of quality-of-life domains and clinical factors in ovarian cancer patients: a Gynecologic Oncology Group study. J Pain Symptom Manage 2010;39(5):839–46.

21. Chase DM, et al. Quality of life and survival in advanced cervical cancer: a Gynecologic Oncology Group Study. Gynecol Oncol 2012. [Epub ahead of print].

22. Temel JS, et al. Early palliative care for patients with metastatic non-small-cell lung cancer. N Engl J Med 2010;363(8):733–42.

23. Von Gruenigen VE, et al. A comparison of complementary and alternative medicine use by gynecology and gynecologic oncology patients. Int J Gynecol Cancer 2001;11(3):205–9.

24. Kennedy J. Herb and supplement use in the US adult population. Clinical Ther 2005;27(11):1847–58.

25. Fouladbakhsh JM, Stommel M. Gender, symptom experience, and use of complementary and alternative medicine practices among cancer survivors in the U.S. cancer population. Oncol Nurs Forum 2010;37(1):E7–15.

26. von Gruenigen VE, et al. Longitudinal assessment of quality of life and lifestyle in newly diagnosed ovarian cancer patients: the roles of surgery and chemotherapy. Gynecol Oncol 2006;103(1):120–6.

27. Astin JA, et al. Mind-body medicine: state of the science, implications for practice. J Am Board Fam Pract 2003;16(2):131–47.

28. Busse JW, et al. Disclosure of natural product use to primary care physicians: a cross-sectional survey of naturopathic clinic attendees. Mayo Clin Proc 2005;80(5): 616–23.

29. Corbin Winslow L, Shapiro H, Physicians want education about complementary and alternative medicine to enhance communication with their patients. Arch Intern Med 2002;162(10):1176–81.

30. Complementary and Alternative Medicine in the United States. Institute of Medicine (US) Committee on the Use of Complementary and Alternative Medicine by the American Public. Washington, DC: National Academies Press (US); 2005.

31. Hughes EF. Overview of complementary, alternative, and integrative medicine. Clin Obstet Gynecol 2001;44(4):774–9.

32. Frenkel M, et al. Integrative medicine consultation service in a comprehensive cancer center: findings and outcomes. Integr Cancer Ther 2010;9(3):276–83.

33. Ang-Lee MK, Moss J, Yuan CS. Herbal medicines and perioperative care. JAMA 2001;286(2):208–16.

34. Rowe DJ, Baker AC. Perioperative risks and benefits of herbal supplements in aesthetic surgery. Aesthet Surg J 2009;29(2):150–7.

35. Mathijssen RH, et al. Effects of St. John's wort on irinotecan metabolism. J Natl Cancer Inst 2002;94(16):1247–9.

36. Breidenbach T, et al. Drug interaction of St John's wort with cyclosporin. Lancet 2000;355(9218):1912.

37. Yue QY, Bergquist C, Gerden B. Safety of St John's wort (Hypericum perforatum). Lancet 2000;355(9203):576–7.

38. Singh DK, et al. Integrative oncology, quality of life and supportive care for gynecological malignancies. In: Karlan B, Bristow R, Li AJ, editors. Gynecologic oncology: clinical practice and surgical atlas. New York: The McGraw-Hill Companies; in press.

39. Hercberg S, et al. The potential role of antioxidant vitamins in preventing cardiovascular diseases and cancers. Nutrition 1998;14(6):513–20.

40. Patterson RE, et al. Vitamin supplements and cancer risk: the epidemiologic evidence. Cancer Causes Control 1997;8(5):786–802.

41. Miller ER 3rd, et al. Meta-analysis: high-dosage vitamin E supplementation may increase all-cause mortality. Ann Intern Med 2005;142(1):37–46.

42. Bardia A, et al. Efficacy of antioxidant supplementation in reducing primary cancer incidence and mortality: systematic review and meta-analysis. Mayo Clin Proc 2008;83(1):23–34.

43. Myung SK, et al. Effects of antioxidant supplements on cancer prevention: meta-analysis of randomized controlled trials. Ann Oncol 2010;21(1):166–79.

44. Bjelakovic G, et al. Antioxidant supplements for prevention of mortality in healthy participants and patients with various diseases. Cochrane Database Syst Rev 2008;2:CD007176.

45. The effect of vitamin E and beta carotene on the incidence of lung cancer and other cancers in male smokers. The Alpha-Tocopherol, Beta Carotene Cancer Prevention Study Group. New Engl J Med 1994;330(15):1029–35.

46. Albanes D, et al. Effects of alpha-tocopherol and beta-carotene supplements on cancer incidence in the Alpha-Tocopherol Beta-Carotene Cancer Prevention Study. The Am J Clin Nutr 1995;62(6 Suppl):1427S–30S.

47. Omenn GS, et al. Effects of a combination of beta carotene and vitamin A on lung cancer and cardiovascular disease. New Engl J Med 1996;334(18):1150–5.

48. Bhutani M, Pathak AK. Re: Should supplemental antioxidant administration be avoided during chemotherapy and radiation therapy? J Natl Cancer Inst 2008; 100(18):1334 [author reply: 1334–5].

49. Simone CB, Simone CB 2nd. Re: Should supplemental antioxidant administration be avoided during chemotherapy and radiation therapy? J Natl Cancer Inst 2008; 100(21):1558–9 [author reply: 1559–60].

50. Block K, et al. Re: Should supplemental antioxidant administration be avoided during chemotherapy and radiation therapy? J Natl Cancer Inst 2009;101(2):124–5 [author reply: 125–6].

51. Lawenda BD, et al. Should supplemental antioxidant administration be avoided during chemotherapy and radiation therapy? J Natl Cancer Inst 2008;100(11): 773–83.

52. Conklin KA. Chemotherapy-associated oxidative stress: impact on chemotherapeutic effectiveness. Integr Cancer Ther 2004;3(4):294–300.

53. D'Andrea GM. Use of antioxidants during chemotherapy and radiotherapy should be avoided. CA Cancer J Clin 2005;55(5):319–21.

54. Block KI, et al. Impact of antioxidant supplementation on chemotherapeutic efficacy: a systematic review of the evidence from randomized controlled trials. Cancer Treatment Rev 2007;33(5):407–18.

55. Meyer F, et al. Interaction between antioxidant vitamin supplementation and cigarette smoking during radiation therapy in relation to long-term effects on recurrence and mortality: a randomized trial among head and neck cancer patients. Int J Cancer 2008;122(7):1679–83.

56. Hilakivi-Clarke L, Andrade JE, Helferich W. Is soy consumption good or bad for the breast? J Nutr 2010;140(12):2326S–4S.

57. Wu AH, et al. Epidemiology of soy exposures and breast cancer risk. Br J Cancer 2008;98(1):9–14.

58. Myung SK, et al. Soy intake and risk of endocrine-related gynaecological cancer: a meta-analysis. BJOG 2009;116(13):1697–705.

59. Horn-Ross PL, et al. Phytoestrogen intake and endometrial cancer risk. J Natl Cancer Inst 2003;95(15):1158–64.

60. Straus SE, Chesney MA. Science and government. Enhanced: in defense of NCCAM. Science 2006;313(5785):303–4.

61. Marcus DM, Grollman AP. Science and government. Review for NCCAM is overdue. Science 2006;313(5785):301–2.

62. Nahrstedt A, Butterweck V. Lessons learned from herbal medicinal products: the example of St. John's Wort (perpendicular). J Nat Prod 2010;73(5):1015–21.

63. Block KI, Jonas WB. "Top of the hierarchy" evidence for integrative medicine: what are the best strategies? Integr Cancer Ther 2006;5(4):277–81.

64. Saxe GA, et al. Biological mediators of effect of diet and stress reduction on prostate cancer. Integr Cancer Ther 2008;7(3):130–8.

65. Ornish D, et al. Increased telomerase activity and comprehensive lifestyle changes: a pilot study. Lancet Oncol 2008;9(11):1048–57.

66. Ornish D, et al. Intensive lifestyle changes may affect the progression of prostate cancer. J Urol 2005;174(3):1065–9 [discussion: 1069–70].

67. Ornish D, et al. Changes in prostate gene expression in men undergoing an intensive nutrition and lifestyle intervention. Proc Natl Acad Sci U S A 2008;105(24):8369–74.

68. Doyle C, et al. Nutrition and physical activity during and after cancer treatment: an American Cancer Society guide for informed choices. CA Cancer J Clin 2006;56(6):323–53.

69. Stevinson C, et al. Physical activity in ovarian cancer survivors: associations with fatigue, sleep, and psychosocial functioning. Int J Gynecol Cancer 2009;19(1):73–8.

70. Donnelly CM, et al. A randomised controlled trial testing the feasibility and efficacy of a physical activity behavioural change intervention in managing fatigue with gynaecological cancer survivors. Gynecol Oncol 2011;122(3):618–24.

71. von Gruenigen VE, et al. Feasibility of a lifestyle intervention for ovarian cancer patients receiving adjuvant chemotherapy. Gynecol Oncol 2011;122(2):328–33.

72. Gallus S, Bosetti C, La Vecchia C. Mediterranean diet and cancer risk. Eur J Cancer Prev 2004;13(5):447–52.

73. Sofi F, et al. Adherence to Mediterranean diet and health status: meta-analysis. BMJ 2008;337:a1344.

74. Trichopoulou A, et al. Adherence to a Mediterranean diet and survival in a Greek population. N Engl J Med 2003;348(26):2599–608.

75. Saura-Calixto F, Goni I. Definition of the Mediterranean diet based on bioactive compounds. Crit Rev Food Sci Nutr 2009;49(2):145–52.

76. Sofi F, et al. Accruing evidence about benefits of adherence to the Mediterranean diet on health: an updated systematic review and meta-analysis. Am J Clin Nutr 2010;92:1189–96.
77. Benetou V, et al. Conformity to traditional Mediterranean diet and cancer incidence: the Greek EPIC cohort. Br J Cancer 2008;99(1):191–5.
78. Couto E, et al. Mediterranean dietary pattern and cancer risk in the EPIC cohort. Br J Cancer 2011;104(9):1493–9.
79. La Vecchia C. Association between Mediterranean dietary patterns and cancer risk. Nutr Rev 2009;67(Suppl 1):S126–9.
80. Kolahdooz F, et al. Meat, fish, and ovarian cancer risk: results from 2 Australian case-control studies, a systematic review, and meta-analysis. Am J Clin Nutr 2010;91(6):1752–63.
81. McCann SE, et al. Risk of human ovarian cancer is related to dietary intake of selected nutrients, phytochemicals and food groups. J Nutr 2003;133(6):1937–42.
82. Garcia-Closas R, et al. The role of diet and nutrition in cervical carcinogenesis: a review of recent evidence. Int J Cancer 2005;117(4):629–37.
83. Garland CF, et al. The role of vitamin D in cancer prevention. Am J Public Health 2006;96(2):252–61.
84. Garland CF, et al. Role of ultraviolet B irradiance and vitamin D in prevention of ovarian cancer. Am J Prev Med 2006;31(6):512–4.
85. Cook LS, et al. A systematic literature review of vitamin D and ovarian cancer. Am J Obstet Gynecol 2010;203(1):70.e1–8.
86. Bakhru A, et al. Casting light on 25-hydroxyvitamin D deficiency in ovarian cancer: A study from the NHANES. Gynecol Oncol 2010;119:314–8.
87. Liu J, Xing J, Fei Y. Green tea (Camellia sinensis) and cancer prevention: a systematic review of randomized trials and epidemiological studies. Chin Med 2008;3:12.
88. Zhang M, Binns CW, Lee AH. Tea consumption and ovarian cancer risk: a case-control study in China. Cancer Epidemiol Biomarkers Prev 2002;11(8):713–8.
89. Larsson SC, Wolk A. Tea consumption and ovarian cancer risk in a population-based cohort. Arch Intern Med 2005;165(22):2683–6.
90. Goel A, Jhurani S, Aggarwal BB. Multi-targeted therapy by curcumin: how spicy is it? Mol Nutr Food Res 2008;52(9):1010–30.
91. Dhillon N, et al. Phase II trial of curcumin in patients with advanced pancreatic cancer. Clinical Cancer Research 2008;14(14):4491–9.
92. McCulloch M, et al. Astragalus-based Chinese herbs and platinum-based chemotherapy for advanced non-small-cell lung cancer: meta-analysis of randomized trials. J Clin Oncol 2006;24(3):419–30.
93. Harikumar KB, Aggarwal BB. Resveratrol: a multitargeted agent for age-associated chronic diseases. Cell Cycle 2008;7(8):1020–35.
94. Gates MA, et al. A prospective study of dietary flavonoid intake and incidence of epithelial ovarian cancer. Int J Cancer 2007;121(10):2225–32.
95. Dolecek TA, et al. Prediagnosis food patterns are associated with length of survival from epithelial ovarian cancer. J Am Diet Assoc 2010;110(3):369–82.
96. Nagle CM, et al. Dietary influences on survival after ovarian cancer. Int J Cancer 2003;106(2):264–9.
97. Grant WB, Mohr SB. Ecological studies of ultraviolet B, vitamin D and cancer since 2000. Ann Epidemiol 2009;19(7):446–54.
98. Zhang M, et al. Green tea consumption enhances survival of epithelial ovarian cancer. Int J Cancer 2004;112(3):465–9.
99. Sieja K, Talerczyk M. Selenium as an element in the treatment of ovarian cancer in women receiving chemotherapy. Gynecol Oncol 2004;93(2):320–7.

100. McTiernan A, Irwin M, Vongruenigen V. Weight, physical activity, diet, and prognosis in breast and gynecologic cancers. J Clin Oncol 2010;28(26):4074–80.

101. Calle EE, et al. Overweight, obesity, and mortality from cancer in a prospectively studied cohort of U.S. adults. N Engl J Med 2003;348(17):1625–38.

102. von Gruenigen VE, et al. Treatment effects, disease recurrence, and survival in obese women with early endometrial carcinoma: a Gynecologic Oncology Group study. Cancer 2006;107(12):2786–91.

103. Moore SC, et al. Physical activity, sedentary behaviours, and the prevention of endometrial cancer. Br J Cancer 2010;103(7):933–8.

104. Cust AE. Physical activity and gynecologic cancer prevention. Recent Results Cancer Res 2011;186:159–85.

105. Pierce JP, et al. Greater survival after breast cancer in physically active women with high vegetable-fruit intake regardless of obesity. J Clin Oncol 2007;25(17):2345–51.

106. Yang EV, Glaser R. Stress-induced immunomodulation: implications for tumorigenesis. Brain Behav Immun 2003;17(Suppl 1):S37–40.

107. Lutgendorf SK, et al. Depressed and anxious mood and T-cell cytokine expressing populations in ovarian cancer patients. Brain Behav Immun 2008;22(6):890–900.

108. Sood AK, et al. Stress hormone-mediated invasion of ovarian cancer cells. Clin Cancer Res 2006;12(2):369–75.

109. Lutgendorf SK, et al. Vascular endothelial growth factor and social support in patients with ovarian carcinoma. Cancer 2002;95(4):808–15.

110. Chrousos GP. Stress and disorders of the stress system. Nat Rev Endocrinol 2009;5(7):374–81.

111. Antoni MH, et al. The influence of bio-behavioural factors on tumour biology: pathways and mechanisms. Nat Rev Cancer 2006;6(3):240–8.

112. Thaker PH, et al. Chronic stress promotes tumor growth and angiogenesis in a mouse model of ovarian carcinoma. Nat Med 2006;12(8):939–44.

113. Lutgendorf SK, Sood AK. Biobehavioral factors and cancer progression: physiological pathways and mechanisms. Psychosom Med 2011;73(9):724–30.

114. Costanzo ES, et al. Psychosocial factors and interleukin-6 among women with advanced ovarian cancer. Cancer 2005;104(2):305–13.

115. Madden KS. Catecholamines, sympathetic innervation, and immunity. Brain Behav Immun 2003;17(Suppl 1):S5–10.

116. Yang EV, et al. Norepinephrine upregulates VEGF, IL-8, and IL-6 expression in human melanoma tumor cell lines: implications for stress-related enhancement of tumor progression. Brain Behav Immun 2009;23(2):267–75.

117. Spiegel D. Effects of psychotherapy on cancer survival. Nat Rev Cancer 2002;2(5):383–9.

118. Lutgendorf SK, Sood AK, Antoni MH. Host factors and cancer progression: biobehavioral signaling pathways and interventions. J Clin Oncol 2010;28(26):4094–9.

119. Hawkley LC, Cacioppo JT. Loneliness and pathways to disease. Brain Behav Immun 2003;17(Suppl 1):S98–105.

120. Sagar SM. Integrative oncology in North America. J Soc Integr Oncol 2006;4(1):27–39.

121. Jacobs GD. The physiology of mind-body interactions: the stress response and the relaxation response. J Altern Complement Med 2001;7(Suppl 1):S83–92.

122. Jacobs GD. Clinical applications of the relaxation response and mind-body interventions. J Altern Complement Med 2001;7(Suppl 1):S93–101.

123. Elkins G, Fisher W, Johnson A. Mind-body therapies in integrative oncology. Curr Treat Options Oncol 2010;11(3-4):128–40.

124. Dusek JA, Benson H. Mind-body medicine: a model of the comparative clinical impact of the acute stress and relaxation responses. Minn Med 2009;92(5):47–50.

125. Ross A, Thomas S. The health benefits of yoga and exercise: a review of comparison studies. J Altern Complement Med 2010;16(1):3–12.

126. Bower JE, et al. Yoga for cancer patients and survivors. Cancer Control 2005;12(3): 165–71.

127. Speca M, et al. A randomized, wait-list controlled clinical trial: the effect of a mindfulness meditation-based stress reduction program on mood and symptoms of stress in cancer outpatients. Psychosom Med 2000;62(5):613–22.

128. Carlson LE, et al. The effects of a mindfulness meditation-based stress reduction program on mood and symptoms of stress in cancer outpatients: 6-month follow-up. Support Care Cancer 2001;9(2):112–23.

129. Musial F, et al. Mindfulness-based stress reduction for integrative cancer care: a summary of evidence. Forsch Komplementmed 2011;18(4):192–202.

130. Mustian KM, Palesh O, Sprod L, et al. Effect of YOCAS yoga on sleep, fatigue, and quality of life: A URCC CCOP randomized, controlled clinical trial among 410 cancer survivors. ASCO Meeting Abstracts 2010;28(15 suppl):9013.

131. Casey C, Chen LM, Rabow MW. Symptom management in gynecologic malignancies. Expert Rev Anticancer Ther 2011;11(7):1077–89.

132. Rutledge TL, et al. Pelvic floor disorders and sexual function in gynecologic cancer survivors: a cohort study. Am J Obstet Gynecol 2010;203(5):514,e1–7.

133. Cassileth BR, Vickers AJ. Massage therapy for symptom control: outcome study at a major cancer center. J Pain Symptom Manage 2004;28(3):244–9.

134. Schmitz KH, et al. Controlled physical activity trials in cancer survivors: a systematic review and meta-analysis. Cancer Epidemiol Biomarkers Prev 2005;14(7):1588–95.

135. Molassiotis A, Sylt P, Diggins H. The management of cancer-related fatigue after chemotherapy with acupuncture and acupressure: a randomised controlled trial. Complement Ther Med 2007;15(4):228–37.

136. Oh B, et al. Impact of medical Qigong on quality of life, fatigue, mood and inflammation in cancer patients: a randomized controlled trial. Ann Oncol 2010; 21(3):608–14.

137. Ezzo JM, et al. Acupuncture-point stimulation for chemotherapy-induced nausea or vomiting. Cochrane Database Syst Rev 2006;2:CD002285.

138. Lee A, Fan LT. Stimulation of the wrist acupuncture point P6 for preventing postoperative nausea and vomiting. Cochrane Database Syst Rev 2009;2: CD003281.

139. Gan TJ, et al. A randomized controlled comparison of electro-acupoint stimulation or ondansetron versus placebo for the prevention of postoperative nausea and vomiting. Anesth Analg 2004;99(4):1070–5.

140. You Q, et al. Vitamin B6 points PC6 injection during acupuncture can relieve nausea and vomiting in patients with ovarian cancer. Int J Gynecol Cancer 2009;19(4):567–71.

141. Manusirivithaya S, et al. Antiemetic effect of ginger in gynecologic oncology patients receiving cisplatin. Int J Gynecol Cancer 2004;14(6):1063–9.

142. Peterson DE, Jones JB, Petit RG 2nd. Randomized, placebo-controlled trial of Saforis for prevention and treatment of oral mucositis in breast cancer patients receiving anthracycline-based chemotherapy. Cancer 2007;109(2):322–31.

143. Listing M, et al. Massage therapy reduces physical discomfort and improves mood disturbances in women with breast cancer. Psychooncology 2009;18(12):1290–9.

144. Kutner JS, et al. Massage therapy versus simple touch to improve pain and mood in patients with advanced cancer: a randomized trial. Ann Intern Med 2008;149(6): 369–79.
145. Dean-Clower E, et al. Acupuncture as palliative therapy for physical symptoms and quality of life for advanced cancer patients. Integr Cancer Ther 2010;9(2):158–67.
146. Alimi D, et al. Analgesic effect of auricular acupuncture for cancer pain: a randomized, blinded, controlled trial. J Clin Oncol 2003;21(22):4120–6.
147. Wade AG, et al. Efficacy of prolonged release melatonin in insomnia patients aged 55–80 years: quality of sleep and next-day alertness outcomes. Curr Med Res Opin 2007;23(10):2597–605.
148. Andrade C, et al. Melatonin in medically ill patients with insomnia: a double-blind, placebo-controlled study. J Clin Psychiatry 2001;62(1):41–5.
149. Sandadi S, et al. The effect of sleep disturbance on quality of life in women with ovarian cancer. Gynecol Oncol 2011;123(2):351–5.
150. Riemann D, Perlis ML. The treatments of chronic insomnia: a review of benzodiazepine receptor agonists and psychological and behavioral therapies. Sleep Med Rev 2009;13(3):205–14.
151. Berger AM, et al. Cancer-related fatigue. N Natl Compr Canc Netw 2010;8(8): 904–31.
152. Mustian KM, et al. Integrative nonpharmacologic behavioral interventions for the management of cancer-related fatigue. Oncologist 2007;12(Suppl 1):52–67.
153. Ettinger DS, et al. Antiemesis. J Natl Compr Canc Netw 2007;5(1):12–33.
154. Raphael J, et al. Cancer pain: part 1: pathophysiology; oncological, pharmacological, and psychological treatments: a perspective from the British Pain Society endorsed by the UK Association of Palliative Medicine and the Royal College of General Practitioners. Pain Med 2010;11(5):742–64.
155. Swarm R, et al. Adult cancer pain. J Natl Compr Canc Netw 2010;8(9):1046–86.
156. Fowler JM, et al. The gynecologic oncology consult: symptom presentation and concurrent symptoms of depression and anxiety. Obstet Gynecol 2004;103(6): 1211–7.
157. Deng G, Cassileth BR. Integrative oncology: complementary therapies for pain, anxiety, and mood disturbance. CA Cancer J Clin 2005;55(2):109–16.
158. Post-White J, et al. Therapeutic massage and healing touch improve symptoms in cancer. Integr Cancer Ther 2003;2(4):332–44.
159. Bardia A, et al. Efficacy of complementary and alternative medicine therapies in relieving cancer pain: a systematic review. J Clin Oncol 2006;24(34):5457–64.

Index

Note: Page numbers of article titles are in **boldface** type.

A

Adenocarcinoma
  cervical, 236–237
  vaginal, 224–225
  vulvar, 218
Alternative therapies
  defined, 286
Antiangiogenesis agents
  in gynecologic malignancies, 136–140

B

β core fragment
  in GTN, 199–200
Basal cell carcinoma
  vulvar, 218
Behavior(s)
  reproductive
    cervical cancer related to, 234–235
Bilateral salpingo-oophorectomy
  in ovarian cancer risk reduction, 167–168
Biologic therapies
  in gynecologic malignancies, **131–144**
    antiangiogenesis agents, 136–140
    cell signaling pathways in, 132–134
    homologous recombination pathways in, 134–135
    molecular targets of interest in, 135
Botanicals
  in cancer prevention, 296–297
BRCA1
  in hereditary breast/ovarian cancer syndrome, 166–170
  in ovarian cancer risk reduction, 167–168
BRCA2
  in hereditary breast/ovarian cancer syndrome, 166–170
  in ovarian cancer risk reduction, 167–168

C

Cancer(s). *See specific types*
Cancer care
  trends in
    in North America, **107–129**. *See also specific cancers*
      methods, 109
      quality of care, 109

Obstet Gynecol Clin N Am 39 (2012) 313–322
http://dx.doi.org/10.1016/S0889-8545(12)00041-1
0889-8545/12/$ – see front matter © 2012 Elsevier Inc. All rights reserved.

obgyn.theclinics.com

Printed and bound by CPI Group (UK) Ltd, Croydon, CR0 4YY

03/10/2024

01040360-0001